Two week loan

REVIEWS IN FOOD AND NUTRITION TOXICITY

Volume 2

REVIEWS IN FOOD AND NUTRITION TOXICITY

Volume 2

Edited by
Victor R. Preedy and Ronald R. Watson

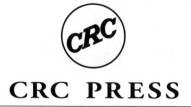

CRC PRESS

Boca Raton   London   New York   Washington, D.C.

Library of Congress Cataloging-in-Publication Data

Reviews in food and nutrition toxicity / edited by Victor R. Preedy and Ronald Watson.
   p. cm.
Includes bibliographical references and index.
ISBN 0-8493-2757-1 (alk. paper)
1. Nutrition policy. I. Preedy, Victor R. II. Watson, Ronald R. (Ronald Ross). III. Title.

TX359.A56 2004
363.8′561—dc22

2004047814

© 2005 CRC Press LLC

No claim to original U.S. Government works
International Standard Book Number 0-8493-2757-1
Library of Congress Card Number 2004047814
Printed in the United States of America 1 2 3 4 5 6 7 8 9 0
Printed on acid-free paper

Preface

This second volume of *Reviews in Food and Nutrition Toxicity* follows directly from the successes of the first volume published last year. The series disseminates important data pertaining to food and nutrition safety and toxicology that are relevant to humans. Chapters in this series will range from, for example, the introduction of toxins in the manufacture or production of artificial food substances to the ingestion of microbial contaminants or toxins and the cellular or physiological changes that arise. This volume features a broad range of topics, including contaminants in beer, the effects of alcohol on the intestine, ciguatera fish poisoning, hepatitis A, β-nitropropionic acid, *Vibrio parahaemolyticus*, bacterial toxins, pesticide toxicity, polyhalogenated and polycyclic aromatic hydrocarbons, and a survey of contamination episodes. Each chapter is written by experts and is accompanied by supporting tables and figures. These concise and informative articles should stimulate a scientific dialogue. Food production processes and nutritional or dietary habits are continually changing, and it is important to learn from past lessons and embrace a multidisciplinary approach. For example, some cellular mechanisms elucidated by studying a particular toxin may also be relevant to other areas of food pathology; therefore, it is the intention of the editors to impart such comprehensive information in a single series, namely *Reviews in Food and Nutrition Toxicity*.

Victor R. Preedy
Ronald R. Watson

About the Editors

Victor R. Preedy, Ph.D., D.Sc., F.R.C.Path., is a professor in the Department of Nutrition and Dietetics, King's College, London. He directs studies regarding protein turnover, cardiology, nutrition, and, in particular, the biochemical aspects of alcoholism. Prof. Preedy graduated in 1974 from the University of Aston with a combined honors degree in biology and physiology with pharmacology. He received his Ph.D. in 1981 in the field of nutrition and metabolism, specializing in protein turnover. In 1992, he received his membership in the Royal College of Pathologists, based on his published works, and in 1993 a D.Sc. degree for his outstanding contribution to the study of protein metabolism. At the time, he was one of the university's youngest recipients of this distinguished award. Prof. Preedy was elected a fellow of the Royal College of Pathologists in 2000. He has published more than 475 articles, which include more than 150 peer-reviewed manuscripts based on original research, and 70 reviews. His current major research interests include the role of alcohol in enteral nutrition, and the molecular mechanisms responsible for alcoholic muscle damage.

Ronald R. Watson, Ph.D., attended the University of Idaho but graduated from Brigham Young University in Provo, Utah, with a degree in Chemistry in 1966. He completed his Ph.D. degree in 1971 in Biochemistry from Michigan State University. His postdoctoral schooling was completed at the Harvard School of Public Health in Nutrition and Microbiology, including a two-year postdoctoral research experience in immunology. He was an assistant Professor of Immunology and did research at the University of Mississippi Medical Center in Jackson from 1973 to 1974. He was an Assistant Professor of Microbiology and Immunology at the Indiana University Medical School from 1974 to 1978 and an Associate Professor at Purdue University in the Department of Food and Nutrition from 1978 to 1982. In 1982, he joined the faculty at the University of Arizona Health Sciences Center in the Department of Family and Community Medicine of the School of Medicine and is also a Professor Health Promotion Sciences in the Mel and Enid Zuckerman Arizona College of Public Health. Prof. Watson is a member of several national and international nutrition, immunology, and cancer societies and research societies on alcoholism. Prof. Watson has edited 35 books on nutrition or foods. He is currently funded by the National Heart Blood and Lung Institute to study nutrition and heart disease during mouse AIDS. He has edited 53 scientific books and 510 research and review articles.

Contributors

Willy Baeyens, Ph.D.
Vrije Universiteit Brussel
Department of Analytical and
 Environmental Chemistry
Brussels, Belgium

Ali Banan, Ph.D.
Rush Medical College
Section of Gastroenterology and
 Nutrition
Chicago, Illinois

Noubar John Bostanian, Ph.D.
Agriculture and Agri-Food Canada
Horticultural Research
Quebec, Canada

George A. Burdock, Ph.D.
Burdock Group
Vero Beach, Florida

Ioana G. Carabin, M.D.
Women in Science
Vero Beach, Florida

Maria Chironna, Ph.D.
University of Bari
Department of Internal Medicine and
 Public Health
Bari, Italy

Nicholas A. Daniels, M.D., MPH
University of California
Department of Medicine
Division of General Internal Medicine
San Francisco, California

Rinne De Bont
Department of Radiotherapy, Nuclear
 Medicine, and Experimental
 Cancerology
Study Center for Carcinogenesis and
 Primary Prevention of Cancer
Ghent University
Gent, Belgium

Marc Elskens, Ph.D.
Vrije Universiteit
Department of Analytical and
 Environmental Chemistry
Brussels, Belgium

Ashkan Farhadi, M.D., M.S.
Rush Medical College
Section of Gastroenterology and
 Nutrition
Chicago, Illinois

Jeremy Z. Fields, Ph.D.
Rush Medical College
Section of Gastroenterology and
 Nutrition
Chicago, Illinois

James C. Griffiths, Ph.D.
Burdock Group
Vero Beach, Florida

Luc Hens, Ph.D.
Vrije Universiteit Brussel
Human Ecology Department
Brussels, Belgium

Yoshitsugi Hokama, M.D.
University of Hawaii
John A. Burns School of Medicine
Honolulu, Hawaii

Ron (L.A.P.) Hoogenboom, Ph.D.
RIKILT
Wageningen, The Netherlands

Ross J. Hunter, B.Sc., M.D.
King's College London
School of Life Sciences
London, United Kingdom

Ali Keshavarzian, M.D.
Rush Medical College
Section of Gastroenterology and
  Nutrition
Chicago, Illinois

Bharti Odhav, Ph.D.
Department of Biotechnology
M.L. Sultan Campus
Durban Institute of Technology
Durban, South Africa

**Victor R. Preedy, Ph.D., D.Sc.,
  F.R.C.Path.**
King's College London
School of Life Sciences
London, United Kingdom

Michele Quarto, M.D.
University of Bari
Department of Internal Medicine and
  Public Health
Bari, Italy

Rajkumar Rajendram, Ph.D.
King's College London
Department of Nutrition and Dietetics
London, United Kingdom

Madhusudan G. Soni, Ph.D.
Burdock Group
Vero Beach, Florida

Nik van Larebeke, M.D., Ph.D.
Department of Radiotherapy, Nuclear
  Medicine, and Experimental
  Cancerology
Study Center for Carcinogenesis and
  Primary Prevention of Cancer
Ghent University
Gent, Belgium

Table of Contents

1 Bacterial Contaminants and Mycotoxins in Beer and Control Strategies

Bharti Odhav

CONTENTS

Abstract   Because beer generally constitutes a relatively inhospitable environment with a pH of 3.8 to 4.3, offering only limited sources of carbohydrates, nitrogen (mainly polypeptides), and certain growth factors, it is usually microbiologically safe. The safety of beer is compromised, however, by the introduction of contaminants into the beer by raw materials, inadequate process control, improper packaging and storage, accidental contamination, or microbiological spoilage. Contaminants introduced through raw materials and inadequate process control generally lead to off-flavors and aroma defects, which lead to serious economic losses. Bacterial spoilage occurs if the beer becomes infected with acetic acid bacteria, *Acetomonas*, coliforms, *Lactobacillus delbruckii*, *Lactobacillus pastorianus*, *Obesumbacterium proteus*, *Pediococcus*, or *Zymomonas* spp., which cause unacceptable byproducts and off-flavors. Mold contamination, on the other hand, affects germination and malt characteristics, and many types of mold are known to produce mycotoxins, which have health implications. Of significance are the aflatoxins, zearalenone, deoxynivalenol, fumonisins, and citrinin. These toxins may be transmitted to beers by the use of contaminated grains during brewing. Surveys indicate that, although a variety of mycotoxins do reach the final product (beer), they are found in limited concentrations. This chapter highlights the contaminants that can be introduced by raw materials or inadequate process control, microbiological spoilage organisms, mycotoxins, and their controls.

INTRODUCTION

Beer and ale are malt beverages produced by brewing. The brewing of beer is a unique mix of art and science that consists of a number of key steps whereby yeasts convert the carbohydrates of grains to ethanol. The expected appearance, flavor, and texture of any alcoholic beverage are the result of a complex but fine balance of hundreds of different chemical compounds (Meilgaard, 1975). Substances that are intentionally or accidentally introduced (contaminants) into the beer bring about changes in the characteristic taste, aroma, or texture, resulting in off-flavors or taints that usually lead to an unacceptable product. The contaminants can be introduced into the beer by raw materials, inadequate process control, improper packaging and storage, accidental contamination, or microbiological spoilage (Engan, 1991). Selection of a beer by the consumer is based on certain expectations and the reputation of the brand; therefore, beers should always maintain a consistent flavor and be microbiologically safe. When these requirements are threatened by the introduction of contaminants from the raw materials used or during processing or storage, the outcome can include substantial economic losses and consumer dissatisfaction. This chapter highlights the contaminants that can be introduced through raw materials or inadequate process control, microbiological spoilage organisms, and their control.

CONTAMINANTS INTRODUCED THROUGH RAW MATERIALS AND INADEQUATE PROCESS CONTROL

MALTING

The process of beer making is initiated with malting followed by mashing, boiling, and fermentation (Figure 1.1). Because most of the carbohydrates in grains used for brewing are in the form of starches and because the fermenting yeasts do not produce amylases to degrade the starches, a necessary part of beer brewing includes the step whereby malt or other exogenous sources of amylase are provided for the hydrolysis

STAGE

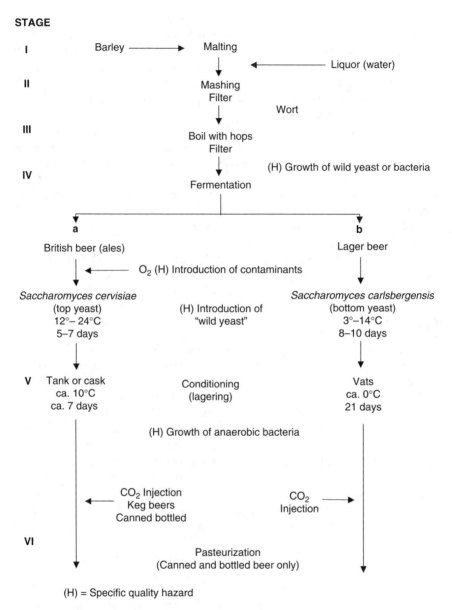

FIGURE 1.1 Beer-making process.

of starches to sugars. The malt is first prepared by allowing the barley grains to germinate. This process serves as a source of amylases. Both β- and α-amylases are involved; the latter acts to liquefy the starch and the former increases sugar formation (Ilori et al., 1991). Malt has an effect on the organoleptic properties of beer, and good-quality malt is essential for maintaining beer quality. During the germination of barley in the malting process, S-methylmethionine (SMM), a precursor of dimethylsulfide

(DMS), is formed which has a tinned sweet-corn/baked-bean/cooked-vegetable flavor (Meilgaard, 1975). This attribute contributes to the overall flavor of certain beers, particularly continental lagers. SMM is heat labile, and the amount remaining in the malt at the end of the malting process is very dependent on the kilning regime. Lager malts are generally kilned to a lesser extent than ale malts; consequently, less of the SMM is destroyed. Excess DMS, described as providing a "blackcurrant" flavor (White, 1977), is undesirable.

Malt has great adsorptive capacity and is easily contaminated, thus both malt and storage areas must be clean, dry, and well ventilated. If stored at high temperature and humidity, malt may develop a grassy, green flavor (Engan, 1991). Pesticide residues on malt can give rise to off-flavors in the final product. Indeed, the sorghum used in certain African countries is the main source of fermentable sugar; colored sorghum such as the red-skinned "bird-proof" varieties used in southern Africa have high polyphenol contents, and the resultant beer brewed from these sorghums may be extremely astringent.

Adjuncts (additional sources of fermentable sugar, such as liquid starch) infected with anaerobic *Clostridium* spp. can become tainted with butyric acid, which has a rancid, sickly flavor (Stenius et al., 1991).

Mashing

The malt is mixed with malt adjuncts, hops, and water. Malt adjuncts include grains, grain products, sugars, and other carbohydrate products to serve as fermentable substances. Hops are added as sources of pyrogallol and catechol tannins, resins, essential oils, and other constituents for the purpose of precipitating unstable proteins during the boiling of wort and to provide for biological stability, bitterness, and aroma. The process by which the malt and barley adjuncts are dissolved and heated and the starches digested is called *mashing*. The soluble part of the mashed material is called *wort*. In some breweries, lactobacilli are introduced into the mash to lower the pH of wort through lactic acid production. Wort and hops are mixed and boiled for 1.5 to 2.5 hours for the purpose of enzyme inactivation, extraction of soluble hop substances, precipitation of coagulable proteins, and control of concentration and sterilization. Following the boiling of wort and hops, the wort is separated, cooled, and fermented.

During boiling, volatile components of the wort are evaporated. The three groups of volatile compounds in the wort are (1) those derived from the metabolic processes that occur in malt during germination, (2) those derived from the hop grist, and (3) those compounds that form as a consequence of thermal processes (malt kilning and the action of the boil itself). The DMS precursor, SMM, is broken down during wort boiling, and DMS is lost by evaporation or oxidation to dimethylsulfoxide, which can be converted at a later stage into DMS by the metabolic action of yeast (Anness and Bamworth, 1982). In an attempt to save energy, boiling times and evaporation rates have often been reduced; however, doing so has led to what have been described as "worty, grassy, cracker-like" flavors (Narziss, 1993).

During the high-temperature stages, Maillard reactions occur. These involve low-molecular-weight and reducing sugars reacting together at high temperature, generating many compounds, including the *N*-heterocycles pyrazine and pyrroles, which have low flavor thresholds and have been described as "roasted/bready." In certain malts used to make dark beers, these flavors are desirable. An increase in the temperature of the boil increases the potential for formation of these compounds, which cause malty off-flavors in beer.

Aged hops can give beer a cheesy off-flavor due to 3-methylbutanoic acid, which originates from the acyl side-chains of alpha-acids (Tressl et al., 1978). Sulfury off-flavors can be derived from hops either from sulfur-containing constituents (thioesters) or as a result of chemical reactions between the normal hop constituent and elemental sulfur from extraneous sources (e.g., used in the field as a fungicide or for sulfuring in the kiln when the hops are dried). The thioesters give cooked cabbage or onion/garlic-like aromas and tastes, while the latter reactions give burned rubber, sulfury flavors (Seaton and Moir, 1987).

FERMENTATION

The fermentation of the sugar-laden wort is carried out by the inoculation of *Saccharomyces cerevisiae*. The freshly fermented product is aged and finished by the addition of CO_2 to a final content of 0.45 to 0.52% before it is ready for commerce. The pasteurization of beer at 140°F (60°C) or higher may be carried out for the purpose of destroying spoilage organisms (O'Conner-Cox et al., 1991).

The flavor and aroma of beer are very complex, being derived from a vast array of components that arise from a number of sources. Not only do malt, hops, and water have an impact on flavor, but so does the synthesis of yeast, which forms byproducts during fermentation and maturation. The most notable of these byproducts are, of course, ethanol and carbon dioxide. In addition, however, a large number of other flavor compounds are produced, such as esters, diacetyl aldehydes, sulfur volatiles, dimethylsulfide, fusel alcohols, organic acids, fatty acids, and nitrogen compounds. Yeast strains vary markedly in their byproducts. Non-flocculent yeasts tend to produce more volatiles than do flocculent strains. Lager yeasts produce more fatty acids and sulfur byproducts than do ale yeasts (Doyle et al., 1997).

If the fermentation is not controlled, an imbalance of flavors can result. Disproportionate amounts of fusel oils can be produced at elevated temperatures, giving beer a pronounced solvent character. Ester production can be influenced by the yeast strain or wort strength. Over-attenuation may give an unbalanced final flavor to the beer, making it dry and astringent with little balancing sweetness. Restricted fermentations, on the other hand, as used in the production of some low-alcohol products, can result in sweet, worty off-flavors because of insufficient gas generation to purge the undesirable wort characteristics. The alternative method of producing low-alcohol products is to remove the alcohol once it has formed; however, in doing so, the esters and higher alcohols may also be removed. The resultant beer can lack these positive yeast-derived flavors and taste thin and watery.

Sulfur compounds, while contributing positively to the overall flavor of beer, can be extremely objectionable if present in excess. The amount of sulfur compounds produced during fermentation is controlled by various factors, among which are yeast strain, metal ion concentrations, source of sulfur, and fermentation conditions.

The most important sulfur compound is hydrogen sulfide, which gives a rotten-egg flavor (Hill and Smith, 2000). Other prominent sulfides (e.g., dimethyltrisulfide, or DMTS), are important contributors to lager beer flavor. When present at levels substantially below threshold (for a particular brand), they add a desirable complexity to the overall flavor; however, in excess of threshold, they give oniony, garlicky notes, which interfere with and alter the aroma profile of the brand.

If aging yeast is used or the yeast is not removed sufficiently early in the process once maturation is complete, then autolysis can occur, causing meaty/yeast-extract-like flavors. A caprylic off-flavor described as "soapy/goaty/fatty" occurs when straight-chain fatty acids produced by yeast during fermentation accumulate in the beer (Clapperton, 1978). The amount produced is dependent upon the yeast strain, oxygen content of the wort, wort composition, and use of oxygen throughout fermentation. Clapperton and Brown (1978) observed that the intensity of this off-flavor could be correlated with the concentration of octanoic acid and decanoic acid.

During fermentation, the vicinal diketones diacetyl and 2,3-pentanedione are produced. Both have a sweet, buttery, butterscotch flavor. Of the two, diacetyl is of more concern to the brewer as it has a taste threshold of only 0.15 ppm, while 2,3-pentanedione has a threshold of 0.9 ppm (Meilgaard, 1975). These diketones are formed as byproducts of amino-acid biosynthesis. Both α-acetolactate and α-acetohydroxybutyrate, the precursors of diacetyl and 2,3-pentanedione, respectively, are excreted by the yeast into the beer. The acetohydroxy acids are then spontaneously decarboxylated to form the vicinal diketones. During maturation, the yeast reduces the vicinal diketones to less flavor-active compounds: diacetyl to acetoin (Meilgaard, 1975) and 2,3-pentanedione to pentanediol.

The beer may then be pasteurized for biological stability, during which it ideally is exposed to the minimum effective pasteurization temperature and held at that temperature only for the time necessary to kill all viable spoilers, then cooled very quickly (O'Connor-Cox et al., 1991). Unfortunately, in practice, this does not always occur. As a result, the flavor of the product can suffer, and cooked vegetable, toffee, bready, dull, grainy, and generally oxidized flavors develop. Over-pasteurization accelerates the changes that occur in beer flavor as it ages.

PACKAGING

Draft beer is packaged in casks or kegs made of stainless steel or aluminum. Beer cans made from steel or aluminum have an internal coating of lacquer. If this is disrupted in a steel can, a metallic flavor will develop, as the iron migrates into the beer. The same can happen with aluminum, but in this case the off-flavor will be sulfury (Andrews, 1987). Lubricants used in the can-making process contain fatty acids, and inadequate removal of these can lead to taints in beers (Hardwick, 1978). Chloroanisoles, which produce a moldy, musty, earthy flavor, have a very low flavor threshold. Packaging materials, bottled beer and processing aids, propylene glycol, and alginate have all been found to contain chloroanisoles (Lambert et al., 1993). Bottles made of glass are unreactive, but the color can cause a "skunky" or "leek-like" off-flavor (Irwin et al., 1993). Beer can also pick up metallic taint from crowns if rust develops (Andrews, 1987).

STORAGE

The conditions under which beer is stored affect the rate at which further changes can occur. Lagers held at 30°C for 12 to 30 days develop a stale flavor (Hashimoto, 1981).

ACCIDENTAL CONTAMINATION

Wherever a potential for contamination exists, it is likely to appear. Metallic taints (Andrews, 1987), "paint-thinner" taints (King et al., 1994), and cardboard taints (Casson, 1984) have been ascribed to external contaminants. The most common off-flavors found in beers and their possible causes are summarized in Table 1.1 (Bennet, 1996).

MICROBIOLOGICAL SPOILAGE

Microbiological spoilage can occur if the wort or beer becomes infected with a spoilage organism or if a change occurs in the normal metabolism of the brewing yeast. The amounts of oxygen and nutrients available determine which microorganisms are capable of spoilage. Wort at pH 5.0 is a complex mixture of carbohydrates and other growth factors. Beer, in comparison, constitutes a relatively inhospitable environment with a pH of 3.8 to 4.3, offering only limited sources of carbohydrates, nitrogen (mainly polypeptides), and certain growth factors. Furthermore, hop bitter compounds have antimicrobial properties (Harms and Nitzsche, 2001), and beer generally contains ethanol, organic acids, fusel oils, and carbon dioxide.

Eight common genera of bacteria will grow in wort or beer (Table 1.2), and these genera can be divided into two groups: wort-spoilage and beer-spoilage. Wort-spoilage bacterial contamination is caused primarily by low pitching rates, unhealthy yeast, impure starter cultures, or the introduction of large quantities of bacteria through unsanitary techniques. Genera causing wort spoilage and odors or off-flavors commonly associated with fermentation with these bacteria include *Obesumbacterium* (parsnip odor), *Aerobacter* (celery), and *Escherichia* (highly phenolic) (Ingledew, 1979). The five predominant groups of bacteria capable of beer spoilage are (1) lactic acid bacteria; (2) acetic acid bacteria; (3) *Zymomonas* spp.; (4) *Obesumbacterium proteus*; and (5) coliforms (Nakakita et al., 2002; Jespersen and Jakobsen, 1996; Brantley and Aranha, 1994).

LACTIC ACID BACTERIA

The Gram-positive bacterial genera *Lactobacillus* and *Pediococcus* are often referred to as lactic acid bacteria because of their propensity to produce lactic acid from simple sugars. These bacteria are capable of growth throughout fermentation, as they are resistant to ethanol, do not require oxygen, and (unlike wort spoilers) flourish at low pH levels. The optimum level for growth is about 5.5, but some strains can survive at pH levels as low as 3.5. Lactic acid bacteria are often contaminants from pitching yeast or from air. They may be the most significant infectious organisms during fermentation and maturation. When lactobacilli grow in beer, the beer

TABLE 1.1
Off-Flavors Found in Beer and Their Possible Causes

Off-Flavors	Descriptor	Possible Cause
Acetaldehyde	Green apples, emulsion paint	Bacterial spoilage (*Zymomonas, Acetobacter, Gluconobacter*) Oxidation
Acetic acid	Acid, vinegar	Bacterial spoilage (e.g., from *Acetobacter, Gluconobacter* spp.)
Acidic	Mineral acid	Abnormally low pH
Astringent	Mouth puckering	Bacterial spoilage (e.g., from *Acetobacter, Gluconobacter* spp.) Over-attenuation Yeast autolysis "Bird-proof" varieties of sorghum used as adjuncts Pesticide residues
Bitter	Harsh	Wild yeast (*Brettanomycess* spp.) Caustic soda detergents
Bready	Old bread	Oxidation Over-pasteurization
Butyric acid	Rancid, sickly (vomit)	Bacterial spoilage (e.g., from *Clostridium, Megasphaera, Pectinatus* spp.)
Carbonation (over/under)	Gassy, flat	Ignorance of gas properties Insufficient equipment
Caprylic	Goaty, fatty, soapy	Yeast strain Wort composition and oxygen content
Cardboard	Cardboard boxes	Oxidation O_2 migration through dispense tubing
Catty	Blackcurrant leaves	Oxidation Malt contamination with paint impurity
Cheesy	Dry cheese rind	Oxidation Bacterial spoilage (e.g., from *Megasphaera* spp.) Aged hops
Cooked vegetables	Parsnip, cabbage	Over-pasteurization/oxidation Bacterial spoilage (*Obesumbacterium proteus*)
Diacetyl	Buttery, butterscotch	Bacterial spoilage (e.g., from *Pediococcus, Lactobocillus*) Inadequate maturation
Dilution	Thin, watery	Alcohol removal Inadequate flushing of tanks and mains
DMS	Baked beans, blackcurrant, tinned sweet corn and tomatoes	Insufficient wort boiling Conversion from DMSO by yeast Bacterial spoilage (*Obesumbacterium proteus*)
Estery	Fruity, solventy	Lack of control (poor oxygenation) in fermentation Wild yeast
Fishy	Fish skin	Quaternary ammonium compounds Use of incompletely cured resin/fiberglass tanks
Grassy	Crushed green leaves	Poorly stored malt Badly manufactured hop pellets
Husky	Barley grain	High pH mash and sparge liquor

TABLE 1.1 (cont.)
Off-Flavors Found in Beer and Their Possible Causes

Off-Flavors	Descriptor	Possible Cause
Honey	Clover honey	Oxidation of lager beer (usually packaged in green bottles)
Hydrogen sulfide	Rotten eggs	Yeast strain
		Fermentation conditions
		Bacterial spoilage (e.g., from *Pectinatus* and *Zymomonas* spp.)
Inky	Bottle ink	Contamination of brewing water
Labox	Cardboardy	Can lacquer absorption of layer-pad volatiles
Lactic acid	Sour astringent	Bacterial spoilage (e.g., from *Pediococcus* and *Lactobacillus* spp.)
Lightstruck	Sunstruck, skunky, leek-like	Light
Metallic	Tinny, inky, rusty	Corrosion, substandard stainless steel vessels
		Lacquer breakdown on steel beer cans
		Additives (e.g., primings)
		Pick-up from kieselguhr on filtration
		Oxidation
		Low pH
Musty	Moldy, earthy	Chloroanisole contamination of packaging
		Propylene glycol alginate
		Mold growth
Oily	Greasy	Contamination with lubricant during canning or kegging
Phenolic	Medicinal, TCP	Bacterial spoilage (e.g., from coliforms)
		Wild yeast
		Raw materials (e.g., malt, liquor)
		Uncured lacquer (e.g., from tank or keg)
		Dispensing tubing
Plastic	Various	Plasticizer leaking from tank linings
		Incomplete can lacquer curing
Rubbery	Car tires	New hoses for tankers
Salty	—	Leakage of coolant
Soapy	Alkaline	Inadequate rinsing of detergent
Spicy	Clove-like	4-vinyl guaiacol from wild yeast (*POF*+)
Sulfuric	Pungent, choking	Additives (e.g., antioxidants, linings)
Sulfury	Cooked vegetables, rubbery	Lacquer breakdown on aluminum cans
		Yeast metabolism
		Bacterial spoilage
		Liquor contamination
Tobacco	Pipe tobacco	Hops stewed or sweated before pelleting
Toffee	Sickly toffees	Oxidation
Worty	Hay-like	Inadequate wort boiling
		Restricted fermentation
Yeasty	Yeast extract, meaty	Yeast autolysis

Source: Adapted from Bennet, S.J.E., in *Foods Taints and Off-Flavours*, Saxby, M.J., Ed., Blackie Academic & Professional, Glasgow, 1996, pp. 290–320.

TABLE 1.2
Common Bacterial Contaminants

Name	Attributes	Classification	Byproducts and Off-Flavors
Acetic acid bacteria	Aerobic Acid tolerant Hop sensitive	Gram-negative Rod-shaped Cocci-shaped Beer spoiler	Surface growth Acidity Vinegar smell Ropiness
Acetomonas	Aerobic Acid tolerant May form chain	Gram-negative Rod-shaped Beer spoiler	Turbidity Apple or cider smell
Coliforms	Aerobic and anaerobic species	Gram-negative Rod-shaped (both long and short) Wort spoiler	Celery odors Phenolic odors
Lactobacillus delbruckii	Facultative aerobe Thermophilic Will not grow in hopped wort	Lactic acid bacteria Gram-positive Rod-shaped Beer spoiler	Acidity
Lactobacillus pastorianus	Anaerobic Hop tolerant Alcohol tolerant	Lactic acid bacteria Gram-positive Rod-shaped Beer spoiler	Acidity Ropiness
Obesumbacterium proteus	Aerobic Very common Present only during early fermentation	Gram-negative Rod-shaped Wort spoiler	Yeast contaminant Parsnip flavors
Pediococcus ("beer *Sarcina*")	Anaerobic Homofermentative Superattentuative Extremely dangerous Nonmotile	Lactic acid bacteria Gram-positive Cocci-shaped Single cells, pairs, and tetrads Beer spoiler	Turbidity Acidity Diacetyl Ropiness Sediment
Zymomonas spp.	Anaerobic Wider range of pH Tolerant to low temperatures Highly motile	Gram-negative Rod-shaped Beer spoiler	Turbidity Rotten apples Hydrogen sulfide Ropiness Acetaldehyde

becomes cloudy. Large amounts of lactic acid and acetic acid are produced, causing souring of the beer (Gaenzle et al., 2001; Hollerova and Kubizniakova, 2001; Sakamoto et al., 2001; Thomas, 2001; O'Mahony et al., 2000). *Pediococcus* is a more common contaminant than *Lactobacillus* and is prevalent at the end of fermentation and during maturation. It is particularly prevalent as a spoilage organism in beers fermented at low temperatures. This organism is one of the most feared because of the difficulty in removing it from the brewery. Contamination is most often from calcified trub deposits. When *Pediococcus* grows in beer, diacetyl is produced, which causes the beer to have a buttery aroma. Some strains are notable for their ability to produce extracellular slime (jelly-like strands) (Goldammer, 2000).

ACETIC ACID BACTERIA

Acetic acid bacteria are particularly known in breweries for their ability to produce acetic acid and, therefore, vinegary off-flavors, turbidity, and ropiness. The surface contamination they cause is often apparent as an oily or moldy film. Acetic acid bacteria are either aerobic or microaerophilic and develop best in wort and beer when exposed to air during early fermentation, usually during racking. Aeration of the beer by rousing or splashing provides it with sufficient oxygen for respiration. The bacteria are therefore unable to grow after the yeast culture has utilized the dissolved oxygen of the wort. Like *Obesumbacterium proteus*, acetic acid bacteria can be transferred with the pitching yeast to the following fermentation. Hough et al. (1982) reported that flies, particularly the fruit fly, spread the infection. No restriction of the growth of acetic acid bacteria is produced by low pH or by hop resins or their isomers.

Acetic acid bacteria spoil beer by converting ethanol into acetic acid. Usually strict aerobes (although some may be microaerophilic), these bacteria are very acid tolerant and are the most common spoilers of draft beer. Two genera have been recognized: *Gluconobacter* and *Acetobacter* (Van Vuuren, 1987). *Gluconobacter* (short Gram-negative rods) range from aerobic to microaerophilic. These bacteria can tolerate conditions of low pH and the ethanol concentrations normally found in beer and grow well at 18°C. Using proline as a nitrogen source, *Gluconobacter* spp. convert ethanol to acetic acid. *Acetobacter* spp., on the other hand, oxidize the acetic acid generated to carbon dioxide and water; consequently, beer infected with acetic acid bacteria has a vinegary flavor, with a lowered pH and ethanol content (O'Connor-Cox et al., 1991).

ZYMOMONAS

Zymomonas anaerobia is a strict anaerobe that grows as motile Gram-negative rods that can tolerate 3.5 to 7 pH and up to 6% ethanol. This bacterium grows optimally at 30°C and can only ferment a narrow range of sugars (e.g., glucose, fructose, and sucrose). Its primary metabolites, ethanol and carbon dioxide, are not a problem; however, its secondary metabolites, hydrogen sulfide and acetaldehyde, are objectionable. Ingledew (1979) observes that *Zymomonas* spp. infections correlate with new construction work. Spoilage with *Zymomonas* spp., while relatively rare, can be a particular problem in breweries that produce primed beers. Contamination by *Zymomonas* in the brewery is very often restricted to the packaging stage, although in some cases it has been traced back to the fermenting stage. Because it is a soil organism, it can gain access to beer through the brushes of the cask washing machines. Infections with *Zymomonas* can result from excavation work in the brewery where the soil had been impregnated with beer.

Pectinatus cerevisiphilus, an obligate anaerobe, spoils beer by producing large amounts of hydrogen sulfide and propionic acid, which is diagnostic of the presence of this bacterium. It produces turbidity, hydrogen sulfide, acetic acid, and propionic acids in wort and packaged beers. The beer becomes turbid with an odor of rotten eggs. The pH optimum is in the range of 4.5 to 6.0, and growth is weak at a beer pH of around 4.0. The temperature range is from 15 to 40°C, with an optimum at about 30°C. Infections are normally encountered at the bottling stage. Suspected infection sources include water and drainage systems, as well as lubricating oil mixed with beer and water. Pasteurization readily kills the bacterium and can also be easily controlled by iodophores and chlorinating agents (Suihko and Haikara, 2001; Motoyama and Ogata, 2000; Satokari et al., 1998; Membre and Tholozan, 1994).

Megasphaera, a Gram-negative motile coccus, produces butanol, butyric acid, valeric acid, and isovaleric acid. The resultant beer has a rancid/cheesy/sickly flavor (Suihko and Haikara, 2001; Ziola et al., 2000; Satokari et al., 1998).

The aroma of beer infected with *Obesumbacterium proteus* has been described as "parsnip." The compound responsible for this is DMS, produced as a secondary metabolite, along with fusel alcohols, acetoin, and volatile fatty acids. The primary metabolites of this Gram-negative, facultatively anaerobic, rod-shaped bacterium are ethanol and lactate. It will not grow at pH less than 3.9. Although rarely spoiling beer, it can grow in pitched wort. The higher temperatures of ale fermentations favor this bacterium.

COLIFORMS

The coliform group of aerobic or facultatively anerobic Gram-negative rods contain the genera *Klebsiella*, *Escherichia*, *Citrobacter*, and *Acinetobacter*. These bacteria require a pH in excess of 4.3 so they do not grow in beer; however, they are able to grow in wort and can spoil it rapidly. Infected wort has been described variously as having a flavor that is "celery like," "sweet," or like "cooked cabbage." These organisms produce diacetyl, sulfur compounds, fusel alcohols, phenolics, and acetaldehyde, which cause a variety of off-flavors. *Enterobacter* and *Citrobacter* are killed at pH 4.4 and 2% alcohol, so organisms found in aging, conditioned, or otherwise finished beer are either *Hafnia* spp. or *Klebsiella* spp. (Tortorello and Reineke, 2000; Tompkins et al., 1996).

WILD YEAST

Wild yeast is any yeast other than the pitching yeast. Wild yeasts can be isolated at all stages of the brewing process from raw materials, wort, pitching yeast, and fermenting beer through to the packaged product and the dispensing system. Wild yeast can produce unintended flavors, including hydrogen sulfide, estery, acidic, fatty acid, and phenolic or medicinal notes. Turbidity is another effect caused by growth of wild yeast that remains after the culture yeast has been removed by filtering or fining. In the presence of air, some wild yeast can grow rapidly and form a film on the surface of the beer which can cause haze. Other effects may include primary yeast fermentation and separation difficulties, significantly lower terminal gravities, and a higher alcohol content in the finished beer. The lower terminal gravities are due to the ability of wild yeast to ferment sugars (such as maltotetraose and dextrins) not used by the primary yeast. Wild yeast infection is usually more of a problem for brewers not having a pure culture yeast propagation system than for those who do. Any yeast, be it wild yeast or the yeast used in beer production, that survives pasteurization can be regarded as a potential problem (Goldammer, 2000).

Various off-flavors are produced by wild yeast contaminants. The most commonly isolated genus is *Saccharomyces*, certain species of which are able to produce phenolic off-flavors. This flavor is produced when phenolic acids are broken down by enzymic decarboxylation or thermal decomposition to their corresponding vinyl derivates; for example, 4-vinyl guaiacol, which has a spicy phenolic flavor and a flavor threshold of 0.2 to 0.3 mg/L, is produced when ferulic acid from the malt is decarboxylated by spoilage yeast or bacteria (Madigan et al., 1994). Whether a particular strain of *Saccharomyces* is able to carry out this reaction or not is controlled by a single dominant gene *POF-1* (POF stands for phenolic off-flavor) (Meaden, 1994). The strains employed by brewers, apart from those used in the production of wheat beer, do not have this gene. *Saccharomyces diastaticus* is able to ferment dextrins and will cause over attenuation and its attendant off-flavors (Schmidt, 1988). *Candida* and *Hansenula* spp. are frequent pitching yeast contaminants, the latter synthesizing large amounts of esters, which impart a fruity flavor to the beer (O'Connor-Cox et al., 1991). Species of *Pichia* can give a sauerkraut off-flavor because of acid formed from the oxidation of ethanol. *Kloeckera* and *Brettanomwes* spp. can both spoil beer in a similar way but are less frequently found.

MOLDS

Beer can pick up a moldy/musty/cellar taint when produced or stored in areas contaminated by various fungi, including powdery mildew, slime molds, *Penicillium* spp., and *Aspergillus* spp. Such molds are often found growing on overlooked areas such as the underside of pipes; they reproduce by spores. Their distribution is aided by good air circulation (Phipps, 1990). In addition to the effects of mold metabolites and other mold metabolites on germination and malt characteristics, the toxins of these molds also have health implications. Mycotoxins may be transmitted to beers from contaminated grains during brewing. Mycotoxins such as aflatoxins, zearalenone, deoxynivalenol, fumonisins, and citrinin could originate from contaminated grains into beer. It is clear from various surveys (Table 1.3) that a variety of mycotoxins reach the final product, beer, but generally in limited concentrations.

Viewed on a worldwide scale, the aflatoxins produced by *Aspergillus flavus* and *A. parasiticus* are the most important of the mycotoxins found in cereals. They not only are toxic but are also potent carcinogens. Other important toxins are produced by various species of *Fusarium* associated with grain, including the estrogenic toxin zearalenone and trichothecenes, which are inhibitors of protein synthesis and are also immunosuppressive, as well as the fumonisins, which if not directly carcinogenic are cancer promoters. Two nephrotoxins that are also important are citrinin and ochratoxin A, produced by *Penicillium verrucosum*.

TABLE 1.3
Incidence of Mycotoxins in Beers from Various Countries

Toxin	Source	Levels	Refs.
Aflatoxins	American and Mexican beers ($N = 24$)	25%	Scott and Lawerence (1997)
Aflatoxins, zearalenone, ochratoxin	Traditional home-brewed beers	200–400 µg/L 2.6–426 µg/L 13–2340 µg/mL	Odhav and Naicker (2002)
Deoxynivalenol	Czechoslovakian beers ($N = 77$)	76%	Ruprich and Ostry (1995)
Fumonisins	Spanish beers ($N = 32$)	44%	Torres et al. (1998)
Fumonisins B_1 and B_2	American beers ($N = 25$) Mexican beers ($N = 3$) Canadian beers ($N = 1$)	86% positive for FB_1 41% positive for FB_2 (.3–12.7 ng/mL)	Hlywka and Bullerman (1999)
Ochratoxin A	26 commercial beers	Not reported	Scott and Kanhere (1995)
Ochratoxin A	Canadian and imported beers ($N = 41$)	63%	Scott and Kanhere (1995)
Ochratoxin A	Imported beers ($N = 107$)	2%	Soleas et al. (2001)
Ochratoxin A_0	Moroccan beers ($N = 5$)	Negative	Filali et al. (2001)
Ochratoxin A plus aflatoxins	Imported beers ($N = 94$) Japanese beers ($N = 22$)	90–95%	Nakajima et al. (1999)
Trichothecenes	Argentinean beers ($N = 50$)	Deoxynivalenol, 44%	Molto et al. (2000)
Trichothecenes, zearalenone	Korean beers ($N = 54$)	Nivalenol, 85%; deoxynivalenol, 19%	Shim et al. (1997)
	Imported beers	Nivalenol, 58%	

CONTROL

The entire brewing process should be monitored. A possible protocol to minimize contaminants is outlined in Table 1.4. Any pieces of equipment or materials used for wort production onward merit particular attention. When spoilage microorganisms are found, appropriate steps should be taken. If pitching yeast is contaminated with wild yeast, it should be discarded, whereas if it is infected with bacteria it can be acid washed (pH 2.1 for 1 to 2 hours; Simpson and Hammond, 1990). Hygiene is of paramount importance, and adequate cleaning and sterilizing programs are imperative. Outside the brewery, in the case of draft beer, close attention should be paid to the hygiene of dispensing equipment and the cellar.

Microbial spoilage can result in significant economic loss, as once a flavor change has occurred it is difficult to rectify the situation. The first obvious control step is to remove and/or destroy the contaminants through sterile filtration or pasteurization. It is possible to remove some metabolites by carbon filtration; however, doing so may also remove some of the desirable flavor attributes. Blending with other beer should be carried out with caution. Effective quality control is essential, and many selective sensitive media have been developed to allow the

TABLE 1.4

Control and Prevention Strategy for Beer Contaminants

Sample	Frequency	Sample Size	Common Contaminants
Water supply	1× per week	100 mL, filtered	Enteric acid, molds
Wort	Every brew	1 mL	Enteric, acetic, and lactic acids; wild yeast
Pitching yeast	Every crop	1 mL	Enteric, acetic, and lactic acids; wild yeast
Fermenting beer, days 1–2	Every tank	1 mL	Enteric, acetic, and lactic acids; wild yeast
Fermenting beer, days 3–5	Every tank	1 mL	Acetic and lactic acids, wild yeast
Storage tank	3× per week	100 mL, filtered	Acetic and lactic acids
Finishing tank	3× per week	100 mL, filtered	Lactic acid
Bottling tank	1× per month	100 mL, filtered	Lactic acid
Bottled beer	Every batch	100 mL, filtered	Acetic and lactic acids
Clean in place (CIP) system rinse water	Every CIP procedure	100 mL, filtered	—
CIP surfaces	Every CIP procedure	Swab	—

Source: Adapted from Kunz, K., *Where and When To Sample for Contaminants*, The Brewing Science Institute, http://www.professionalbrewer.com.

detection and quantification of contaminants. After beer is packaged (with the exception of bottle-conditioned and cask products), the occurrence of any micro-organism is undesirable. Rapid tests are available to detect contamination, such as the determination of adenosine triphosphate (ATP) based on a luciferin–luciferase system. ATP bioluminescence can also be used to monitor the sterility of vessels (Simpson and Hammond, 1990).

The conditions under which a beer is brewed or dispensed can also increase the likelihood of microbial spoilage and should, if possible, be controlled; for example, low-density polythene dispensing tubing lets through more oxygen required for the growth of acetic acid bacteria than does polyvinylchloride or co-extruded nylon piping (Casson, 1984).

CONCLUSION

The safety of beer, in microbiological terms, has been recognized for centuries, and it was often considered to be safer than water when traveling in "high-risk" areas. The selection of beer by the consumer is based on certain expectations and the reputation of the brand; therefore, beers should always maintain a consistent flavor and be microbiologically safe. If this balance is perturbed by the introduction of contaminants either from the raw materials or during processing or storage, then substantial economic losses could result, as well as consumer dissatisfaction. Most contaminants that are introduced into the beers (including bacteria and wild yeast) make beer unpalatable rather than unsafe, except for mycotoxins. It is clear from the surveys conducted that, although a variety of mycotoxins reach the final product, they are generally present in limited concentrations. It is impossible to assess the real importance of mycotoxins in beer to human health, but the risk of disease does exist, so all contaminants that could enter beer must be prevented or controlled.

ACKNOWLEDGMENTS

I would like to thank Ms. B. Jeena for her editorial assistance with the manuscript.

REFERENCES

Andrew, D.A. (1987) Beer off-flavours: their cause, effect and prevention, *Brew. Guardian*, 116: 14–21.

Anness, B.J. and Bamworth, C.W. (1982) Dimethyl sulphide: a review, *J. Inst. Brew.*, 88: 244–252.

Bennet, S.J.E. (1996) Off-flavours in alcoholic beverages, in *Foods Taints and Off-Flavours*, Saxby, M.J., Ed., Blackie Academic & Professional, Glasgow, pp. 290–320.

Brantley, J.D. and Aranha, H. (1994) Comparison of the retention of different beer spoilage organisms by membrane filters, *Tech. Q. Master Brew. Assoc. Am.*, 31: 121–122.

Casson, D. (1984) Interactions in beer dispense systems, *Brew. Guardian*, 113: 7–14.

Clapperton, J.F. (1978) Fatty acids contributing to caprylic flavour in beer: the use of profile and threshold data in flavour research, *J. Inst. Brew.*, 84: 107–112.

Clapperton, J.F. and Brown, D.G.W. (1978) Caprylic flavour as a feature of beer flavour, *J. Inst. Brew.*, 84: 90–92.

Doyle, M.P., Beuchat, L.R., and Montville, T.J., Eds. (1997) *Food Microbiology: Fundamentals and Frontiers*, American Society for Microbiology, Washington, D.C., p. 784.

Engan, S. (1991) Off-flavours in beers, *Brauwelt Int.*, 3: 217–223.

Filali, A., Ouammi, L., Betbeder, A.M., Baudrimont, I., Soulaymani, R., Benayada, A., and Creppy, E.E. (2001) Ochratoxin A in beverages from Morocco: a preliminary survey, *Food Add. Contam.*, 18: 565–568.

Gaenzle, M.G., Ulmer, H.M., and Vogel, R.F. (2001) High-pressure inactivation of *Lactobacillus plantarum* in a model beer system, *J. Food Sci.*, 66: 1174–1181.

Goldammer, T. (2000) Beer spoilage, in *The Brewers' Handbook: The Complete Book to Brewing Beer*, KVP Publishers, Clifton, VA, pp. 353–366.

Hardwick, W.A. (1978) Two-piece cans: some flavour problems caused by manufacturing materials or practices, *Tech. Q. Master Brew. Assoc. Am.*, 15: 23–25.

Harms, D. and Nitzsche, F. (2001) High performance separation of unmodified and reduced hop and beer bitter compounds by single high performance liquid chromatography method, *J. Am. Soc. Brew. Chem.*, 59: 28–31.

Hashimoto, N. (1981) Flavour stability of packaged beers, in *Brewing Science*, Pollock, J.R., Ed., Academic Press, London, pp. 347–405.

Hill, P.G. and Smith, R.M. (2000) Determination of sulphur compounds in beer using headspace solid-phase micro-extraction and gas chromatography with pulsed flame photometric detection, *J. Chromatogr. A*, 872: 203–213.

Hlywka, J.J. and Bullerman, L.B. (1999) Occurrence of fumonisin B1 and B2 in beer, *Food Add. Contam.*, 16: 319–324.

Hollerova, I. and Kubizniakova, P. (2001) Monitoring Gram-positive bacterial contamination in Czech breweries, *J. Inst. Brew.*, 107: 355–358.

Hough, J.S., Briggs, D.E., Stevens, R., and Young, I.W. (1982) *Malting and Brewing Science*, Vol. 2: *Hopped Wort and Beer*, 2nd ed., Chapman & Hall, London.

Ilori, M.O., Fessehatzion, B., Olajuyigbe, O.A., Babalola, G.O., and Ogundiwin, J.O. (1991) Effect of malting and brewing processes on the microorganisms associated with sorghum grains and malt, *Tech. Q. Master Brew. Assoc. Am.*, 28: 45–49.

Ingledew, W.M. (1979) Effect of bacterial contamination on beer: a review, *J. Am. Soc. Brew. Chem.*, 37: 145–150.

Irwin, A.J., Bordeleau, L., and Barker, R.L. (1993) Model studies and flavour: threshold determination of 3-methyl-2-butene-1-thiol in beer, *J. Am. Soc. Brew. Chem.*, 51: 1–3.

Jespersen, L. and Jakobsen, M. (1996) Specific spoilage organisms in breweries and laboratory media for their detection, *Int. J. Food Microbiol.*, 33: 139–155.

King A.W., Meads, D.J., and Vernel, C. (1994) Identification of a beer flavour taint originating from contamination during transportation of packaging materials, *Proc. Conv. Inst. Brew.*, 23: 198.

Lambert, D.E., Shaw, K.J., and Whitfield, F.B. (1993) Lacquered aluminum cans as an indirect source of 2,4.6-trichloroanisole in beer, *Chem. Ind.*, 12: 461–462.

Madigan, D., McMurrough, I., and Smith, M.R. (1994) Rapid determination of 4-vinyl guaiacol and ferulic acid in beers and worts by high-performance liquid chromatography, *J. Am. Soc. Brew. Chem.*, 52: 152–155.

Meaden, P. (1994) Padding out the POF gene, *Ferment*, 7: 229–230.

Meilgaard, M.C. (1975) Flavour chemistry of beer. Part II. Flavour and threshold of 239 aroma volatiles, *Tech. Q. Master Brew. Assoc. Am.*, 12: 151–168.

Membre, J.M. and Tholozan, J.L. (1994) Modeling growth and off-flavours production of spoiled beer bacteria, *Pectinatus frisingensis*, *J. Appl. Bacteriol.*, 77: 456–460.

Molto, G., Samar, M.M., Resnik, S., Martinez, E.J., and Pacin, A. (2000) Occurrence of trichothecenes in Argentinean beer: a preliminary exposure assessment, *Food Add. Contam.*, 9: 809–813.

Motoyama, Y. and Ogata, T. (2000) Detection of *Pectinatus* spp. by PCR using 16S–23S rDNA spacer regions, *J. Am. Soc. Brew. Chem.*, 58: 4–7.

Nakajima, M., Tsubouchi, H., and Miyabe, M. (1999) A survey of ochratoxin A and aflatoxins in domestic and imported beers in Japan by immunoaffinity and liquid chromatography, *J. AOAC Int.*, 82: 897–902.

Nakakita, Y., Takahashi, T., Tsuchiya, Y., Watari, J., and Shinotsuka, K. (2002) A strategy for detection of all beer-spoilage bacteria, *J. Am. Soc. Brew. Chem.*, 60: 63–67.

Narziss, L. (1993) Modern wort boiling, in *Proc. Conv. Institute of Brewing*, Central and South African Section, Feb. 28–March 4, Johannesburg, South Africa, pp. 195–212.

O'Conner-Cox, E.S.C., Yui, P.M., and Ingledew, W.M. (1991) Pasteurization: thermal death of microbes in brewing, *Tech. Q. Master Brew. Assoc. Am.*, 28: 67–77.

Odhav, B. and Naicker, V. (2002) Mycotoxins in South African traditionally brewed beers, *Food Add. Contam.*, 19: 55–61.

O'Mahony, A., O'Sullivan, T., Walsh, Y., Vaughan, A., Maher, M., Fitzgerald, G.F., and van Sinderen, D. (2000) Characterisation of antimicrobial producing lactic acid bacteria from malted barley, *J. Inst. Brew.*, 106: 403–410.

Phipps, M.E. (1990) Brewing mold control, *Brew. Dig.*, 65: 28–29.

Ruprich, J. and Ostry, V. (1995) Determination of the mycotoxin deoxynivalenol in beer by commercial ELISA tests and estimation of the exposure dose from beer for the population in the Czech Republic, *Centre Eur. J. Public Health*, 3: 224–229.

Sakamoto, K., Margolles, A., van Veen, H.W., and Konings, W.N. (2001) Hop resistance in the beer spoilage bacterium *Lactobacillus brevis* is mediated by the ATP-binding cassette multi-drug transporter HorA, *J. Bacteriol.*, 183: 5371–5375.

Satokari, R., Juvonen, R., Mallison, K., von Wright, A., and Haikara, A. (1998) Detection of beer spoilage bacteria *Megasphaera* and *Pectinatus* by polymerase chain reaction and colorimetric microplate hybridization, *Int. J. Food Microbiol.*, 45: 119–127.

Schmidt, H.J. (1988) Beer defects caused by microorganisms, *Brauwelt Int.*, 1: 72–74.

Scott, P.M. and Kanhere, S.R. (1995) Determination of ochratoxin A in beer, *Food Add. Contam.*, 12: 591–598.

Scott, P.M. and Lawerence, G.A. (1997) Determination of aflatoxins in beer, *J. AOAC Int.*, 80: 1229–1234.

Seaton, J.C. and Moir, M. (1987) Sulphur compounds and their impact on beer flavour, in *European Brewing Convention Monograph III: Symposium on Hops*, Weihenstephan, Sept. 18, Verlag, Nuremberg, Germany, pp. 130–145.

Shim, W.B., Kim, J.C., Seo, J.A., and Lee, Y.W. (1997) Natural occurrence of trichothecenes and zearalenone in Korean and imported beers, *Food Add. Contam.*, 14: 1–5.

Simpson, W.J. and Hammond, J.R.M. (1990) A practical guide to the acid washing of brewer's yeast, *Ferment*, 3: 363–365.

Soleas, G.J., Yan, J., and Goldberg, D.M. (2001) Assay of ochratoxin A in wine and beer by high-pressure liquid chromatography photodiode assay and gas chromatography mass selective detection, *J. Agric. Food Chem.*, 6: 33–40.

Stenius, V., Majamaa, E., Haikora, A., Henriksson, E., and Virtanen, H. (1991) Beer off-flavours originating from anaerobic spore-forming bacteria in brewery adjuncts, in *Proc. of European Brewing Convention*, 23rd Congress, Lisbon, Oxford University Press, London, pp. 483–490.

Suihko, M.L. and Haikara, A. (2001) Characterization of *Pectinatus* and *Megasphaera* strains by automated ribotyping, *J. Inst. Brew.*, 107: 175–184.

Thomas, K. (2001) Fight your foes, feed your friends: lactic acid bacteria in brewing, *Brew. Int.*, 1: 62–64.

Tompkins, T.A., Stewart, R., Savard, L., Russell, I., and Dowhanick, T.M. (1996) RAPD–PCR characterization of brewery yeast and beer spoilage bacteria, *J. Am. Soc. Brew. Chem.*, 54: 91–96.

Torres, M.R., Sanchis, V., and Ramos, A.J. (1998) Occurrence of fumonisins in Spanish beers analysed by an enzyme-linked immunosorbent assay method, *Int. J. Food Microbiol.*, 39: 139–143.

Tortorello, M.L. and Reineke, K.F. (2000) Direct enumeration of *Escherichia coli* and enteric bacteria in water, beverages and sprouts by 16S rRNA *in situ* hybridization, *Food Microbiol.*, 17: 305–313.

Tressl, F., Friese, R.L., Fedesack, F., and Koppler, H. (1978) Studies of the volatile composition of hops during storage, *J. Agric. Food Chem.*, 26: 1426–1430.

Van Vuuren, H.J.J. (1987) Gram-negative spoilage bacteria, in *Brewing Microbiology*, Priest, F.G. and Campbell, I., Eds., Elsevier, London.

White, F.H. (1977) The origin and control of dimethyl sulfide in beer, *Brew. Dig.*, 52: 38–50.

Ziola, B., Gee, L., Berg, N.N., and Lee, S.Y. (2000) Serogroups of the beer spoilage bacterium *Megasphaera cerevisiae* correlate with the molecular weight of the major EDTA-extractable surface protein, *Can. J. Microbiol.*, 46: 95–100.

2 Alcohol and Intestinal Permeability: Implications for Human Toxicity

*Ashkan Farhadi, Jeremy Z. Fields,
Ali Banan, and Ali Keshavarzian*

CONTENTS

Abstract   Whatever the reason for alcohol ingestion (and there are many, such as a food, social lubricant, or religious, ritual, or psychotropic drug), alcohol remains a toxin that can affect virtually every cell in the human body. It is not surprising, then, that alcohol-related effects on the mind and body represent one of the most important worldwide health problems today. In this article, we consider in detail how alcohol modifies diet and nutrient absorption and, conversely, how foods in the diet affect alcohol absorption and metabolism. In addition, we discuss how alcohol exerts its toxic effects on the gastrointestinal tract, particularly disruption of the gastrointestinal barrier, and how this disturbance might contribute to several systemic disorders, including alcoholic liver disease.

Abbreviations   adenosine triphosphate (ATP); alcoholic liver disease (ALD); chromium ethylenediaminetetraacetic acid (Cr-EDTA); colon cancer cell monolayer (Caco-2 cells); constitutive nitric oxide synthase enzyme (cNOS); cyclic guanosine monophosphate (cGMP); cyclooxygenase-2 (COX-2); ethyl alcohol (EtOH); gastrointestinal (GI); immunoglobulin M (IgM); inducible nitric oxide synthase enzyme (iNOS); interleukin-2 (IL-2); lipopolysaccharide (LPS); liver disease (LD); lymph node (LN); nitric oxide (NO); nitric oxide synthase (NOS); peroxynitrite (ONOO$^-$); polyethylene glycol (PEG); reactive oxygen species (ROS); tumor necrosis factor-α (TNF-α)

Key Words   *alcohol, alcoholic liver disease, endotoxin, food, intestinal absorption, intestinal permeability, toxicity*

INTRODUCTION

Alcohol was used by humans as a beverage or an adjunct to the ingestion of food even in ancient civilizations, and wine drinking has long played important social and religious roles (Nencini, 1997). In the modern world, alcohol is still used in these ways, but we are more aware of the downside of the use of alcohol. Alcohol is a causal or contributing factor in thousands of motor vehicle accidents (22,000

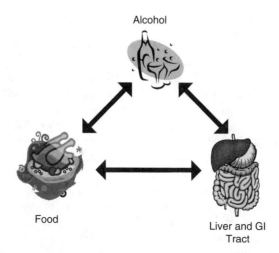

FIGURE 2.1 The dynamic interactions among alcohol, gastrointestinal tract, and food modulate several gastrointestinal tract physiologic and absorptive properties.

deaths and $148 billion in costs related to alcohol-involved crashes per year in the United States alone) (Miller and Blincoe, 1994). On top of that, alcohol-related medical problems are important health problems worldwide. Although alcohol can affect virtually every cell in the human body, the effect of alcohol has only been widely studied in a few organ systems, such as the liver and brain. More recently, alcohol researchers have begun to direct their inquiries toward the effects of alcohol on other systems, including the intestinal tract. In this chapter, we will review what is known about the effects of alcohol on the intestinal tract (Figure 2.1).

ALCOHOL AS A FOOD

Alcohol is widely used either with meals or between meals for a variety of reasons: (1) to enhance the taste of other foods, (2) for its psychotropic effects, and (3) for social and religious reasons. It can also be a source of calories, particularly for those who consume a lot of it. Each gram of pure ethyl alcohol contains 7 kcal/g. Each drink of alcohol (1.5 oz. of whiskey, 3.5 oz. of wine, and 12 oz. of beer are each considered to be roughly about 1 drink) contains 99 to 146 kcal, about the same number of calories as 2 to 3 slices of bread. Thus, it is not surprising that some researchers believe that alcohol should be considered as a food (Forsander, 1994). Other researchers believe that alcohol does not satisfy the definition of a food, in part because animals do not decrease their nutrient-derived calories when they receive alcohol-derived calories (Gill et al., 1996). Giner and Meguid (1996), however, reported that replacing 50% of calories with ethanol in rat diets resulted in a decrease in food intake of 16% if ethanol was supplied through the intragastric route and 9% if ethanol was supplied intravenously.

ALCOHOL MODIFICATION OF DIET

The data on the effect of alcohol on dietary constituents are controversial. In a large cross-sectional study, Kesse et al. (2001) showed that increasing alcohol consumption in humans was associated with higher total energy intake and higher intake of protein and fat. This was associated with a decrease in carbohydrates, vegetables, and dairy products in these populations (Kesse et al., 2001). Data from the U.S. Department of Agriculture's Nationwide Food Consumption Survey (Windham et al., 1983) showed that the average daily nutrient intake was similar in drinkers and non-drinkers, but the energy/calorie intake was higher among the drinkers. This study also showed that the nutrient density of the diet of non-drinkers was significantly lower than that for drinkers. Interestingly, an animal study showed that consumption of a 20% alcohol solution as the only source of drinking water resulted in a reduction in weight gain in rats. This reduction was not associated with a decreased energy intake but with an increased energy expenditure in these animal through increases in alcohol metabolism and postprandial thermogenesis (Larue-Achagiotis et al., 1990). A similar outcome was reported for humans, showing that, despite higher calorie intakes in alcoholics, these alcohol drinkers were not more obese than non-drinkers (Jones et al., 1982). It seems that consumption of excess calories at low levels of alcohol intake in drinkers is offset by higher basal metabolic rates (Camargo et al., 1987); however, the excess calorie intake by heavy drinkers might result in higher adiposity.

ALCOHOL MODIFICATION OF ABSORPTION

Alcohol modulates the digestion and absorption of various compounds in the intestine. Several animal and human studies have already shown the effect of alcohol on the handling of nutrients, vitamins, water, electrolytes, and drugs, but this area is complex and controversial. Overall, *acute* exposure of intestine to ethanol appears to result in morphological alterations, including subepithelial fluid accumulation, exfoliation of enterocytes, and vascular congestion (Buell et al., 1983), or functional alteration of enterocytes which is mainly seen as a reduction in the adenosine triphosphate (ATP) content of the cells and inhibition of cellular metabolism and transport (Money et al., 1990; Krasner et al., 1976a; Dinda and Beck, 1977; Dinda et al., 1975). These changes, however, are usually not associated with changes in intestinal absorption of nutrients. Pfeiffer et al. (1993) showed that adding ethanol to a nutrient solution did not significantly affect the net absorption of nutrients in the upper intestine, but perfusion of a 4% ethanol solution into the duodenal and jejunal portion of the intestine decreased water and sodium secretion and increased the rate of absorption of nitrogen and fatty acids. Mekhjian and May (1977) also showed that acute perfusion of 2 to 10% ethanol solutions into the jejunum or ileum did not significantly alter sodium or water transport. Higher doses of alcohol (5000 μmol/L), however, resulted in increases in albumin in jejunal fluid, suggestive of an increase in membrane permeability (Lavo et al., 1992).

The effect of *chronic* alcohol ingestion on gastrointestinal absorptive function is even more complex. Also, compared to acute exposure, chronic ethanol exposure is more associated with changes in enterocyte function than with structure. Merino et al. (1997) showed that hydrophilic molecules are absorbed much faster in intestine of chronic alcohol-fed rats, while the rate of absorption of lipophilic homologs does not change. In a study by Rossi et al. (1980), chronic alcohol-fed rats showed a 40% increase in fecal fat excretion compared to pair-fed controls.

Mucosal water handling is also significantly affected by chronic alcohol consumption. In a study by Krasner et al. (1976b) of 10 patients with acute-on-chronic alcoholism, the absorption of water and Na^+ and Cl^- was significantly lower in alcoholics compared to controls. Chronic alcohol-fed rats had decreased Na^+-stimulated glucose and glycine uptakes without affecting Na^+-independent solute transport in intestine. On the other hand, absorption of bovine serum albumin and gamma-globulin was markedly augmented. These observations suggest that chronic ethanol intake affects the uptake of organic solutes and macromolecules in the rat intestine rather than inorganic solutes (Kaur et al., 1993), a finding that is discussed in greater detail in the following section on barrier integrity. It appears that folate deficiency, a state that is usually linked with alcoholism, contributes to the changes in absorption of water and electrolytes associated with chronic alcohol consumption. The administration of a folate-deficient diet and ethanol for 2 weeks produced a marked reduction in sodium and water absorption or a small net secretion. The administration of ethanol with a folate-supplemented diet produced significant but less pronounced changes in sodium and water transport compared to controls; thus, a folate-deficient diet might contribute to the diarrhea observed in a significant proportion of alcoholics (Mekhjian et al., 1977).

Ethanol can also modulate the rate of absorption, metabolism, and elimination of several drugs. It decreases the rate of absorption and increases elimination of propranolol (Grabowski et al., 1980). Chronic alcoholism has always been linked to thiamine deficiency. Ironically, acute exposure to 1% ethanol significantly increased active transport of thiamine by approximately fourfold in a study by Holler et al. (1975). In addition, chronic alcohol exposure does not change the thiamin absorption properties of intestine; however, the major mechanism contributing to ethanol-induced thiamin deficiency in chronic alcoholics would be the alteration of thiamin metabolism and reduction of the metabolically active form of the vitamin (Ba et al., 1996).

Celada et al. (1978) showed that acute ingestion of ethanol does not influence the absorption of inorganic iron, but it significantly diminishes the absorption of heme iron. Polache et al. (1996) showed that the maximum transport of methionine decreases dramatically in the chronic alcohol-fed rat. The effect of alcohol on intestinal absorption may be biphasic; for example, at low concentrations, ethanol increases estradiol absorption while at high concentrations it inhibits estrone absorption (Martins and Dada, 1982).

DIETARY MODIFICATION OF ALCOHOL METABOLISM

Several studies have suggested that food modulates alcohol pharmacokinetics (Whitmire et al., 2002; Hahn et al., 1994; Jones and Jonsson, 1994; Lin et al., 1976; Sedman et al., 1976). These studies suggest that simultaneous ingestion of ethanol with meals results in a lower peak concentration and greater lag time to peak blood alcohol concentrations, which results in a smaller area under the curve for blood alcohol vs. time. This raises the question that this effect may be due to changes in absorption of ethanol from the gastrointestinal tract or increases in its systemic elimination. The change in gastrointestinal absorption might be due to delayed gastric emptying, which affects alcohol pharmacokinetics in several ways: (1) it increases the exposure of ethanol to gastric mucosal alcohol dehydrogenase; (2) it decreases the transit of alcohol to a highly absorbable area of small intestine; and (3) the gradual absorption of ethanol permits higher clearance of ethanol from portal blood by the liver (i.e., first-pass effect). In addition, food constituents can interact with alcohol and decrease the luminal concentration of ethanol. Increases in alcohol elimination might be due to increased hepatic blood flow associated with meal intake or stimulation of alcohol-metabolizing enzymes in the liver (Ramchandani et al., 2001). Not all foods decrease blood alcohol levels; for example, salty food increased blood alcohol level in one human study (Talbot and LaGrange, 1999).

ALCOHOL AS A TOXIN

The gastrointestinal (GI) tract is the only organ in humans that can be affected by both local and systemic effects of ingested alcohol. Alcohol affects GI structure and function through several different mechanisms (Figure 2.2). The structural damage from alcohol can present as a wide spectrum of mucosal damage such as ulcer, erosion, bleeding, and edema or even damage at the cellular and subcellular level, such as damage to the cell membrane, mitochondria, and cytoskeleton. The functional disturbances that usually follow structural damage can manifest as disrupted GI motility (Keshavarzian et al., 1986a,b, 1990), abnormal secretion and absorption, and disturbances in barrier function. In this section, we will concentrate on the detrimental effects of alcohol on the GI barrier, with a major emphasis on the effect of alcohol on intestinal permeability and the consequences of barrier disruption.

INTESTINAL BARRIER

The intestinal barrier is the largest interface between the body and the external environment (Farhadi et al., 2003). This barrier protects the internal milieu against exposure to harmful materials including microorganisms, toxins, and antigens and at the same time permits the passage of nutrients from the intestinal lumen into the circulation. Not surprisingly, then, the presence of an intact intestinal barrier is essential in maintaining health and preventing tissue injury in several organ systems (Farhadi et al., 2003). Barrier protection includes both immunogenic mechanisms and non-immunogenic mechanisms (Figure 2.3). The immunogenic components include immunoglobulins, lymphocytes (luminal, interepithelial, intraepithelial, and submucosal), macrophages, neutrophils, mast cells, basophils, and Langerhans cells. The non-immunogenic component of the intestinal barrier consists of multiple layers that regulate the transport of materials from lumen to blood, including the unstirred water layer, the mucous coat, epithelial and paracellular routes, basement membranes,

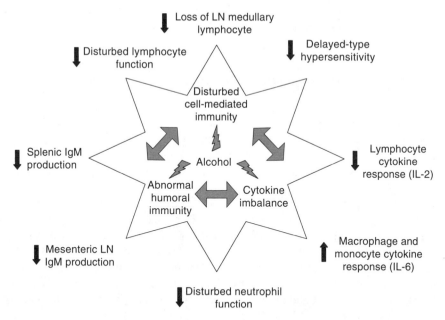

FIGURE 2.2 Various effects of alcohol on immunogenic components of the intestinal barrier disturb both the cell-mediated and humoral immune systems.

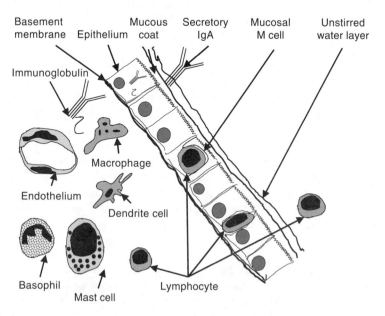

FIGURE 2.3 Components of the gastrointestinal barrier system. (From Farhadi, A. et al., *J. Gastroenterol. Hepatol.*, 18(5), 479–497. With permission.)

the lamina propria matrix, capillary and lymphatic endothelium, and eventually GI blood flow. It appears that alcohol can affect both immunogenic and non-immunogenic barrier functions.

Effect of Alcohol on Immunogenic Barrier

Several studies have shown the suppressive effect of ethanol on the GI immune system that can result in increased risk of infection, a finding that has been widely tested in a rat thermal injury model. Thermal injury in the rat is associated with immunosuppression and increased risk of bacterial translocation and infection. Using this model, researchers were able to better investigate the effect of alcohol on the GI and systemic immune systems. Acute ethanol exposure potentiates the immunosuppression associated with burn injury, and this effect is dose dependent (Messingham et al., 2000). This immunosuppression is associated with an imbalance of cytokines and changes in the population and function of blood cells (neutrophils, lymphocytes, and macrophages), eventually resulting in disturbances of the cell-mediated and humoral immune systems. Acute and chronic ethanol exposure before thermal injury was associated with more severe immunosuppression associated with thermal injury alone (Choudhry et al., 2002; Tabata et al., 2002; Napolitano et al., 1995; Kawakami et al., 1990).

Alcohol and cytokines

Chronic ethanol exposure in the rat decreased the cytokine responses of lymphocytes (Wang et al., 1994), particularly interleukin-2 (IL-2) production (Choudhry et al., 2000). On the other hand production of IL-6 by macrophages is stimulated by either burn or ethanol, independently or synergistically. Increases in IL-6 in the rat burn model were associated with suppression of cell-mediated immunity, increases in hepatic reactive oxygen species (ROS), and overall mortality (Colantoni et al., 2000; Faunce et al., 1997; Kawakami et al., 1991). Blocking of IL-6 function by corticosteroids or IL-6 antibody, which improves cellular immune responses, is another clue that IL-6 is important in the pathogenesis of immunosuppression induced by ethanol in the burn/ethanol rat model (Fontanilla et al., 2000; Faunce et al., 1997, 1998).

Alcohol and cellular immunity

Chronic exposure to ethanol results in suppression of cell-mediated immunity that is associated with loss of medullary lymphocytes in the mesenteric lymph node (LN) in rats in 1 week (Sibley et al., 1995), disturbed lymphocyte and splenocyte proliferation, and decreased delayed-type hypersensitivity (Choudhry et al., 2000; Faunce et al., 1997, 1998; Kawakami et al., 1991).

Alcohol and humoral immunity

Immunoglobulin M (IgM) production is affected by both burns and ethanol exposure; however, ethanol dominantly decreases mesenteric lymph-node IgM production while burns decrease splenic IgM production (Tabata and Meyer, 1995). This might explain the synergistic effect of burns and ethanol on the humoral immune system in the burn/ethanol rat model.

Alcohol and neutrophil function

Acute ethanol exposure transiently suppresses chemotactic functions of granulocytes (Kawakami et al., 1989; Patel et al., 1996). Woodman et al. (1996) also showed that, in pigs, acute alcohol intoxication at the time of trauma decreased neutrophil and lymphocyte function, plasma cortisol, and the response to endotoxin challenge. In this study, ethanol resulted in neutropenia after trauma. The mechanism by which ethanol affects the immune system is still not well understood. Some observers believe that the immunotoxic effects of chronic ethanol ingestion are partly the result of nutritional deficiencies associated with chronic ethanol use (Watzl and Watson, 1993; Watzl et al., 1993); however this cannot explain the effect of acute ethanol exposure on the immune system that was noted in rat models.

Effect of Alcohol on Non-Immunogenic Intestinal Barrier

Alcohol and non-immunogenic barrier components

Alcohol may affect all components of the non-immunogenic GI barrier. For example, the unstirred water layer is influenced by acute exposure to ethanol, and the passive permeability properties of this layer toward certain lipids declines (Thomson et al., 1984). Ethanol is also able to disrupt gastric surfactants by changing the hydrophobic properties of phospholipid components (Mosnier et al., 1993). In addition, the gastric mucous layer, which is an important barrier against acid and pepsin, can be easily penetrated by alcohol, causing high concentrations of this toxin adjacent to epithelial mucosa (Matuz, 1992). Among all non-immunogenic barrier components, however, mucosal epithelium is the one that is particularly affected and has been studied extensively for years.

The integrity of the intestinal barrier depends on both healthy epithelial cells and on an intact paracellular pathway, which appears to be the main route for permeation of macromolecules such as endotoxin (Hollander, 1992). This pathway is a complex array of structures that includes tight junctions between gut epithelial cells. This dynamic conduit is highly regulated and is able to change its size under various physiological and pathological conditions (Madara, 1990). One of the main cellular structures essential for the integrity of this conduit is the cytoskeleton, a complex array of protein filaments extending throughout the cytosol and attaching to the cell membrane (Small, 1988; Alvia, 1987). The cytoskeleton not only is essential for the paracellular pathway but is also pivotal for maintaining the normal structure, transport, and functional integrity of all eukaryotic cells, including GI epithelium (MacRae, 1992; Small, 1988; Steinert and Room, 1988; Alvia, 1987; Bretscher, 1987). Hence, the cytoskeleton is a critical structure for maintaining intestinal barrier function and can be a potential target in ethyl alcohol (EtOH)-induced gut leakiness.

Role of cytoskeletons in barrier integrity

The cytoskeleton includes three types of protein filaments: actin filaments, microtubules, and intermediate filaments, formed, respectively, from actin, tubulin, and a family of related proteins (vimentin, laminin). Of these three filaments, microtubules and actin are the largest and provide the greatest structural support. Not surprisingly, disruption of these filaments affects cell structure and function (Banan et al., 2000d, 2001a,b,e). Disruption of microtubules and actin by either oxidants (Banan et al., 2000a, 2001c,d) or EtOH (Banan et al., 1996, 2000b, 2001d) causes monolayer barrier disruption.

Nitric oxide, nitric oxide synthase, and the intestinal barrier

Nitric oxide (NO) is a key mediator in normal cellular processes in many organs, including normal intestinal cells and barrier function (Kanwar et al., 1994; Kubes, 1992), but excess NO is a culprit in barrier dysfunction (Alican and Kubes, 1996; Boughton-Smith et al., 1993), including EtOH-induced barrier dysfunction (Banan et al., 1996, 2000b). NO is a labile free radical made from L-arginine by nitric oxide synthase (NOS). Two major isoforms of NOS have been identified: a constitutive enzyme (cNOS) that is Ca^{2+} dependent and an inducible form (iNOS) that is Ca^{2+} independent. Both are present in enterocytes; iNOS is also present in inflammatory cells, and its expression and activity can be induced by endotoxin, cytokines, or EtOH.

A great deal of what is known about the involvement of NO in intestinal epithelial physiology and pathophysiology has been based on research studies that have used intestinal cell monolayers, especially monolayers made of Caco-2 cells. This cell line has been widely used to study the mechanism of intestinal barrier function in general and of NO pathways in particular (Banan et al., 2000c; Unno et al., 1997). NO regulates GI physiology by modulating both epithelial cells and the microcir- culation (Alican and Kubes, 1996; Whittle, 1994; Kubes, 1992; Kubes and Granger, 1992). A low level of NO, which is normally synthesized by cNOS, is important for maintaining normal mucosal barrier function. L-NAME, which inhibits both cNOS and iNOS and prevents normal NO production, increases intestinal epithelial (Alican and Kubes, 1996) and microvascular (Kubes and Granger, 1992) permeability in animals. In contrast, overproduction of NO by iNOS disrupts barrier function, and prevention of NO overproduction in rat and in monolayers restores normal barrier integrity (Colgan, 1998). In addition, in a study using Caco-2 cells transfected with iNOS antisense oligonucleotides, an injurious dose of EtOH did not upregulate iNOS or disrupt monolayer barrier integrity. This clearly indicates that the effect of EtOH on barrier integrity is not simply a solvent effect and must be mediated by a specific (iNOS-driven) intracellular pathway.

How NO overproduction causes damage is an important question that needs to be addressed. It has been suggested that the main mechanism by which NO over- production induces intestinal barrier dysfunction is oxidation (and nitration) of cytoskeletal proteins (Banan et al., 1996, 2000b, 2001b). NO-mediated oxidation of cellular proteins is most likely due to its metabolite, peroxynitrite ($ONOO^-$), which is a product of the reaction of NO with superoxide radicals (Grisham et al., 1999; Beckman et al., 1990). Peroxynitrite oxidizes and damages proteins by reacting with their amino acid residues, such as cysteine. For example, nitration of phenolic amino acid residues produces nitrotyrosine, a stable footprint of $ONOO^-$ reactions and thus an index of $ONOO^-$ formation (Kimura et al., 1998). Indeed, EtOH disrupts the monolayer barrier through upregulation of iNOS and increases in NO and $ONOO^-$ formation. Not surprisingly, donors of NO and $ONOO^-$ mimic these effects (Banan et al., 1996, 2000b).

High levels of NO can cause loss of intestinal barrier integrity by other potential mechanisms besides protein nitration. These include activation of cyclic guanosine monophosphate (cGMP) pathways and ATP depletion (Liu and Sundqvist, 1997; Alican and Kubes, 1996); however, these alternative mechanisms are unlikely to mediate many of the effects of EtOH. Oxidation and nitration of epithelial proteins, which are the end result of NO overproduction, can disturb cell function in several ways. The nitration and oxidation of proteins and other cellular compartments are usually irreversible reactions and result in functional impairment and/or barrier disruption.

It should be mentioned that EtOH dose-dependently and markedly disrupts barrier integrity without causing cell death. This supports the idea that the effects of EtOH are not merely due to a solvent effect (i.e., non-specific toxicity). Indeed, pretreatment of monolayers with colchicine exaggerated EtOH-induced barrier disruption, while a microtubule stabilizer, taxol, attenuated the effects of EtOH. Thus, depolymerization of microtubules appears to be key to EtOH-induced loss of barrier integrity.

Interestingly, one of the products of NO overproduction is nitrosylation. In contrast to *nitration* of amino acids, which is irreversible and can cause depolymerization of cytoskeletal proteins, protein S-*nitrosylation* is reversible and might even protect proteins from oxidative damage (Dalle-Donne et al., 2001). The importance of this accessory pathway in ethanol-induced epithelial damage is still unclear and hyper-activation of this pathway might contribute to cytoprotection of cells against oxidative stress under special circumstances.

NF-κB, intestinal barrier, and alcohol

Inducible NOS upregulation causes NO overproduction and loss of intestinal barrier integrity after exposure of cells to EtOH (Banan et al., 1996, 2000b), but how does EtOH upregulate intestinal iNOS? It seems to be via activation of NF-κB. It is now known that cytokine-induced iNOS upregulation in astrocytes, macrophages, and hepatocytes (Moon et al., 1999) depends on the activation of NF-κB. Indeed, NF-κB appears to regulate many important cellular genes involved in inflammatory processes such as cytokines (IL-8, tumor necrosis factor-α), cyclooxygenase-2 (COX-2), and iNOS (Jobin et al., 1999).

Intestinal permeability as a gauge to assess intestinal barrier integrity

A direct method to assess intestinal barrier integrity quantitatively is measurement of intestinal permeability. Detecting bacterial translocation to mesenteric lymph nodes, liver, and spleen is a qualitative measure of intestinal barrier integrity. Several methods are available to measure intestinal permeability to macromolecules. *In vitro* models include using a monolayer cell culture or an Ussing chamber. *In vivo* methods include the use of macromolecular or sugar probes. Urinary measurement of these probes can easily be done after an oral dose. Sugar probes include sucrose, mannitol, cellubiose, lactulose, and sucralose and are commonly used. Differently sized polyethylene glycols (PEGs), saccharides, polysucrose 15000, ^{14}C-mannitol, and ^{51}Cr-EDTA are other probes designed to measure intestinal permeability in humans.

Alcohol and intestinal permeability

Many reports have shown that EtOH consumption substantially disturbs intestinal mucosal structure and function in both humans and animals (Keshavarzian et al., 1996; Dinda and Beck, 1984; Beck and Dinda, 1981; Rubin et al., 1972), but studies on intestinal permeability are more limited (Parlesak et al., 2000; Keshavarzian et al., 1994). Acute EtOH increased intestinal permeability to macromolecules in both humans and animals in some studies (Worthington, 1980) but not all (Keshavarzian et al., 1994). The effects of exposure to chronic EtOH on intestinal permeability are even less well established. Chronic EtOH increased intestinal permeability to macro-molecules in the rat (Robinson et al., 1981; Worthington et al., 1978). In their rat model, Kinoshita et al. (1989) showed that 3 weeks of alcohol exposure resulted in increased IgA antibody formation to food antigens, particularly from Peyer's patches; however, the effect of chronic EtOH use in humans is less clear, and the two original reports provide conflicting data. One study (Bjarnson et al., 1984) evaluated intestinal permeability using Cr-EDTA in 36 unselected alcoholics and reported that alcoholics had increased gut leakiness, but the authors did not stratify their analysis based on the presence or absence of liver disease. We evaluated intestinal permeability using urinary lactulose/mannitol in 18 alcoholics without liver disease and found normal intestinal permeability (Keshavarzian et al., 1994). We later studied three groups of drinking subjects: (1) alcoholics with liver disease, (2) alcoholics with a comparable history of alcoholism but without liver disease, and (3) patients with non-alcoholic liver disease with liver disease severity comparable to that of the alcoholic liver disease (ALD) group (Keshavarzian et al., 1999). Our data suggested that intestinal permeability (leaky gut) is greater than control subjects only for alcoholics with liver disease. Gut leakiness was probably not due to the presence of liver disease because non-alcoholics with equally severe liver disease had normal intestinal per-meability. More recently, Parlesak et al. (2000) studied alcoholics with liver disease and found that they exhibited increased permeation to large molecules (PEG-1000 to PEG-10000).

The presence of gut leakiness can also contribute to modulation of immunogenic barrier components, as well. For example, monocytes from alcoholics with and without liver disease behave differently (Criado-Jimenez et al., 1995; Hunt and Goldin, 1992). Unstimulated monocytes from alcoholics without liver disease or from non-alcoholic subjects had low NO levels that were significantly increased by endotoxin (LPS). In contrast, unstimulated monocytes from ALD patients produced high baseline NO levels, similar to levels in LPS-stimulated monocytes from controls or alcoholics without LD. Leaky gut is thus a highly plausible mechanism to explain the susceptibility of alcoholics to ALD.

CONSEQUENCE OF ALCOHOL-INDUCED BARRIER DYSFUNCTION

The intestinal mucosal epithelium is a highly selective barrier that permits the absorp-tion of nutrients from the gut lumen into the circulation and normally restricts the passage of harmful and potentially toxic compounds such as bacteria or products of the luminal microflora (e.g., endotoxin) (Hollander, 1992; Madara, 1990). It is thus not surprising that diminished intestinal barrier integrity has been implicated in a wide range of illnesses, such as inflammatory bowel disease, systemic disease such as cancer, and even hepatic encephalopathy (Madara, 1990; Gardiner et al., 1995).

Barrier Dysfunction and Diseases

The intestinal mucosa is incessantly exposed to a huge burden of proinflammatory luminal antigens. Normally, the epithelium allows only small amounts of these antigens to cross the mucosa. This passage might be through cellular or paracellular epithelial pathways or mucosal M-cells. These antigens interact with and activate local and systemic immune system. This activation is well controlled by the immune regulatory system and results in maintenance of a balance between antigen exposure and immune activation that is necessary for protection of barrier integrity. Disproportionate penetration of luminal antigens and/or immune dysregulation may inappropriately activate the immune system, leading to GI or systemic inflammatory disorders. Whether abnormal intestinal permeability is the cause or effect is not clear in many of these situations. Several other GI diseases are also associated with abnormal intestinal permeability including inflammatory bowel diseases, celiac disease, food allergy, and extraintestinal disorders such as acute pancreatitis, abdominal trauma, total parental nutrition, eczema, urticaria–angiedema, psoriasis and dermatitis herpetiformis, hepatobiliary disorders, alcoholic liver disease, collagen–vascular disorders, renal failure, sarcoidosis, and cardiopulmonary bypass.

Alcoholic Liver Disease

One of the most common and serious complications of heavy drinking — a major health problem in the United States that accounts for 15% of total healthcare costs annually (O'Conner and Schottenfeld, 1998) — is alcoholic liver disease (Maher, 2002a; Grant et al., 1988), with a 20% mortality rate (Maher, 2002b). The mechanisms linking EtOH consumption to ALD are not well established, however. Because only a subgroup (~30%) of alcoholics develops ALD (Grant et al., 1988), co-factors other than EtOH must be involved. Several potential co-factors have been suggested, including hepatitis C infection and hemochromatosis trait, but none is present in most ALD cases.

Alcoholic liver disease and endotoxin

A more likely co-factor culprit in the pathogenesis of ALD is gut-derived endotoxin. Indeed, a variety of recent clinical observations and data on experimental EtOH-induced liver damage strongly suggest that endotoxin is a key co-factor (Criado-Jimenez et al., 1995; Nanji et al., 1993; Hunt and Goldin, 1992; Bode et al., 1987; Nolan, 1975). For example:

- Alcoholics with ALD have high serum endotoxin level, and serum endotoxin levels correlate with ALD severity (Bigatello et al., 1987).
- Monocytes from alcoholics with ALD appear to be primed for producing cytokines and oxidants (reactive oxygen and nitrogen species), and this priming seems to be due to endotoxin (McClain and Cohen, 1989; Bigatello et al., 1987).

- Rats with EtOH-induced liver damage have high endotoxin levels in the portal vein, and a strong correlation exists between endotoxin levels and the severity of liver damage in these rats (Nanji et al., 1993).
- Lowering serum endotoxin level by oral administration of non-absorbable antibiotics (Adachi et al., 1995) or *Lactobacillus* (Nanji et al., 1994) attenuated EtOH-induced liver damage in these rats.
- Neither EtOH alone nor endotoxin alone (at least not low endotoxin levels) causes severe liver injury but a combination of these two agents is sufficient to cause significant liver damage.
- Endotoxin can prime and activate macrophages (Küpffer cells) in rats chronically exposed to EtOH so that they overproduce cytokines such as TNF, IL-6, and IL-8 (Hill et al., 1997); these cytokines not only injure hepatocytes directly but can also initiate a hepatic necro-inflammatory cascade, which includes migration of leukocytes, including neutrophils, into the liver (Nanji et al., 1995; Lumeng and Crabb, 2001). These leukocytes produce injurious products, especially oxidants such as NO and ONOO-, which can cause liver cell necrosis.

The EtOH–endotoxin synergy, along with other direct metabolic effects of EtOH on the liver (e.g., hypoxia, perturbation of NO-dependent pathways) not only can initiate liver injury but can also create a vicious cycle that sustains a chronic necro-inflammatory process and hastens the onset of liver failure.

Source of endotoxemia

Although endotoxin appears to be an important co-factor in the pathogenesis of ALD, a question remains regarding the etiology of abnormally high blood endotoxin levels (endotoxemia). Endotoxin, which is generated by intestinal bacteria in the gut lumen, can permeate into the portal circulation and then the liver, where it is taken up and eliminated by Küpffer cells, important cells for preventing endotoxemia. Although, the mechanism for endotoxemia in alcoholics is not well established, it can theoretically be due to increased production of endotoxin by abnormal gut flora, increased permeation of endotoxin through the intestinal wall (gut leakiness), shunting of blood away from the liver (as seen in advanced liver damage with portal hypertension), or defective Küpffer cell function. Even if shunting of the blood away from the liver and Küpffer cell dysfunction contribute to endotoxemia in ALD, these factors may not be the sole contributing factors in this scenario. Bacteria producing abnormally high levels of toxin or gut leakiness allowing abnormally high permeability to endotoxin are probably key contributors.

Shunting of the blood away from the liver can be an important factor for endotoxemia in patients with advanced liver disease but clearly is not a factor for initiation of liver damage without portal hypertension. Abnormal intestinal flora is also a less likely cause of endotoxemia as it is not present in most alcoholics (Keshavarzian and Fields, 1999) and because ALD can be initiated in rats having normal intestinal flora. Abnormal intestinal permeability (leaky gut), on the other hand, is a very plausible cause for endotoxemia. In fact, a leaky gut has been suggested to be a major factor for endotoxemia in ALD (Lumeng and Crabb, 2001).

It has recently been shown that intestinal leakiness is present in alcoholics with liver disease but not in alcoholics without liver disease (Keshavarzian et al., 1999). It should be noted that intestinal leakiness would still be extremely important in the pathogenesis of ALD even if other mechanisms, such as defective Küpffer cell function or increased endotoxin production, were contributing factors in pathological endotoxemia. Even in these situations, if gut leakiness can be controlled, then the amount of endotoxin that can permeate the intestinal wall will be limited; therefore, Küpffer cells would be exposed to a lower endotoxin levels, levels they could handle even if their function were defective due to EtOH use.

"Leaky-Prone" vs. "Leaky-Resistant" Gut

Leaky gut is a term that has been used in the literature for years to explain intestinal hyperpermeability to macromolecules that are usually not absorbable; however, based on recent studies, this phenomenon is not a static condition. In fact, intestinal permeability is a highly dynamic process and may be adjusted according to various stimuli (Farhadi et al., 2003). Considering the various components of the intestinal barrier and the various regulatory mechanisms that control this barrier, it is not surprising that a wide variation exists in intestinal permeability from one individual to the other, based on different genetic and environmental factors. Thus, the response of each individual to the stimuli that stress barrier integrity could be somewhat unique. This makes sense if we assume that exposing the population to such a stressful stimulus could result in dividing the population into "leaky-prone" or "leaky-resistant" individuals, depending on their baseline level of intestinal barrier integrity and the severity of the stressor. Alcohol is one of these stressors. When used on a regular basis for a long period of time, it can result in separation of the population into two subpopulations that are either hyperpermeable to macromolecules (leaky prone) or are not hyperpermeable to macromolecules (leaky resistant) (Figure 2.4). Whether this property of the intestine can result in progression toward ALD over the long term in those with leaky-prone intestines or can prevent ALD in those with leaky-resistant intestines should be investigated in a long-term cohort study.

SUMMARY

Alcohol, a constituent of meals for a large proportion of the world's population, affects almost all cells in the body; in particular, it affects the gastrointestinal tract in both direct and systemic ways and causes disturbances in various GI functions, including motility, digestion, absorption, and barrier function. The latter is particularly important in protection of the body from various harmful bacterial and antigen exposures. Disturbing this barrier predisposes the body to several systemic disorders and alcoholic liver disease. It seems that individuals respond differently to exposure to alcohol based on how their intestinal barriers handle stressors such as alcohol. Based on this theory, individuals are either leaky prone or leaky resistant, and this intestinal barrier property might determine the pathogenesis of ALD in the long run.

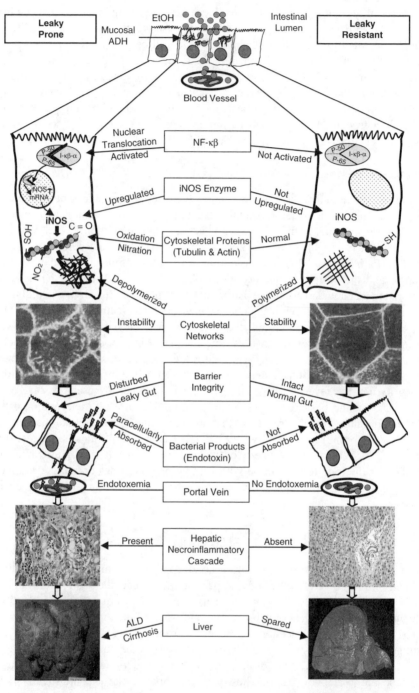

FIGURE 2.4 Proposed pathophysiology of alcoholic liver disease in susceptible alcoholics.

ACKNOWLEDGMENTS

This research was supported in part by a grant from Rush University Medical Center, Department of Internal Medicine, and by two National Health Institute (NIH) R01 Research Grants (AA1374501A1 [AK] and NIDDK60511 [AB]). The authors also want to acknowledge and thank the patients and volunteers who participated in our research only for their good will and also to express our appreciation to our colleagues who assisted us doing this research, particularly Lei Zhang, Dr. Shriram Jakate, and Mrs. Megan Bakaites.

REFERENCES

Adachi, Y., Moore, L.E., Bradford, B.U., Gao, W., and Thurman, R.G. (1995) Antibiotics prevent liver injury in rats following long-term exposure to ethanol, *Gastroenterology*, 108: 218–224.

Alican, I. and Kubes, P. (1996) A critical role for nitric oxide in intestinal barrier function and dysfunction, *Am. J. Physiol.*, 270: G225–G237.

Alvia, J. (1987) Microtubule function, *Life Sci.*, 50: 327–333.

Ba, A., Seri, B.V., and Han, S.H. (1996) Thiamine administration during chronic alcohol intake in pregnant and lactating rats: effects on the offspring neurobehavioural development, *Alcohol Alcohol.*, 31: 27–40.

Banan, A., Choudhary, S., Zhang, Y., and Keshavarzian, A. (1999) Ethanol-induced barrier dysfunction and its prevention by growth factors in human intestinal monolayers: evidence for oxidative and cytoskeletal mechanisms, *J. Pharmacol. Exp. Therap.*, 291: 1075–1085.

Banan, A., Choudhary, S., Zhang, Y., and Keshavarzian, A. (2000a) Role of the microtubule cytoskeleton in protection by epidermal growth factor and transforming growth factor-α against oxidant-induced barrier disruption in a human colonic cell line, *Free Radical Biol. Med.*, 28: 727–738.

Banan, A., Fields, J.Z., Zhang, Y., and Keshavarzian, A. (2000b) Nitric oxide and its metabolites mediate EtOH-induced microtubule disruption and intestinal barrier dysfunction, *J. Pharmacol. Exp. Therap.*, 294: 997–1008.

Banan, A., Smith, G.S., Kokoska, E.R., and Miller, T.A. (2000c) Role of cytoskeleton in prostaglandin-induced protection against ethanol in a small intestinal epithelial cell line, IEC-6, *J. Surg. Res.*, 88: 104–113.

Banan, A., Zhang, Y., Losurdo, J., and Keshavarzian, A. (2000d) Carbonylation and disassembly of the F-actin cytoskeleton in oxidant-induced barrier dysfunction and its prevention by epidermal growth factor and transforming growth factor-α in a human intestinal cell line, *Gut*, 46: 830–837.

Banan, A., Fields, J.Z., Zhang, Y., and Keshavarzian, A. (2001a) iNOS upregulation and cytoskeletal nitration explain how oxidants disrupt the cytoskeleton and increase permeability of monolayers of intestinal epithelia, *Am. J. Physiol. (GI Liver)*, 280: G1234–G1246.

Banan, A., Fields, J.Z., Zhang, Y., and Keshavarzian, A. (2001b) β1 Isoform of protein kinase C mediates epidermal growth factor-induced protection of the microtubule cytoskeleton and intestinal monolayer barrier function against oxidant injury, *Am. J. Physiol. (GI Liver)*, 281: G833–G847.

Banan, A., Fields, J.Z., Zhang, Y., and Keshavarzian, A. (2001c) Targeted molecular inhibition of PLC-γ prevents EGF-mediated protection of microtubule cytoskeleton and intestinal barrier function, *Am. J. Physiol. (GI Liver)*, 281: G412–G423.

Banan, A., Fitzpatrick, L., Zhang, Y., and Keshavarzian, A. (2001d) OPC-compounds prevent oxidant-induced carbonylation and depolymerization of the cytoskeleton and intestinal barrier hyperpermeability, *Free Radical Biol. Med.*, 30, 287–298.

Banan, A., Zhang, Y., Fields, J.Z., and Keshavarzian, A. (2001e) Key role of PKC and calcium homeostasis in epidermal growth factor-induced protection of the microtubule cytoskeleton and intestinal barrier against oxidant injury, *Am. J. Physiol. (GI Liver)*, 280: G828–G843.

Beck, I.T. and Dinda, P.D. (1981) Acute exposure of small intestine to ethanol, *Dig. Dis. Sci.*, 26: 817–838.

Beckman, J.S., Beckman, T.W., Chen, J., Marshall, P.A., and Freeman, B.A. (1990) Apparent hydroxyl radical production by peroxynitrite: implications for endothelial injury from nitric oxide and superoxide, *Proc. Natl. Acad. Sci. USA*, 87: 1620–1624.

Bigatello, L.M., Broitman, S.A., Fattori, L., Di, Paoli, M., Pontello, M., Bevilacqua, G., and Nespoli, A. (1987) Endotoxemia, encephalopathy, and mortality in cirrhotic patients, *Am. J. Gastroenterol.*, 82: 11–15.

Bjarnson, B., Ward, R., and Peters, T.J. (1984) The leaky gut of alcoholism: possible route of entry for toxic compounds, *Lancet*, 1: 179–182.

Bode, C., Kugler, V., and Bode, J.C. (1987) Endotoxemia in patients with alcoholic and nonalcoholic cirrhosis and in subjects with no evidence of chronic liver disease following acute alcohol excess, *J. Hepatol.*, 4: 8–14.

Boughton-Smith, N.K., Evans, S.M., Laszlo, F., Whittle, B.J., and Moncada, S. (1993) The induction of nitric oxide synthases and intestinal vascular permeability by endotoxin in the rat, *Br. J. Pharmacol.*, 110: 1189–1195.

Bretscher, M.S. (1987) How animal cells move, *Science*, 257: 72–90.

Buell, M.G., Dinda, P.K., and Beck, I.T. (1983) Effect of ethanol on morphology and total, capillary, and shunted blood flow of different anatomical layers of dog jejunum, *Dig. Dis. Sci.*, 28(11): 1005–1017.

Camargo, C.A., Jr., Vranizan, K.M., Dreon, D.M., Frey-Hewitt, B., and Wood P.D. (1987) Alcohol, calorie intake, and adiposity in overweight men, *J. Am. Coll. Nutr.*, 6: 271–278.

Celada, A., Rudolf, H., and Donath, A. (1978) Effect of a single ingestion of alcohol on iron absorption, *Am. J. Hematol.*, 5: 225–237.

Choudhry, M.A., Fazal, N., Goto, M., Gamelli, R.L., and Sayeed, M.M. (2002) Gut-associated lymphoid T cell suppression enhances bacterial translocation in alcohol and burn injury, *Am. J. Physiol. (GI Liver)*, 282: G937–G347.

Choudhry, M.A., Messingham, K.A., Namak, S., Colantoni, A., Fontanilla, C.V., Duffner, L.A., Sayeed, M.M., and Kovacs, E.J. (2000) Ethanol exacerbates T cell dysfunction after thermal injury, *Alcohol*, 21: 239–243.

Colantoni, A., Duffner, L.A., De Maria, N., Fontanilla, C.V., Messingham, K.A., Van, Thiel, D.H., and Kovacs, E.J. (2000) Dose-dependent effect of ethanol on hepatic oxidative stress and interleukin-6 production after burn injury in the mouse, *Alcohol. Clin. Exp. Res.*, 24: 1443–1448.

Colgan, S. (1998) Nitric oxide and intestinal epithelia: just say NO, *Gastroenterology*, 3: 601–603.

Criado-Jimenez, M., Rivas-Cabanero, L., Martin-Oterino, J.A., Lopez-Novoa, J.M., and Sanchez-Rodriguez, A. (1995) Nitric oxide production by mononuclear leukocytes in alcoholic cirrhosis, *J. Mol. Med.*, 73: 31–33.

Dalle-Donne, I., Rossi, R, Milzani, A., Simplicio, D.P., and Colombo, R. (2001) The actin cytoskeleton response to oxidants: from small heat shock protein phosphorylation to changes in the redox state of actin itself, *Free Radical Biol. Med.*, 31: 1624–1632.

Dinda, P.K. and Beck, I.T. (1977) On the mechanism of the inhibitory effect of ethanol on intestinal glucose and water absorption, *Am. J. Dig. Dis.*, 22: 529–533.

Dinda, P.K. and Beck, I.T. (1984) Effects of ethanol on cytoplasmic peptidases of the jejunal epithelial cell of the hamster, *Dig. Dis. Sci.*, 29: 46–55.

Dinda, P.K., Beck, I.T., Beck, M., and McElligott, T.F. (1975) Effect of ethanol on sodium-dependent glucose transport in the small intestine of the hamster, *Gastroenterology*, 68: 1517–1526.

Farhadi, A., Banan, A., Fields, J., and Keshavarzian, A. (2003) The intestinal barrier: an interface between health and disease, *J. Gastroenterol. Hepatol.*, 18, 479–497.

Faunce, D.E., Gregory, M.S., and Kovacs, E.J. (1997) Effects of acute ethanol exposure on cellular immune responses in a murine model of thermal injury, *J. Leukocyte Biol.*, 62: 733–740.

Faunce, D.E., Gregory, M.S., and Kovacs, E.J. (1998) Acute ethanol exposure prior to thermal injury results in decreased T-cell responses mediated in part by increased production of IL-6, *Shock*, 10: 135–140.

Fontanilla, C.V., Faunce, D.E., Gregory, M.S., Messingham, K.A., Durbin, E.A., Duffner, L.A., and Kovacs, E.J. (2000) Anti-interleukin-6 antibody treatment restores cell-mediated immune function in mice with acute ethanol exposure before burn trauma, *Alcohol. Clin. Exp. Res.*, 24: 1392–1399.

Forsander, O.A. (1994) Hypothesis: factors involved in the mechanisms regulating food intake affect alcohol consumption, *Alcohol Alcohol.*, 29: 503–512.

Gardiner, K.R., Halliday, M.I., and Barclay, G.R. (1995) Significance of systemic endotoxemia in inflammatory bowel disease, *Gut*, 36: 897–901.

Gill, K., Amit, Z., and Smith, B.R. (1996) Alcohol as a food: a commentary on Richter, *Physiol. Behav.*, 60: 1485–1490.

Giner, M. and Meguid, M.M. (1993) Effect of intragastric and intravenous ethanol on food intake in rats, *Physiol. Behav.*, 54: 399–401.

Grabowski, B.S., Cady, W.J., Young, W.W., and Emery, J.F. (1980) Effects of acute alcohol administration on propranolol absorption, *Int. J. Clin. Pharmacol. Ther. Toxicol.*, 18: 317–319.

Grant, B.F., Dufour, M.C., and Harford, T.C. (1988) Epidemiology of alcoholic liver disease, *Semin. Liver Dis.*, 8: 12–25.

Grisham, M.B., Jourdheuil, D., and Wink, D.A. (1999) Nitric oxide. I. Physiological chemistry of nitric oxide and its metabolites: implications in inflammation, *Am. J. Physiol. (GI Liver)*, 39: G315–G321.

Hahn, R.G., Norberg, A., Gabrielsson, J., Danielsson, A., and Jones, A.W. (1994) Eating a meal increases the clearance of ethanol given by intravenous infusion, *Alcohol Alcohol.*, 29: 673–677.

Hill, D., Shedlofsky, S., McClain, C., Diehl, A., and Tsukamoto, H. (1997) Cytokines and liver disease, in *Cytokines in Health and Disease*, 2nd ed. (rev. exp.), Remick, D.R. and Friedland, J.S., Eds., Marcel Dekker, New York, pp. 401–425.

Hollander, D. (1992) The intestinal permeability barrier: a hypothesis as to its regulation and involvement in Crohn's disease, *Scand. J. Gastroenterol.*, 27: 721–726.

Holler, H., Schaller, K., and Werth, R. (1975) Thiamine absorption in the rat. III. Effect of ethyl alcohol on active absorption of thiamine *in vitro*, *Int. J. Vit. Nutr. Res.*, 45: 138–143.

Hunt, N.C. and Goldin, R.D. (1992) Nitric oxide production by monocytes in alcoholic liver disease, *J. Hepatol.*, 14: 146–150.

Jobin, C., Bradham, C.A., Russo, M.P., Juma, B., Narula, A.S., Brenner, D.A., and Sartor, B. (1999) Curcumin blocks cytokine-mediated NF-κB activation and proinflammatory gene expression by inhibiting inhibitory factor I-κB kinase activity, *J. Immunol.*, 163: 3474–3483.

Jones, A.W. and Jonsson, K.A. (1994) Food-induced lowering of blood-ethanol profiles and increased rate of elimination immediately after a meal, *J. Forensic Sci.*, 39: 1084–1093.

Jones, B.R., Barrett-Connor, E., Criqui, M.H., and Holdbrook, M.J. (1982) A community study of calorie and nutrient intake in drinkers and nondrinkers of alcohol, *Am. J. Clin. Nutr.*, 35: 135–139.

Kanwar, S., Wallace, J., Befus, D., and Kubes, P. (1994) Nitric oxide synthesis inhibition increases epithelial permeability via mast cells, *Am. J. Physiol.*, 266: G222–G229.

Kaur, J., Jaswal, V.M., Nagpaul, J.P., and Mahmood, A. (1993) Effect of chronic ethanol administration on the absorptive functions of the rat small intestine, *Alcohol*, 10: 299–302.

Kawakami, M., Meyer, A.A., Johnson, M.C., and Rezvani, A.H. (1989) Immunologic consequences of acute ethanol ingestion in rats, *J. Surg. Res.*, 47: 412–417.

Kawakami, M., Meyer, A.A., Johnson, M.C., deSerres, S., and Peterson, H.D. (1990) Chronic ethanol exposure before injury produces greater immune dysfunction after thermal injury in rats, *J. Trauma*, 30: 27–31.

Kawakami, M., Switzer, B.R., Herzog, S.R., and Meyer, A.A. (1991) Immune suppression after acute ethanol ingestion and thermal injury, *J. Surg. Res.*, 51: 210–215.

Keshavarzian, A. and Fields, J.Z. (1996) Gastrointestinal motility disorders induced by ethanol, in *Ethanol and the Gastrointestinal Tract*, Preedy, V.R. and Watson R.R., Eds., CRC Press, Boca Raton, FL, pp. 235–253.

Keshavarzian, A. and Fields, J.Z. (1999) Alcohol: "ice-breaker," yes; "gut barrier-breaker," maybe, *Am. J. Gastroenterol.*, 95: 1124–1125.

Keshavarzian, A., Iber, F.L., Dangleis, M.D., and Cornish, R. (1986a) Intestinal-transit and lactose intolerance in chronic alcoholics, *Am. J. Clin. Nutr.*, 44: 70.

Keshavarzian, A., Iber, F.L., Greer, P., and Wobbleton, J. (1986b) Gastric emptying of solid meal in male chronic alcoholics, *Alcohol. Clin. Exp. Res.*, 10: 432.

Keshavarzian, A., Polepalle, C., Iber, F.L., and Durkin, M. (1990) Esophageal motor disorder in alcoholics: result of alcoholism or withdrawal?, *Alcoholism*, 14: 561.

Keshavarzian, A., Fields, J., Vaeth, J., and Holmes, E. (1994) The differing effects of acute and chronic alcohol on gastric and intestinal permeability, *Am. J. Gastroenterol.*, 89(12): 2205–2211.

Keshavarzian, A., Holmes, E.W., Patel, N., Iber, F.L., Fields, J.Z., and Pethkar, S. (1999) Leaky gut in alcoholic cirrhosis: a possible mechanism for alcohol-induced liver damage, *Am. J. Gastroenterol.*, 94: 200–207.

Kesse, E., Clavel-Chapelon, F., Slimani, N., van Liere, M., and E3N Group (2001) Do eating habits differ according to alcohol consumption? Results of a study of the French cohort of the European Prospective Investigation into Cancer and Nutrition (E3N-EPIC), *Am. J. Clin. Nutr.*, 74: 322–327.

Kimura, H., Hokari, R., Miura, S., Shigematsu, T., Hirokawa, M., Akiba, Y., Kurose, I., Higuchi, H., Fujimori, H., Tsuzuki, Y., Serizawa, H., and Ishii, H. (1998) Increased expression of an inducible isoform of nitric oxide synthase and the formation of peroxynitrite in colonic mucosa of patients with active ulcerative colitis, *Gut*, 42: 180–187.

Kinoshita, A., Yamada, K., and Hayakawa, T. (1989) Hypoxic injury of rat cortical neurons in primary cell cultures: introduction of a modified method to create the hypoxic state, *Exp. Cell Biol.*, 57: 310–314.

Krasner, N., Carmichael, H.A., Russell, R.I., Thompson, G.G., and Cochran, K.M. (1976a) Alcohol and absorption from the small intestine: effect of ethanol on ATP and ATPase activities in guinea-pig jejunum, *Gut*, 17: 249–251.

Krasner, N., Cochran, K.M., Russell, R.I., Carmichael, H.A., and Thompson, G.G. (1976b) Alcohol and absorption from the small intestine: impairment of absorption from the small intestine in alcoholics, *Gut*, 17: 245–248.

Kubes, P. (1992) Nitric oxide modulates epithelial permeability in the feline small intestine, *Am. J. Physiol.*, 262: G1138–G1142.

Kubes, P. and Granger, N. (1992) Nitric oxide modulates microvascular permeability, *Am. J. Physiol.*, 262: H611–H615.

Larue-Achagiotis, C., Poussard, A.M., and Louis-Sylvestre, J. (1990) Alcohol drinking, food and fluid intakes and body weight gain in rats, *Physiol. Behav.*, 47: 545–548.

Lavo, B., Colombel, J.F., Knutsson, L., and Hallgren, R. (1992) Acute exposure of small intestine to ethanol induces mucosal leakage and prostaglandin E2 synthesis, *Gastroenterology*, 102: 468–473.

Lianos, E.A. and Guglielmi, K. (1998) Regulatory interactions between inducible nitric oxide synthase and eicosanoids in glomerular immune injury, *Kidney Int.*, 53: 645–653.

Lin, Y., Weidler, D.J., Garg, D.C., and Wagner, J.G. (1976) Effects of solid food on blood levels of alcohol in man, *Res. Comm. Chem. Pathol. Pharmacol.*, 13: 713–722.

Liu, S.M. and Sundqvist, T. (1997). Nitric oxide and cGMP regulate endothelial permeability and F-actin distribution in hydrogen-peroxide-treated endothelial cells, *Exp. Cell Res.*, 235: 238–244.

Lumeng, L. and Crabb, D.W. (2001) Alcoholic liver disease, *Curr. Opin. Gastroenterol.*, 17: 211–220.

Luna, E.J. and Hitt, A.L. (1992) Cytoskeleton-plasma membrane interactions, *Science*, 258: 955–964.

MacRae, T.H. (1992) Towards an understanding of microtubule function and cell organization: an overview, *Biochem. Cell Biol.*, 170: 835–841.

Madara, J.L. (1990) Pathobiology of the intestinal epithelial barrier, *Am. J. Pathol.*, 137: 1273–1281.

Maher, J.J. (2002a) Alcoholic steatosis and steatohepatitis, *Semin. Gastrointest. Dis.*, 13: 31–39.

Maher, J.J. (2002b) Treatment of alcoholic hepatitis, *J. Gastroenterol. Hepatol.*, 17: 448–455.

Martins, O.O. and Dada, O.A. (1982) The effect of alcohol on the *in vitro* absorption of estradiol and estrone sulphate in rat intestine, *J. Steroid Biochem.*, 16: 265–268.

Matuz, J. (1992) Role of mucus in mucosal protection through ethanol and pepsin damage models, *Acta Physiol. Hungarian*, 80(1–4): 189–194.

McClain, C.J. and Cohen, D.A. (1989) Increased tumor necrosis factor by monocytes in alcoholic hepatitis, *Hepatology*, 9: 349–351.

Mekhjian, H.S. and May, E.S. (1977) Acute and chronic effects of ethanol on fluid transport in the human small intestine, *Gastroenterology*, 72: 1280–1286.

Merino, V., Martin-Algarra, R.V., Rocher, A., Garrigues, T.M., Freixas, J., and Polache, A. (1997) Effects of ethanol on intestinal absorption of drugs. I. *In situ* studies with ciprofloxacin analogs in normal and chronic alcohol-fed rats, *Alcohol. Clin. Exp. Res.*, 21: 326–333.

Messingham, K.A., Fontanilla, C.V., Colantoni, A., Duffner, L.A., and Kovacs, E.J. (2000) Cellular immunity after ethanol exposure and burn injury: dose and time dependence, *Alcohol*, 22: 35–44.

Miller, T.R. and Blincoe, L.J. (1994) Incidence and cost of alcohol-involved crashes in the United States, *Accid. Anal. Prev.*, 26: 583–591.

Money, S.R., Petroianu, A., Kimura, K., and Jaffe, B.M. (1990) The effects of short-term ethanol exposure on the canine jejunal handling of calcium and glucose, *Surgery*, 107: 167–171.

Moon, R.M., Parikh, A.A., Pritts, T.A., Fischer, J.E., Cottongim, S., Szabo, C., Salzman, A.L., and Hasselgren, P.O. (1999) Complement component C3 production in IL-1β-stimulated human intestinal epithelial cells is blocked by NF-κB inhibitors and by transfection with Ser 32/36 mutant I-κBα, *J. Surg. Res.*, 82: 48–55.

Mosnier, P., Rayssiguier, Y., Motta, C., Pelissier, E., and Bommelaer, G. (1993) Effect of ethanol on rat gastric surfactant: a fluorescence polarization study, *Gastroenterology*, 104: 179–184.

Nanji, A.A., Khettry, U., Sadrzadeh, S.M., and Yamanaka, T. (1993) Severity of liver injury in experimental alcoholic liver disease: correlation with plasma endotoxin, prostaglandin E2, leukotriene B4, and thromboxane B2, *Am. J. Pathol.*, 142: 367–373.

Nanji, A., Khettry, U., and Hossein-Sadrzadeh, S.M. (1994) *Lactobacillus* feeding reduces endotoxemia and severity of experimental alcoholic liver (disease), *Proc. Soc. Exp. Biol. Med.*, 205: 243–247.

Nanji, A., Greenberg, S., Tahan, S., Fogt, F., Loscalzo, J., Hossein-Sadrzadeh, S.M., Xie, J., and Stamler, J. (1995) Nitric oxide production in experimental alcoholic liver disease in the rat: role in protection from injury, *Gastroenterology*, 109: 899–907.

Napolitano, L.M., Koruda, M.J., Zimmerman, K., McCowan, K., Chang, J., and Meyer, A.A. (1995) Chronic ethanol intake and burn injury: evidence for synergistic alteration in gut and immune integrity, *J. Trauma*, 38: 198–207,

Nencini, P. (1997) The rules of drug taking: wine and poppy derivatives in the ancient world, general introduction, *Subst. Use Misuse*, 32: 89–96.

Nolan, J.P. (1975) The role of endotoxin in liver injury, *Gastroenterology*, 69: 1346–1356.

O'Conner, P.G. and Schottenfeld, R.S. (1998) Patients with alcohol problems, *N. Engl. J. Med.*, 9: 592–601.

Parlesak, A., Schafer, C., Schutz, T., Bode, J.C., and Bode, C. (2000) Increased intestinal permeability to macromolecules and endotoxemia in patients with chronic alcohol abuse in different stages of alcohol-induced liver disease, *J. Hepatol.*, 32: 742–747.

Patel, M., Keshavarzian, A., Kottapalli, V., Badie, B., Winship, D., and Fields, J.Z. (1996) Human neutrophil functions are inhibited *in vitro* by clinically relevant ethanol concentrations, *Alcohol. Clin. Exp. Res.*, 20: 275–283.

Pfeiffer, A., Schmidt, T., Vidon, N., and Kaess, H. (1993) Effect of ethanol on absorption of a nutrient solution in the upper human intestine, *Scand. J. Gastroenterol.*, 28: 515–521.

Polache, A., Martin-Algarra, R.V., and Guerri, C. (1996) Effects of chronic alcohol consumption on enzyme activities and active methionine absorption in the small intestine of pregnant rats, *Alcohol. Clin. Exp. Res.*, 20: 1237–1242.

Ramchandani, V.A., Kwo, P.Y., and Li, T.K. (2001) Effect of food and food composition on alcohol elimination rates in healthy men and women, *J. Clin. Pharmacol.*, 41(12): 1345–1350.

Robinson, G.M., Orrego, H., Israel, Y., Devenyi, P., and Kapur, B.M. (1981) Low-molecular-weight polyethylene glycol as a probe of gastrointestinal permeability of alcohol ingestion, *Dig. Dis. Sci.*, 26: 971–977.

Rossi, M.A., Zucoloto, S., and Carillo, S.V. (1980) Impairment of fat absorption induced by alcohol in rats, *Int. J. Vit. Nutr. Res.*, 50: 315–320.

Rubin, E., Rybak, B.J., Lindenbaum, J., Gerson, G., and Walker, C.S. (1972) Ultrastructural changes in the small intestine induced by ethanol, *Gastroenterology*, 63: 801–814.

Sedman, A.J., Wilkinson, P.K., Sakmar, E., Weidler, D.J., and Wagner, J.G. (1976) Food effects on absorption and metabolism of alcohol, *J. Stud. Alcohol*, 37: 1197–1214.

Sibley, D.A., Fuseler, J., Slukvin, I., and Jerrells, T.R. (1995) Ethanol-induced depletion of lymphocytes from the mesenteric lymph nodes of C57B1/6 mice is associated with RNA but not DNA degradation, *Alcohol. Clin. Exp. Res.*, 19: 324–331.

Small, J.V. (1988) The actin cytoskeleton, *Electron Microsc. Rev.*, 1: 155–174.

Steinert, P.M. and Room, D.R. (1988) Molecular and cellular biology of intermediate filaments, *Annu. Rev. Biochem.*, 57: 593–625.

Tabata, T. and Meyer, A.A. (1995) Immunoglobulin M synthesis after burn injury: the effects of chronic ethanol on postinjury synthesis, *J. Burn Care Rehab.*, 16: 400–406.

Tabata, T., Tani, T., Endo, Y., and Hanasawa, K. (2002) Bacterial translocation and peptidoglycan translocation by acute ethanol administration, *J. Gastroenterol.*, 37: 726–731.

Talbot, R. and LaGrange, L. (1999) The effects of salty and nonsalty food on peak breath alcohol concentration and divided attention task performance in women, *Subst. Abuse*, 20: 77–84.

Thomson, A.B., Man, S.F., and Shnitka, T. (1984) Effect of ethanol on intestinal uptake of fatty acids, fatty alcohols, and cholesterol, *Dig. Dis. Sci.*, 29: 631–642.

Unno, N., Menconi, M.J., Smith, M., Aguirre, D.E., and Fink, M.P. (1997) Hyperpermeability of intestinal epithelial monolayers induced by NO: effect of low extracellular pH, *Am. J. Physiol.*, 272: G923–G934.

Wang, Y., Huang, D.S., Giger, P.T., and Watson, R.R. (1994) Influence of chronic dietary ethanol on cytokine production by murine splenocytes and thymocytes, *Alcohol. Clin. Exp. Res.*, 18: 64–70.

Watzl, B. and Watson, R.R. (1993) Role of nutrients in alcohol-induced immunomodulation, *Alcohol Alcohol.*, 28: 89–95.

Watzl, B., Lopez, M., Shahbazian, M., Chen, G., Colombo, L.L., Huang, D., Way, D., and Watson, R.R. (1993) Diet and ethanol modulate immune responses in young C57BL/6 mice, *Alcohol. Clin. Exp. Res.*, 17: 623–630.

Whitmire, D., Cornelius, L., and Whitmire, P. (2002) Effects of food on ethanol metabolism, *Drug Metab. Drug Inter.*, 19: 83–96.

Whittle, B., Jr. (1994) Nitric oxide, in *Gastrointestinal Physiology and Pathology of the Gastrointestinal Tract*, Johnson, L.R., Ed., Raven, New York, pp. 267–294.

Windham, C.T., Wyse, B.W., and Hansen, R.G. (1983) Alcohol consumption and nutrient density of diets in the Nationwide Food Consumption Survey, *J. Am. Dietetic Assoc.*, 82: 364–370, 373.

Woodman, G.E., Fabian, T.C., Croce, M.A., and Proctor, K.G. (1996) Acute ethanol intoxication and endotoxemia after trauma, *J. Trauma*, 41: 61–72.

Worthington, B.S. (1980) Changes in intestinal passive permeation induced by alcohol, *Serum*, 95: 507–518.

Worthington, B.S., Meserole, L., and Syrotuck, J.A. (1978) Effect of daily ethanol ingestion on intestinal permeability to macromolecules, *Dig. Dis. Sci.*, 23: 23–32.

3 Ciguatera Fish Poisoning: Features, Tissue, and Body Effects

Yoshitsugi Hokama

CONTENTS

0-8493-2757-1/05/$0.00+$1.50

INTRODUCTION

Fish poisoning probably dates back to antiquity. It was cited in Homer's *Odyssey* (800 B.C.) and was observed during the time of Alexander the Great (356–323 B.C.), whose armies were forbidden to eat fish in order to avoid the accompanying sickness and malaise that could threaten his conquests (Halstead, 1988). Ciguatera fish poisoning was described as early as 1606 in the South Pacific island chain of New Hebrides (Helfrich, 1964). A similar outbreak there and in nearby New Caledonia was reported by the famous English navigator Captain James Cook in 1774 (Cook et al., 1977), who described the clinical symptoms of his sick crew — symptoms that coincide with clinical manifestations described today for ciguatera fish poisoning (Bagnis, 1968; Engleberg et al., 1983). In addition, viscera from the same fishes given to Cook's crew were also given to pigs, causing their deaths (Cook et al., 1977).

The term *ciguatera* originated in the Caribbean area to designate intoxication induced by the ingestion of the marine snail, *Turbo livona pica* (called *cigua*), as described by a Cuban ichthyologist. Today, the term is widely accepted to denote a particular type of fish poisoning that results from ingestion of certain fishes (primarily reef fishes) encountered around islands in the Caribbean, the Pacific, and elsewhere in the tropical regions. Current information points to at least one of the many polyether toxins, such as okadaic acid, palytoxin, or maitotoxin, which are structurally closely associated with ciguatoxin (CTX), as also being associated with ciguatera (Yasumoto and Murata, 1993; Murakami et al., 1982). The characteristic clinical symptoms are described in Table 3.1 and are discussed further in the clinical section.

Since the 1970s, much progress has been made in ciguatera research by several investigators (Hokama et al., 1977, 1998a,b; Nukina et al., 1984; Yasumoto et al., 1977, 1979a,b, 1984; Banner 1974; Scheuer et al., 1967). These areas, covered in this chapter, include: (1) biology; (2) chemistry, including the closely related polyethers;

TABLE 3.1
Clinical Symptoms Associated with Ciguatera Fish Poisoning

Category or System	Symptoms
Digestive	Nausea often followed by vomiting; diarrhea; painful defecation; abdominal pain and cramps. Symptoms generally abate after 24 hours, leaving an asthenic and dehydrated patient.
Neurological	Dysethesia, principally with sensitivity to cold, temperature reversal; paresthesia, painful tingling of the palms of hands and soles of feet on contact with cold water; superficial hyperesthesia with sensation of burning and electrical discharge; mydriasis often present; patellar and Achilles reflexes sometimes diminished. Neurological symptoms generally persist for 1 week; it is not unusual to see contact dysethesia lasting a month.
Cardiovascular	Pulse slow (35 to 50 beats/minute) and often irregular; low arterial pressure (heart sounds distant). EKG may show dysrhythmia, from sinus bradycardia (slow heart beat) to bursts of supraventricular or ventricular extra systoles (rapid systolic heart beat). Ventricular tachycardia, excessively rapid action of the heart, may also occur. A first atricular–ventricular (A-V) block may also be observed. Cardiovascular disorders usually disappear in 48 to 72 hours and may be mistaken for a heart attack. Toxins from carnivorous fishes tend to cause cardiovascular problems.
General	Asthenia, making it difficult to walk and keeping patient in bed for several days; arthralgia, especially of knee, ankle, shoulder, and elbow; dorsolumbar stiffness; myalgia, especially leg muscles; headache; marked and constant chilliness but no problems of thermal regulation; lipothymia and dizziness; itching 2 to 3 days after onset, which may persist for many days; oliguria, sometimes during the first 48 hours.

Source: Adapted from Bagnis, R., *Haw. Med. J.*, 20, 25–28, 1968.

(3) pharmacology; (4) clinical aspects; (5) epidemiology; (6) immunological analysis, or the testing or detection of the major toxin ciguatoxin and its related polyether toxins, and other biological testing methods for assessing ciguatoxin and related polyethers; (7) pathology; and (8) therapy.

This chapter covers one of the common foodborne diseases associated with consumption of fishes off the coral reefs and near-shore environments of the oceans in the tropics and, in some instances, the semitropics to depths of 60 meters. The region is circumglobal between the Tropic of Cancer and the Tropic of Capricorn.

Seafood poisoning encompasses a broad spectrum of a variety of low-molecular-weight marine toxins. Some of the better known seafood poisonings include: (1) paralytic shellfish poisoning, (2) scombroid, (3) pufferfish poisoning, (4) anamnestic poisoning, (5) ciguatera poisoning, and (6) diarrhetic shellfish poisoning. Paralytic shellfish poisoning (PSP) is associated with dinoflagellates producing saxitoxins and gonyautoxins, which accumulate in shellfishes during heavy dinoflagellate blooms at a certain time of the year (Shimizu, 1982; Oshima et al., 1977). Scombroid poisoning results from the spoilage of fish tissues due to bacterial contamination and subsequent production of the enzyme decarboxylase, which converts amino acids to amines (e.g., histidine to histamine), thus inducing clinical changes mimicking histamine-like attacks. This poisoning is associated with poor and inadequate fish preservation and storage processes (Taylor et al., 1984). Pufferfish poisoning is associated with tetrodotoxin (TTX) found in fishes in the order *Tetraodontoidea* and in certain crustacea (Fuhrman, 1986) and is probably of bacterial origin (Yotsu et al., 1987). Tetrodotoxin is also found in the newt and certain species of octopus. Anamnestic shellfish poisoning (ASP) is caused by domoic acid and was first reported in a mussel poisoning outbreak in St. Andrews Island, Canada, in late 1987 (Perl et al., 1990). The neuroexcitotoxin (domoic acid) produced by *Pseudonitizches* was identified as the causative factor. Diarrhetic shellfish poisoning (DSP) causes severe diarrhea in patients consuming shellfish or fish containing okadaic acid or its analogs (Murakami, 1982; Yasumoto et al., 1980a,b). The emphasis in this chapter is on the seafood poisoning known as ciguatera, which is becoming a major problem as fish consumption in the United States increases and the fishing industries from endemic areas (tropics, semitropics, and temperate zones) increase their export and distribution of various palatable fishes worldwide (see Table 3.1).

MAJOR FEATURES

BIOLOGY

Fish poisoning outbreaks occurred throughout the tropical regions of the Pacific before, during, and after World War II. It became a serious problem for the military during the war because outbreaks of ciguatera occurred among the fishing population of the troops stationed in various areas endemic for ciguatera poisoning. The areas included Midway, Wake, Guam, Johnson Island, French Polynesia, and New Caledonia, as well as the Pacific islands of the Marshalls and the Marianas. Other tropical areas of the world with ciguatera included the Caribbean, Gulf of Mexico, and Indian Ocean. In the post-war years, investigators from the University of Hawaii, Japan, and Tahiti went in search of the etiological factor causing ciguatera fish poisoning.

Banner et al. (1960) were pioneers in the study of the ecology and biology of ciguatera fish poisoning. Randall (1958), in his investigations of toxic fish, showed that all fish of the same species in the same area were not necessarily carriers of the toxin; therefore, the toxin was not produced by the fish species, and the toxin in the fish must have been derived from their food source. This was the beginning of the development of the food chain concept shown in Figure 3.1. The sequence of this concept follows this scheme: Dinoflagellates or other sources (bacteria, invertebrates, macroalgae) are consumed by herbivores or omnivores, which, in turn, are eaten by carnivores that store the toxins. Humans and other mammals develop ciguatera poisoning as a result of eating the contaminated fish.

The etiology of ciguatera fish poisoning was established when Yasumoto et al. (1980a) discovered that a dinoflagellate resembling a *Diplopsalis* sp. was the initiator of the food chain disease. Later, the organism was correctly identified as *Gambierdiscus toxicus*, a new species of the family Dinophyceae (Adachi and Fukuyo, 1979). The species was named after its origin of discovery, the French Polynesian Islands

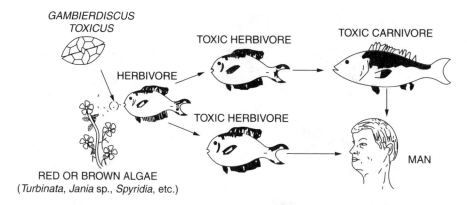

FIGURE 3.1 Transmission path of ciguatera toxin from the marine dinoflagellate *Gambierdiscus toxicus* through herbivorous and carnivorous fishes to humans.

of Gambier in the South Pacific (Yasumoto et al., 1980b; Adachi and Fukuyo, 1979). Present-day studies have confirmed the validity of the food chain concept. Campbell et al. (1987) reported an outbreak of ciguatera poisoning in a species of herbivore (*Ctenochaetus* sp., kole). Examinations of gut smears stained with anti-CTX fluorescence dye showed that 95% of the gut contents contained numerous *G. toxicus*. All tissues tested positive for ciguatoxin in the stick enzyme immunoassay (S-EIA). Yasumoto et al. (1980a) earlier demonstrated *G. toxicus* in the gut of herbivores. More recently, chemically characterized congeners of ciguatoxin were found in moray eel tissue (Satake et al., 1998). The precursor for these two oxidized congeners appear to be CTX3C, characterized and obtained from *G. toxicus* (Satake et al., 1993; LeGrand et al., 1992).

Gambierdiscus toxicus, a benthic organism that has been collected from the natural environment, yields both ciguatoxin and maitotoxin, but when cultured in the laboratory ciguatoxin production is essentially nil. Maitotoxin, a water-soluble, polyhydroxy-containing compound and one of the most potent toxins (0.125 μg/kg, LD_{100} in mouse), was obtained in moderate yields (Yasumoto et al., 1976). The inability of *G. toxicus* to produce ciguatoxin in culture may be due to its symbiotic relationship with the red-brown alga in nature. *Gambierdiscus toxicus* was found in large blooms at certain times of the year. Among the macroalgae associated with *G. toxicus* were *Turbinaria*, *Jania*, *Sypridia*, and *Bryopsis* species (Ichinotsubo et al., 1994; Taylor et al., 1984; Shimizu, 1982; Yasumoto et al., 1979). Other organisms of significant interest involved in ciguatera fish poisoning (Yasumoto et al., 1987) include *Prorocentrum* species and coral (*Halichondria* spp.), which produce okadaic acid and its congeners, and, recently, *Ostreopsis* spp. that show evidence of palytoxin (Usami et al., 1995), which was originally discovered in *Palythoa* (Moore and Scheuer, 1971).

The geographical distribution of *G. toxicus* is circumglobal and primarily in the tropics. It has been found in the Pacific and Caribbean by numerous investigators (Brusle, 1997). The growth of *G. toxicus* in nature is subject to changes in the environment. Heavy growth (40,000 cells per liter seawater) in the environment is

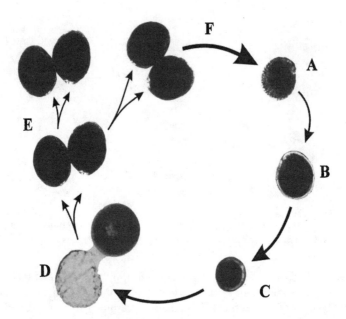

FIGURE 3.2 Life cycle of *Gambierdiscus toxicus*. (A) Motile, free-swimming *G. toxicus*. (B) Precyst: immobile, dark, dense, intracellular pigment; initial secretion of mucoid sheath. (C) Cyst: adherence to Petri dish bottom; thick, mucoid sheath; dark, centrally located pigment. (D) Exocyst: emergence from thick mucoid wall. (E) Division of exocyst: about 20 divisions per exocyst. (F) Conditions unknown, 4 to 6 months.

spotty; in some areas, growth has been nonexistent, while in other areas growth has been low to moderate (100 to 1000 cells per liter). Proper amounts of sunlight, temperature (24 ± 4°C), salinity, and appropriate nutrients are necessary for growth. Salinity of less than 2.8% generally shows no growth; that is, the presence of freshwater is deleterious for *G. toxicus* growth. No cyclic pattern for growth was observed after monthly collections of *G. toxicus* from Waianae Boat Harbor, Hawaii, for the duration of 2 years (Hokama et al., 1996a), during which the physical parameters (dissolved oxygen, salinity, pH, temperature, and water) remained constant. The only significant finding was the lack of growth of the associated macroalga (*Bryopsis* sp.), which made it difficult to find *G. toxicus* during this period of no algal growth. An example of *G. toxicus* of Waianae Boat Harbor and its life cycle are shown in Figure 3.2. The asexual life cycle of *G. toxicus* was examined *in vivo* and *in vitro* (Hokama et al., 1996a). *G. toxicus* was initially cultured successfully by Yasumoto et al. (1979); since then, numerous laboratories have grown *G. toxicus* for biological and chemical studies. A comprehensive compilation of *G. toxicus* and other dinoflagellate literature is presented by Brusle (1997).

In recent studies using scanning electron microscopy (SEM), *Gambierdiscus* species have been morphologically characterized, and a total of six species of *Gambierdiscus* have been identified, including *Gambierdiscus toxicus* Adachi et Fukuyo 1979, *G. belizanus* Faust 1995, *G. yasumotoi* Holmes 1998, and three new species in 1999: *G. polynesiensis* sp. nov., *G. ausrales* sp. nov., and *G. pacificus* sp.

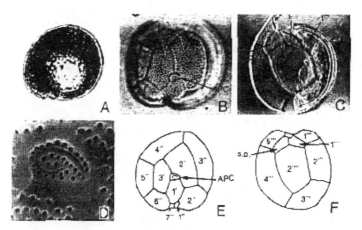

FIGURE 3.3 (A) Microscopic view of *G. toxicus* Adachi et Fukuyo. (B) SEM of ventral area. (C) SEM of dorsal area. (D) Enlarged SEM of APC region. (E) Theca of ventral area. (F) Theca of dorsal area. (From Fukuyo, Y. et al., Eds., *Red Tide Organisms in Japan: An Illustrated Taxonomic Guide*, Uchida Rokakuho, Tokyo, Japan, 1990, pp. 114–115. With permission.)

nov. (Hokama and Yoshikawa-Ebesu, 2001). Adachi and Fukuyo (1979) produced a scanning microscopic description of *Gambierdiscus toxicus*, the first known dinoflagellate to produce ciguatoxin in wildlife (Figure 3.3).

Based on microscopic and scanning electron microscopy, *Gambierdiscus toxicus* Adachi et Fukuyo 1979 has been described as follows (Fukuyo et al., 1990):

Cells large, lenticulate, 24–60 μm in length, 42–140 μm in transdiameter, and 45–155 μm in dorsoventral diameter. In apical view, cells rounded to ellipsoidal, compressed anterioposteriorly. Cingulum deep, narrow, ascending, both ends entering into deep sulcal hollow. Plate formula APC, 3, 7", 6c, 8s, 5", 2". Apical pore complex (APC) triangular, with a fishhook-shaped apical pore. First and seventh precingular plates fairly small, lying just above sulcus. First antapical and sulcal posterior plates long pentagonal, lying symmetrically concerning dorsoventral axis. Second antapical plate large, occupying antapex. Thecal plates densely porous. Numerous small yellow-brown chromatophores and one large transparent globule present.

CHEMISTRY

The isolation, purification, and determination of the structure of the causative factor associated with ciguatera fish poisoning have constituted a tedious and long-term study, initiated in Hawaii by Scheuer et al. (Tachibana et al., 1987; Nukina et al., 1984, 1986; Scheuer et al., 1967). A major obstacle in the structural determination has been an ample source of natural material that is scarce even in the most toxic fish, *Gymnothorax javanicus* (one moray eel liver yields about 1 μg purified ciguatoxin). Nevertheless, following the first isolation and characterization in 1967 (Scheuer et al., 1967), purified ciguatoxin (0.45 μg/kg, IP LD_{50} in mouse) was

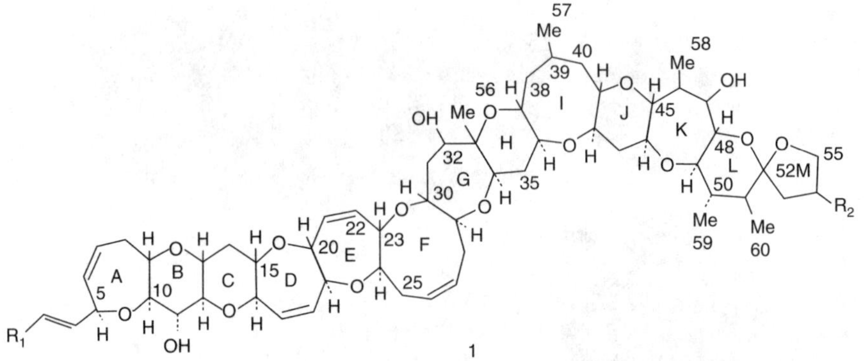

CTX1B $R_1 = HOCH_2CH(OH)-$ (From moray eel liver)

$R_2 = OH$

CTX4B $R_1 = CH_2 = CH-$ (From *Gambierdiscus toxicus*)

$R_2 = H$

FIGURE 3.4 Structures of ciguatoxin from *G. toxicus* (CTX4B) and moray eel liver (CTX1B). (From Yasumoto, T. and Murata, M., *Chem. Rev.*, 93, 1897–1909, 1993. With permission.)

obtained and the structure determined (Nukina et al., 1984; Scheuer et al., 1967; Banner et al., 1960). This ciguatoxin was found to be a polyether of a lipid nature consisting of several hydroxyl groups, soluble in organic solvents (chloroform, diethyl ether, methanol, ethanol, 2-propanol, and acetone), with a molecular weight of 1111.7 ± 0.3 and an empirical formula of $C_{59}H_{85}NO_{19}$ (Nukina et al., 1986). The polyether nature of ciguatoxin was noted following the demonstration by Yasumoto et al. (1980a,b) that a compound (toxin PII) isolated from *Prorocentrum lima* had all the biological and thin-layer chromatography (TLC) characteristics of ciguatoxin; however, this compound was later identified as okadaic acid, a polyether that was earlier isolated from a sponge (*Halichondria okadai*) by Scheuer's group (Tachibana et al., 1981), and brevetoxin (Lin et al., 1987a,b). Many of the dinoflagellate toxins (brevetoxin, okadaic acid, maitotoxin, and ciguatoxin) appear to have the same effect on various electrolytes (Na^+, K^+, Ca^{++}), although the precise mechanisms have not all been determined. In the late 1980s and early 1990s, the structures of ciguatoxin from moray eel tissues and *G. toxicus* cultures were determined and reported by Yasumoto and Murata (1993); the initial report was presented in 1990 by Murata et al. Figure 3.4 shows the structure of CTX1B (from moray eel tissues) and CTX4B (from *G. toxicus*).

The yield from 125 kg of *Gymnothorax javanicus* viscera was 0.35 mg of pure CTX (MW, 1111.5843 ± 0.0053) with a formula of $C_{60}H_{86}O_{19}$. Several thousand liters of *G. toxicus* culture yielded 0.74 μg of pure CTX4B (the less polar congener of CTX), with a molecular weight of 1061.584 and the formula $C_{60}H_{85}O_{16}$ (Yasumoto and Murata 1993; LeGrand et al., 1992; Murata et al., 1990). Prior to the isolation and identification of CTX4B from cultured *G. toxicus*, gambiertoxin was only isolated from collecting wild, natural growing *G. toxicus*. Yasumoto and colleagues (Yasumoto and Murata, 1993; LeGrand et al., 1992; Murata et al., 1990) have reported approximately 19 or more ciguatoxins that are associated with either ciguatera fish poisoning in fish or *G. toxicus* from the Pacific. The 1 major and 10 minor ciguatoxins (polyether isolates) from *G. toxicus* were referred to as gambiertoxins, while the 3 major and numerous minor ciguatoxins from 3 species of fish were called ciguatoxins. Table 3.2 shows the number of ciguatoxin congeners characterized to date.

TABLE 3.2
Ciguatoxins from Various Species of Fish and *Gambierdiscus toxicus*

Code No.	Molecular Weight	*G. toxicus*	*Scarus gibbus* (Flesh)	*Lutjanus bohar* (Viscera)	*Gymnothorax javanicus* (Viscera)	*Caranx latus* (Caribbean)[a]
1A	—					
1B (CTX)	1111			♦	♦	
	1023	•				
1C	—		•	•	•	
2A1	1057				•	
2A2	1095			•	•	
2A3	1057				•	
2B1	1061			•	•	
2B2	1095			•	•	
2C	1061				•	
	1095				•	
3A	—		•		•	
3B	1077		♦			
3C	1085	•				
3C	1080[a]				•	
3C	1062[a]				•	
3C	1023	•			•	
3D	941	•				
	1095	•				
	1023	•			•	
	1061	•				
	1023	•				
4A	1061	•	•			
4B (GT-4B)	1061	•	•			
4C	—	♦				
C-CTX-1	1142[b]					•
C-CTX-2	1142[b]					•

[a] Recent CTX congeners isolated from moral eel tissues; see Lewis et al. (1991).

[b] Electrophysiological studies (neuromuscular and cardiac tissues) show that Caribbean C-CTX resembles Pacific CTX, with some differences detected; see Vernoux and Lewis (1997).

Note: •, Stereoisomer; ♦, major toxic fraction.

Other polyether compounds isolated from *G. toxicus* were of significance. Gambieric acids isolated from the culture medium have shown potent antifungal properties (Nagai et al., 1993) and weak toxic properties. A drawback is that yields from *G. toxicus* culture medium are poor; yields of these toxins are very limited and generally are obtained only in the low microgram quantities. Nevertheless, if they can be synthesized in the laboratory, their use against fungal diseases would be of great significance.

Lewis et al. (1991) have also isolated, purified, and determined ciguatoxin structures from moray eel, confirming the findings of Murata et al. (1990). All of these chemical studies have demonstrated the diversity of ciguatoxins that contribute to the clinical entity referred to as ciguatera poisoning. Also contributing to this variability are the genetic and ethnic backgrounds of the individuals consuming ciguatoxin-contaminated fishes. Thus, the diverse clinical findings in ciguatera fish poisoning appear to be consistent with the variation of chemical structures described in the study of ciguatoxin chemistry in the marine environment (Yasumoto and Murata, 1993; LeGrand et al., 1992). Furthermore, the isolation, purification, and structural determination of ciguatoxin represented a major breakthrough in ciguatera research, making possible the potential synthesis of ciguatoxin and the preparation of epitopes for better immunological assay developments.

Two ciguatoxins were recently isolated in the Caribbean from horse-eye jack (*Caranx latus*), a species associated with ciguatera poisoning (Vernoux and Lewis, 1997). These two ciguatoxins were considered diastereomers and differed from CTX1B, the major toxin isolated from moray eel viscera (Murata et al., 1990). Whether these toxins were related to the numerous minor ciguatoxins of *Gymnothorax* spp. and *Lutjanus* spp. remains to be determined. Caribbean ciguatoxin was found to show similar biological toxicity in the mouse. At this date, it is much too early to conclude that Caribbean ciguatoxin differs significantly from Pacific ciguatoxin. Immunologically, studies with sheep anti-CTX and antibody prepared with ciguatoxin coupled to human serum albumin reacted very well with tissues of *Lutjanus*, a species involved in a large ciguatera outbreak in the Caribbean (Lewis et al., 1981).

Recently, two new ciguatoxin analogs, 2,3-dihydroxy CTX3C and 51-hydroxy CTX3C, were isolated from moray eel *Gymnothorax javanicus* by Satake et al. (1998). The precursor CTX3C is a minor analog originating as a component of *G. toxicus*. Synthesis of CTX1B is currently being attempted by two laboratories in Japan, with one laboratory starting at the west sphere and the other at the east sphere of the CTX1B molecule (see Figure 3.4). Both synthetic spheres (the west consisting of the A, B, and C rings; the east consisting of the J, K, L, and M rings) have been tested with the monoclonal antibody to ciguatoxin (MAb-CTX). Only the east rings J, K, L, and M have shown activity with the S-EIA procedure (Sasaki et al., 1995).

Recently, synthesis of ciguatoxin has been achieved by Hirama et al. (2001) using a highly convergent strategic approach in which the chemoselective ring-closing metathesis reaction is key. This approach has enabled the total synthesis of ciguatoxin CTX3C (natural toxin isolated from *G. toxicus* culture). This monumental achievement will enable researchers to find answers to biological roles of ciguatoxin. During the synthesis process, the ABC fragment was conjugated to protein (BSA), and the monoclonal antibody was prepared and reacted with CTX3C, as determined by a surface plasmon resistance spectroscopic method (Nagumo et al., 2001). Earlier, Pauillac et al. (2000) prepared mouse antibody to CTX1 by immunizing mice with fragment JKLM (the east sphere of ciguatoxin). These antibodies will be useful in developing assays for ciguatoxin detection in contaminated fish and food products and in human sera assessment in ciguatera outbreaks.

PHARMACOLOGY

In an earlier pharmacological study (an assessment of ciguatera fish poison with rabbit intestine suspended in Tyrode's solution), the resulting contraction of muscle was shown to be greater when the blood was initially primed with ciguatera fish poison prior to the addition of acetylcholine plus blood with glucose (Li, 1965a,b). Because no information regarding preparation of the ciguatera fish poison was provided, the data appear questionable in light of today's information on the chemistry of ciguatoxin. Subsequently, Rayner (1972) used a partially purified ciguatoxin preparation to show that the physiological effect of ciguatera fish poison was not due to an anticholinesterase action; instead, the action of ciguatoxin is related to the voltage-dependent sodium channel. Ciguatoxin is a novel type of Na^+ channel toxin. The primary receptor site of ciguatoxin action is the fifth domain of the Na^+ channel, similar in this respect to the primary receptor site of brevetoxin (Lombert et al, 1987). Ciguatoxin and brevetoxin (PbTx) share a common receptor site on the neuronal voltage-dependent Na^+ channel (Catterall, 1992), although ciguatoxin has 20 to 50 times greater affinity for the Na^+ channel than brevetoxin. Whereas the varied clinical symptoms of ciguatera would suggest the involvement of different toxins (Hokama and Miyahara 1986; Bagnis, 1968), ciguatoxin alone exerts its action on many tissue target sites. In nervous tissues, ciguatoxin causes a tetrodotoxin-sensitive increase in sodium ion permeability and depolarization of the resting membrane (Rayner, 1972). Depending on the magnitude of the depolarization, the consequence can be an increase in excitability of the neuronal membrane or a depolarizing type of conduction block at high concentrations.

Lower doses of ciguatoxin have marked effects on both the respiratory and cardiovascular systems. Although ciguatoxin has some neuromuscular blocking properties, the respiratory arrest induced by a lethal dose results primarily from depression of the central respiratory center (Cheng et al., 1969). In the cardiovascular system, the effect is often biphasic: hypotension with bradycardia followed by hypertension and tachycardia (Li, 1965a,b). The hypotension and accompanying bradycardia are readily antagonized by the anticholinergic agents atropine, hexamethonium, and hemicholinium, whereas the tachycardia and hypertension are mediated by the sympathetic nervous system and suppressed by the adrenergic blockers propranolol and reserpine (LeGrand et al., 1982).

The effects of ciguatoxin on smooth muscles are quite complex and dependent on the predominant autonomic innervation and the postsynaptic receptor function. For example, in isolated guinea pig tissues, ciguatoxin enhances the inhibition of the taenia caecum (Miyahara et al., 1985) and excitation of the vas deferens (Ohizumi et al., 1981). These effects are associated with norepinephrine release and antagonized by guanethidine, propranolol, reserpine, and tetrodotoxin. In contrast, ciguatoxin induces a sustained contraction of the ileum that is potentiated by eserine and completely blocked by atropine (LeGrand et al., 1982; Ohizumi et al., 1981). Similar affects on excitation and inhibition are observed in other tissues. Ciguatoxin contracts the thoracic aortic strip of the rabbit (LeGrand et al., 1982) and relaxes the spontaneously contracting rat jejunum (Miyahara et al., 1985). Many of these effects of ciguatoxin can best be explained by the depolarization of nerve terminals and the resultant release of neurotransmitters.

Recent examination of various crude methanol-soluble extracts of a herbivore (*Ctenochaetus strigosus*) and a carnivore (*Seriola dumerili*) demonstrated that the pharmacological use of guinea pig tissues (atrium and taenia caecum) *in vitro* was of great value in the characterization of ciguatoxin-like or maitotoxin-like toxins. *C. strigosus* flesh extracts showed maitotoxin characteristics, whereas *S. dumerili* extracts showed ciguatoxin-like activity in the atrium and taenia caecum studies (Miyahara et al., 1985).

In electrophysiological studies with rats and human patients affected with ciguatera fish poisoning, Cameron et al. (1991a,b) obtained findings indirectly suggesting that ciguatoxin acts on mammalian nerves by prolonging sodium channel actions. The paradoxical sensory discomfort experienced in paresthesia and dysethesia are most likely a result of an exaggerated and intense nerve depolarization occurring in peripheral small myelinated A-delta and, in particular, C-polymodal nociceptor fibers (Cameron et al., 1991a,b).

EPIDEMIOLOGY

Geographic Distribution

As indicated in the introduction, ciguatera fish poisoning is found worldwide between latitudes 35°N and 35°S. The major endemic areas where most studies have been done are the Caribbean and the Pacific Islands, including the lands adjacent to the Indian Ocean and the Gulf of Mexico. Archipelagos of the tropics considered to be safe from ciguatera poisoning are scarce and probably nonexistent. The travels of ships today and the periodic destructive hurricanes in the Pacific and Caribbean have contributed to the distribution and increase of the toxic dinoflagellate *Gambierdiscus toxicus* (Rigby and Hallegraff, 1996; Bagnis and LeGrand, 1987). For example, the presence of *G. toxicus* in the state of Hawaii may be attributed to troop transports and warships traveling from endemic areas of the Pacific to Pearl Harbor during World War II; cysts or dinoflagellates may have been carried on the bottoms and sides of these ships and in ballast water released from the ships. Two major hurricanes in the state of Hawaii, Iwa (1982) and Iniki (1991), have further contributed to ciguatera. The increase in knowledge of ciguatera in recent years has also heightened awareness of the problem.

Incidence

Ciguatera have been reported throughout the world. French Polynesia has been extensively studied by Bagnis and LeGrand (1987). Also in French Polynesia,

TABLE 3.3

Incidence of Ciguatera Fish Poisoning in French Polynesia, the Micronesian Islands, and Other Areas

Country	Cases/100,000	Period	Ref.
Federated States of Micronesia	4.8	1982–1987	SPC (1990)
Marshall Islands	234.6	1982–1987	SPC (1990), Randall (1980)
Northern Mariana Islands	74.8	1982–1987	SPC (1990)
Palau	2.4	1982–1987	SPC (1990)
French Polynesia	807	1960–1984	Danielson and Danielson (1985), Bagnis et al. (1985)
Australia	100	—	Bagnis et al. (1979)
Society	500		
Tuamotu	1700		
Marquesas	4300		
Gambier	22,700		
State of Hawaii	7.8	1970–1995	Department of Health (unpublished data)
Puerto Rico	8–11	1996	Demotta et al. (1996)

Yasumoto et al. (1979) discovered the culprit involved, *Gambierdiscus toxicus*. Ciguatera fish poisoning has been recognized in most of these epidemiological surveys, in which it is believed that only 20% of the total cases have been reported. In the Pacific, the epidemiology of ciguatera fish poisoning has received considerable attention because of the efforts of the South Pacific Commission (SPC).

The countries compiled in Table 3.3 comprise what is probably the most studied areas for the incidence of ciguatera fish poisoning. The Federated States of Micronesia, Palau, Puerto Rico, and Hawaii share a relatively low incidence of toxicity from fish in contrast to French Polynesia. In parts of the Central Pacific, the incidence of ciguatera fish poisoning is generally higher than in Hawaii, but much lower than in the French Archipelagos (SPC, 1990; Danielson and Danielson, 1985). The incidence of ciguatera fish poisoning in the region of the Indian Ocean is relatively low and nonexistent for some islands, such as Madagascar, Comores, Ceylon, and Indonesia. A recent incident of interest, however, occurred in Madagascar, where 98 out of 500 people died after eating the flesh of a shark. Clinical symptoms were not definitive for ciguatera fish poisoning, but, with limited tissues, two new liposoluble compounds, designated carchatoxin A and B, were isolated (Demotta et al., 1996; Boisier et al., 1995; Habermehl et al., 1994; Lewis 1986; Bagnis et al., 1985a,b).

Reunion Island would appear to be unfavorable for toxic algae growth, but its rate of intoxication for ciguatera fish poisoning is the highest, with 13.4 cases per

100,000 fish. This finding may be due to imported fishes (Lewis, 1986). In the Caribbean, ciguatera fish poisoning varies with the islands involved. The incidence of ciguatera fish poisoning was found to be low to moderate in Puerto Rico (Demotta et al., 1996), high in St. Barthelemy (Bourdeau, 1986), and high in the Virgin Islands (Morris et al., 1982). Ciguatera fish poisoning toxicities are also relatively high in the Dominican Republic and Cuba. Countries such as the United States and Canada have reported sporadic cases of ciguatera poisoning. In the United States, the major states reporting ciguatera fish poisoning are Hawaii and Florida. Other state reports have resulted from importation of fish from endemic areas such as the Caribbean and in some instances from the Pacific. Ciguatera outbreaks from fish poisoning also occur among tourists returning after consuming toxic fish in endemic areas.

Fish Associated with Ciguatera Poisoning

Ciguateric fish are generally restricted to species feeding on algae or detritus around tropical reefs (Quod, 1992), especially surgeonfish (Acanthuridae) and parrotfish (Scaridae). Carnivores such as snappers (Lutjanidae), jacks (Carangidae), wrasses (Labridae), groupers, sea bass, rock cod (Serranidae), moray eels (Muraenidae), triggerfish (Balistidae), and barracudas (Sphyraenidae) prey on the herbivores (Bourdeau, 1986). For example, an outbreak of toxicity on the island of Kauai occurred when a large bloom of *Gambierdiscus toxicus* among the green alga *Bryopsis* contaminated the surgeonfish, *Ctenochaetus strigosus*, causing an outbreak of ciguatera fish poisoning following consumption of the *C. strigosus*. *G. toxicus* was found in 95% of the gut contents of the surgeonfish when examined with sheep anti-CTX fluorescent-labeled antibody (Campbell et al., 1987). The fish reportedly involved in ciguatera fish poisoning are compiled in Table 3.4. These fish represent the major sources of ciguatera fish poisoning in those regions of the tropics where they are present. In all of the regions reported, the families of fish causing ciguatera are similar and include moray eels, snappers, groupers, wrasses, barracuda, amberjacks, jacks, surgeonfish, and triggerfish, representing primarily tropical reef fishes.

DETECTION METHODS

BIOASSAY

It is imperative to have an assay with specificity, sensitivity, and simplicity of application if it is to be used to confirm ciguatera poisoning in humans consuming fish following isolation of the chemical or biological entity responsible for initiation of the toxicity. For this purpose, various invertebrate and vertebrate animals have been utilized for bioassays (Banner et al., 1960). Later, when extraction procedures were developed and the toxins were shown to be lipids, chemical procedures using fluorescent markers were utilized for the isolation and purification of the toxic principles. Purification of ciguatoxins allowed development of immunological procedures (Hokama, 1985a,b, 1990).

Banner et al. (1960) examined a number of animal species, from the lower forms to mammals, including: Protozoa, ciliates, Arthropoda (Crustacea and Insecta), Mollusca, Echinodermata, Chordata, Amphibia, Reptilia, Aves, and Mammalia; these animals were fed pieces of raw flesh by voluntary and force feeding and in some cases were fed residues of alcoholic extracts. In feeding experiments with crayfish, significant physiological changes were observed, ranging from paralysis to death. The African land snail gave questionable results. The oral feeding of raw and dried toxic *Lutjanus bohar* showed variable reactions in the mouse. The 36 other species used demonstrated no responses; in light of current knowledge of the chemistry and concentration of ciguatoxin in fish tissue, these results obtained by Banner et al. (1960) were to be expected. Oral administration of raw or dried toxic fish flesh to mammals required a larger dose of samples over long periods to demonstrate any effect.

Based on the mouse bioassay for paralytic shellfish poisoning, Banner et al. (1960) turned to intraperitoneal injection of toxic fish extracts in mice with some success; however, because humans become intoxicated via the oral route, they turned to the mongoose (*Herpestes mungo*) for the feeding assay. The mongoose can be fed up to 15% of its body weight of raw fish, dried fish, or oil extracts of fish incorporated with raw eggs. Unlike cats, mongooses retain all of the food consumed; cats tend to regurgitate fish tissue, so the accuracy of the amounts eaten is questionable at times.

The clinical response to toxic fish following consumption by the mongoose showed similarities to that of humans. The responses were classified into five stages for a single feeding that was followed for 48 hours: no reaction, 0; slight weakness and flexing of the forelimbs, 1; slight motor ataxia, pronounced flexion of the forelimbs, and weakness of the hind limbs, 2; moderate motor ataxia, weakness, and partial paralysis of limbs and muscles, 3; acute motor ataxia and extreme weakness, limited movement, or coma, 4; and death, 5. All responses were accompanied by loosely formed stool (diarrhea); responses 3, 4, and 5 were sometimes accompanied by extensive salivation and trembling. Although in acute cases symptoms were neurological, no histological changes were observed upon postmortem examination with light microscopy. Postmortem examination revealed some animals with gastric ulcers, but this phenomenon was also noted earlier in natural, wild, untreated mongooses.

Animals used in ciguatera poisoning bioassays include cat, mongoose, chicken, mouse, mosquito, and fish. Cats (*Feliscatus*) have been shown to be highly sensitive to toxic fishes, and kittens have been used previously as animal models in bacterial food poisoning; however, for humane reasons, the use of cats has been discouraged in the United States. Nevertheless, in earlier studies in other countries (Tahiti, Japan), cats were used because of their sensitivity to toxic fish which permitted the use of small fish samples without extraction procedures. Hypersalivation in cats was one of the significant physiological reactions to ciguateric fish, but regurgitation of the fish samples caused difficulties in obtaining accurate results. In addition, maintaining proper and clean housing facilities was also a problem (Bagnis et al., 1985a,b; Banner et al., 1960; Hessel, 1960).

Chicks (*Gallus gallus* and *G. domesticus*) were used as an assay method for ciguatera poisoning assessment by administration of fish extracts via intravenous (IV), intraperitoneal (IP), or intramuscular (IM) methods (Kosaki and Anderson, 1968). Administration of extracts by intramuscular injection in hens demonstrated

TABLE 3.4
Fishes Implicated in Ciguatera Poisoning from Various Regions

Geographical Region	Fish
American Samoa	*Lutjanus bohar* (snapper)
	Sphyraena (barracuda)
	Carcharhinidae (shark)
	Groupers and others
Australia	*Scomberomorus regalis* (narrow-barred Spanish mackerel), other *Scomberomorus* species
	Scomberoides commeroniarus (giant dart)
	Sphyraena jello (barracuda)
	Plectropomus (coral trout)
	Epinephalus (flowery cod spotted cod, cod, grouper, wire-netting cod)
	Lutjanus sebae (red emperor)
	L. bohar (red snapper)
	Lethriones nebulosa (yellow sweet lip)
	Seriola lalandi (yellowtail king fish)
	Seriola (kingfish)
	Caranx (trevally)
	C. ignobilis (lowly trevally)
	Cephalopholis miniatus (coral cod)
	Cheilinus trilobatis (maori wrasse)
	Choerodon venustus (venus tusk fish)
	Trachinatus (dart)
	Paracesio perdiryi (southern fuselier)
	Lates calcarifer (barramundii)
Caribbean (Virgin Islands)	*Lutjanus* (snapper) and others
Florida	*Caranx* (jack)
	Sphyraena (barracuda)

pathomorphological changes in the nervous system (Rayner, 1972). The oral administration of toxic fish tissues or extracts to chicks induced hypersalivation, loss in weight, drop in rectal temperature, and acute motor ataxia. Chicks appeared to be two to five times more sensitive to toxic fish than mice.

Chicks have proven to be satisfactory animal models for both feeding and injection assays for fish poisoning. They are readily available, easy to manage, relatively small in size, and unlikely to regurgitate. They are highly sensitive to fish toxins, and the effects of the toxin are cumulative; however, some negative aspects regarding the use of chicks (e.g., nonspecificity and unusual sensitivity to various toxins) have been pointed out by several investigators, including those using the chick assay themselves (Kosaki and Anderson, 1968).

The effects of crude ciguatera toxin extracts fed to red snapper (*Lutjanus bohar*) were first determined by Banner et al. (1966). In this study over a long period, it was demonstrated that the toxin accumulated and was retained in the tissues of the snapper with no adverse effect to the fish; however, fish fed both ciguatoxin and

TABLE 3.4 (cont.)
Fishes Implicated in Ciguatera Poisoning from Various Regions

Geographical Region	Fish
Florida, cont.	Groupers, snappers, kingfish
	Seriola dumerili (amberjack)
	Dolphin fish (dorado)
	Scomberomorus (mackerels)
	Others
French Polynesia	*Sphyraena barracuda*
	Plectropomus leopardes (grouper)
	Lutjanus (snapper)
	Cheilinus undulatus (wrasse)
	Ctenochaetus striatus (surgeonfish)
	Gymnothorax (moray eel)
	Others (80 fishes in 27 families implicated)
Hawaii	*Carangoides* (jack)
	Seriola dumerili (amberjack)
	Cheilinus rhodochrous (wrasse)
	Ctenochaetus strigosus (surgeonfish)
	Cephalopholis argus (grouper)
	Aphareus furca (black snapper)
	Scarus (parrotfish)
	Mulloidichthys (weke, goatfish)
	Gymnothorax (moray eel)
	Acanthurus (surgeonfish)
	Mugil cephalus (mullet)
	Others (39 species implicated in Hawaii)

Source: Adapted from Hokama, Y. and Yoshikawa-Ebesu, J., *J. Toxicol. Tox. Rev.*, 20(2), 85–139, 2001.

maitotoxin showed behavioral changes. Maitotoxin was the probable cause of the behavioral change, as experiments with *Gambierdiscus toxicus*-fed fish showed pathomorphological changes in the liver of, for example, *Serranus cabrilla* (Amade et al., 1990). Feeding experiments to various fish species were difficult to assess because the dinoflagellate *G. toxicus* can produce several toxins in addition to CTX4B and CTX4C, maitotoxin, and several minor polyether toxins (LeGrand et al., 1992). Consequently, to attribute tissue changes only to ciguatoxin alone may be misleading. The results could also depend upon the species of fish used for a particular assay; the use of freshwater and nontoxic reef fish (not exposed to *G. toxicus* in nature) could contribute to misleading results. More recent studies using fish and dinoflagellate extracts have demonstrated that fish are sensitive to IP administration but less so than the mouse.

Mosquitoes (*Aede aegyptii*) have been used extensively in French Polynesia to assess crude ciguatera fish extract for toxicity (Bagnis et al., 1987). Crude fish extracts are injected into the intrathoracic cavity of the mosquito. The LD_{50} of the extract toxicity is expressed as gram fish extract per mosquito. Significant correlations between toxicity in mosquito, mouse, and cat and toxicity in humans have been shown (Bagnis et al., 1985a,b). Not considering the extraction preparation for each fish, the mosquito test is time consuming but cost saving. It was considered the most reliable bioassay in French Polynesia. Unfortunately, however, as with all bioassays, unless pure material is tested the test has no specificity; thus, the effects of CTX1 alone cannot be demonstrated in this way in a crude mixture of unrelated toxins.

Invertebrates have been used in assay systems for qualitative and semiquantitative assessment of fish toxicity. One advantage of their use is that their testing requires only small amounts of materials. The invertebrates utilized by some investigators have included: (1) brine shrimp, (2) crayfish, (3) flies, and (4) mosquitoes (Amade et al., 1990; Bagnis et al., 1985a,b, 1987; Kimura et al., 1982a,b; Hashimoto, 1979; Granade et al., 1976; Kosaki and Anderson, 1968; Banner et al., 1966). In these procedures, technique is critical to the success of using these assay organisms.

IN VITRO BIOASSAY

Mouse Bioassay

Currently, the mouse toxicity assay is the accepted method for evaluating ciguatoxin toxicity in fish extracts. Mice have been the primary animal used to assess ciguatera fish poisoning. Because oral feeding in both mice and rats showed no promise, investigators have used the intraperitoneal route in the mouse assay. In their purification studies using the IP mouse assay, Banner et al. (1960) showed that the active toxin was in the diethyl ether fraction and not the polar, water-soluble fraction. Eventually, most investigators began to use a standardized procedure for the mouse toxicity assay with the formulation: $MU = 2.3 \log (1 + 1/t)$, where t = hours, and 1 mouse unit (MU) is the concentration of toxic extract injected IP that kills a 20-g mouse in 24 hours. It has been found that in highly purified moray eel CTX1B, 1 MU = 7–8 ng.

With crude fish extracts, the general procedure is as follows: Swiss-Webster mice weighing 20 to 25 g are utilized to assess the toxicity of fish extracts; 100 mg of crude fish extract is resuspended in 1 mL of 1% Tween 60 in saline and injected IP into mice. Symptoms displayed by the mouse are observed at .5, 1, 2, 4, 6, 8, 24, and 48 hours after injection and rated on a scale of 0 to 5 according to toxicity (Table 3.5).

The estimation of ciguatoxin by MU from known cases of ciguatera fishes obtained from the Hawaii Department of Health and other laboratories ranges from 7 to 9 ng (Yasumoto et al., 1995; Kimura et al., 1982a,b). The mouse test, like the other bioassays, has a lack of *specificity*, as any toxic factor in fish extracts to which the mouse is sensitive will cause death.

Guinea Pig Atrial Assay

The *in vitro* bioassay to assess marine toxins has attracted great interest in the past decade because of its sensitivity and the use of minimal amounts of material;

TABLE 3.5
Mouse Toxicity Assay Scoring

Toxicity	Description of Visible Clinical Symptoms in Mouse After Extract Injection
0	No ill effect
1	15 to 60 minutes: muscle contraction in lower back area (flexion), increased respiration, immobile (inactive), recovery
2	Same as 1, but recovery in 2 to 3 hours; pilo-erection
3	Same as 2, but recovery in 12 to 24 hours; muscle contraction, paralysis in extremities (usually hind legs), rapid and irregular breathing, immobile, closed eyes, pilo-erection, slight cyanosis (tail)
4	Symptoms same as in 3, but death within 24 to 48 hours[a]
5	Symptoms same as 3 and 4, but death in less than 6 hours

[a] A mouse unit is defined here as the amount of toxin required to cause the death of a 20-g mouse within 24 hours; 7 to 9 ng ciguatoxin in a 100-mg sample of crude extract/mouse was injected intraperitoneally (estimated from Department of Health confirmed ciguateric fish extracts).

however, these test systems require special physiological instrumentation and tissue culture techniques (Hokama and Miyahara, 1986; Miyahara et al., 1985). Nevertheless, these assays give some measure of specificity, as the actions are at the sites of the sodium channel of neuroblastoma cells or guinea pig atrial tissue (Manger et al., 1995; Miyahara et al., 1985).

For the guinea pig atrial assay (Miyahara et al., 1985; Kimura et al., 1982a,b), 100 mg of each fish extract is resuspended in 1 mL of Krebs–carbonate solution; 100 μL of the suspension is tested on the guinea pig atria in 25 mL of Krebs solution. Subsequent inotropic and chronotropic actions are noted in addition to the pharmacological response of the extract to tetrodotoxin (TTX), verapamil, and the adrenergic blockers propranolol and phentolamine. The inhibitors (TTX and verapamil) and the adrenergic blockers are given after inotropic responses at 12.5 μL of a 10^{-3}-M concentration (Miyahara et al., 1985).

The guinea pig atrial *in vitro* assay, in spite of the specialized techniques involved (including dissection of the atria, left and right, from the heart), is an excellent means of studying marine toxins, especially crude marine toxin extracts. Once inotropic standard patterns are obtained for each pure toxin and the effects of various chemical inhibitors are ascertained, the inotropic patterns of crude fish extracts with inhibitors can be compared with the standardized patterns of the pure samples. Thus, CTX1B and other ciguatoxin-like toxins (okadaic acid and brevetoxin) show similar inhibition with tetrodotoxin; that is, ciguatoxin, okadaic acid, and brevetoxin can be readily distinguished from palytoxin and maitotoxin. Sodium channel effector toxins can be distinguished from calcium channel effectors by use of appropriate inhibitors to the inotropic response. Figure 3.5 presents the classical inotropic patterns of pure ciguatoxin, okadaic acid, palytoxin, and brevetoxin with or without TTX inhibition.

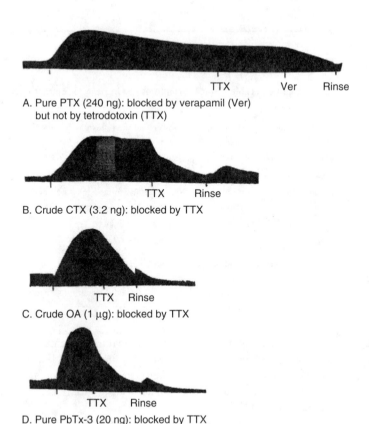

A. Pure PTX (240 ng): blocked by verapamil (Ver)
   but not by tetrodotoxin (TTX)

B. Crude CTX (3.2 ng): blocked by TTX

C. Crude OA (1 µg): blocked by TTX

D. Pure PbTx-3 (20 ng): blocked by TTX

FIGURE 3.5 Inotropic patterns for PTX, CTX, OA, and PbTx-3 in the guinea pig atrial assay.

IN VITRO CELL ASSAY

Neuroblastoma Assay

Directed cytotoxicity to sodium channels of neuroblastoma cells has been established
for purified ciguatoxin, brevetoxin, saxitotoxin, and crude seafood extracts, including
finfish extracts from the Caribbean as well as from the Pacific (Manger et al., 1995).
Mouse neuroblastoma (Neuro-2a, ATCC) were grown in RPMI complete medium
supplemented with 10% heat-inactivated fetal bovine serum, 2 mM glutamine, 1 mM
sodium pyruvate, 50 µg/mL streptomycin, and 50 units/mL penicillin. Actively growing cultures were maintained at 37°C in a humidified 5% CO_2 atmosphere. For
bioassay, 96-well plates were seeded with 1×10^5 neuroblastoma cells in 200 µL
growth medium and incubated for 24 hours. Culture wells then received 10 µL each
of the test sample, 10 mM ouabain, and 1 mM veratridine. Toxin samples were tested
in replicates of 4 at various concentrations of the sample. A minimum of 15 wells
were processed as ouabain/veratridine controls, and 5 wells were evaluated as
untreated control (cells only). Purified brevetoxin (PbTx-1) was included as a positive
control of sodium-channel-enhancing activity in conjunction with ciguatoxic finfish

extract assays. Nonspecific cell activity was assessed by the addition of samples and PbTx-1, but no ouabain and veratridine.

Cultures were then incubated for either 4 or 22 hours for detection of sodium-channel-enhancing activity, or 24 to 48 hours to assess sodium channel inhibitory activity. MTT (3-[4,5-dimethylthiazol-2-yl]-2.5-diphenyl-tetrazolium) was used to assess cytotoxicity by replacing the overlying medium with 60 μL of a 1:6 dilution of MTT stock (5 mg/mL PBS, pH 7.4) in complete culture medium. Plates were then incubated for 15 minutes at 37°C or until sufficient formazan deposits were observed in untreated control wells. The overlying medium was then replaced in each well with 100 μL of DMSO and the plates read at 570 nm in an enzyme-linked immunosorbent assay (ELISA) plate reader. This procedure measures the viable active cells via mitochondrial dehydrogenase reduction of the colorless MTT to formazan to give a purplish color read at 570 nm.

The ID_{50} (infectious dose 50%) PbTx-1 was detected at 250 pg and the ID_{50} for purified ciguatoxins was detected at 1 pg for CTX1 and 3 pg for CTX3C after 7 hours of incubation. CTX1 was isolated from moray eel livers and CTX3C from *G. toxicus* culture as a minor component. This cell bioassay is of value for marine toxin studies and may replace mouse assays when the use of live animals for experimental studies is prohibited. Measures of specificity and sensitivity for sodium channel activator or inhibitor compounds were excellent. In this respect, it was very similar to the guinea pig experiments but appeared to have a greater sensitivity.

Radiolabeled Binding Assay

Because ciguatoxin and brevetoxin share a common receptor in the sodium channel (domain 5), although with different affinities (CTX1 > PbTx), the use of labeled brevetoxin (3H-PbTx-B) allows ciguatoxin to be quantitated by competitive binding assay with sodium-channel-containing proteins. This has been demonstrated by several investigators (Trainer et al., 1995) using isolated rat brain synaptosome with 3H-PbTx-B and the CTX3C congener of CTX1B isolated from *Gambierdiscus toxicus* (Trainer et al., 1995). This procedure requires a small amount of fish extract, the method is rapid and simple, and it has a high sensitivity. Although the method may be useful for research, it may be impractical for large-scale fish screening because of the required use of a beta counter and radiolabeled compounds.

IMMUNOASSAY

Radioimmunoassay

The first successful detection of a low-molecular-weight polyether toxin, ciguatoxin, directly from contaminated fish tissues was reported in 1977 using a radioimmunoassay (RIA) with sheep antibody prepared with purified moray eel ciguatoxin conjugated to human serum albumin (HSA) as carrier (Hokama et al., 1977). Subsequently, the RIA was used to screen 5529 *Seriola dumerili* (kahala), a species associated with ciguatera outbreaks, in the State of Hawaii from 1979 through part of 1981 (Kimura et al., 1982a,b). The 15% of fish testing borderline or positive were discarded, and the remaining 85% of the fish, which scored negative, were sold commercially with no false negatives. Although the RIA procedure proved effective, its complexity and cost factors suggested seeking alternative immunological ciguatera screening methods.

Enzyme Immunoassay

An enzyme immunoassay (EIA) was subsequently established using sheep anti-ciguatoxin (anti-CTX) coupled to horseradish peroxidase (HRP), based on the same principle used in the RIA (Hokama et al., 1977). This method, although economically satisfactory because the need for expensive isotope counting instruments was eliminated, was found to be tedious. Consequently, this EIA method was abandoned and followed by the stick enzyme immunoassay (S-EIA) employing sheep anti-CTX and monoclonal antibody to ciguatoxin (MAb-CTX) coupled to horseradish peroxidase. This method has been used extensively for surveys of ciguatera-endemic areas and clinical confirmation of documented ciguatera fish poisoning for the State of Hawaii Department of Health (HDOH) (Hokama et al., 1985a,b, 1987a,b, 1989, 1990).

Immunobead Assay

The application of colored polystyrene particles coated with MAb-CTX as markers for direct detection of ciguatoxin adsorbed onto bamboo paddles coated with organic correction fluid was instituted in 1990. In this solid-phase immunobead assay (SPIA), the organic correction fluid coat bound both polar and non-polar components onto the bamboo paddle sticks. Numerous documented ciguateric fish from the DOH and reef fishes surveyed in Hawaii were assessed using this procedure (Ganal et al., 1993; Hokama et al., 1993).

Summary

Table 3.6 is a compilation of data regarding ciguatera-poisoning-implicated fish tested by RIA, S-EIA, and SPIA. The data include findings for fish implicated in ciguatera poisoning as compiled by the HDOH as well as routinely tested Hawaiian reef fish generally associated with ciguatera poisoning. The major species tested included *Ctenochaetus strigosus* (kole) and *Seriola dumerili* (kahala). Ciguatera poisoning in patients was clinically documented by physicians or epidemiologists from the HDOH. Of the total 176 ciguatera-implicated fish tested with these assays, 171 (97.2%) were found to be borderline or positive, while 5 (2.8%) were found to be negative (false negative). These procedures demonstrated a high degree of sensitivity with both sheep anti-CTX and MAb-CTX. On the other hand, the examination of Hawaiian reef fish of unknown toxicity demonstrated only a fair to moderate degree of specificity with the MAb-CTX in the S-EIA and SPIA procedures (45.0 to 51.4% specificity for the unknown fish). This is due in part to nonspecific binding to the coated bamboo stick. This moderate specificity has limited the commercial use of these tests; however, following extraction, 70% of the borderline and positive extracts of unknown fish tested by the mouse and guinea pig assays proved to be toxic. The sheep anti-CTX proved to give the best results in specificity (85.3 to 97.8%) and sensitivity (95.6%)

TABLE 3.6

Compilation of the Assessments of Test Procedures Prior to the Membrane Immunobead Assay[a]

Procedure	Antibody Used	Source of Sample	Total Number of Fish	Results Borderline/ Positive	Negative
Radioimmuno-assay (RIA)	Sheep anti-CTX	Hawaii Dept. of Health	46	44 (95.6%)	2 (4.4%)
		Routine samples (*S. dumerili*)	5596	824 (14.7%)	4772 (85.3%)
		Other species	766	17 (2.2%)	749 (97.8%)
Stick-enzyme immunoassay (S-EIA)	Sheep anti-CTX	Hawaii Dept. of Health	16	16 (100%)	—
		Routine samples (various species)	574	212 (36.9%)	362 (63.1%)
	MAb-CTX	Hawaii Dept. of Health	83	81 (96.8%)	2 (2.4%)
		Routine samples (*C. strigosus*)	712	392 (55%)	320 (45%)
		Routine samples (*S. dumerili*)	168	82 (49%)	86 (51%)
		Other species	3539	1720 (48.6%)	1819 (51.4%)
Solid-phase immunobead assay (SPIA)	MAb-CTX	Hawaii Dept. of Health	31	30 (96.8%)	1 (3.2%)
		Routine samples (various species)	482	261 (54.1%)	221 (45.9%)

[a] MIA data are presented in detail in Tables 3.7 and 3.8.

in the RIA procedure for assessment of *S. dumerili* and other reef fishes. The lack of a higher specificity suggested the need to continue searching for a better solid-phase medium for binding ciguatoxin and related polyethers.

MEMBRANE IMMUNOBEAD ASSAY

The membrane immunobead assay (MIA) technique is based on the same immuno-logical principles used to develop the SPIA (Hokama, 1990); it uses a monoclonal antibody to purified moray eel ciguatoxin (CTX1), colored polystyrene beads, and a hydrophobic membrane laminated onto a solid plastic support. The membrane binds only to lipids and generally not to polar or aqueous soluble compounds, unlike the correction-fluid-coated sticks. The polyether toxins bind to the hydrophobic polyvinylidene fluoride (PVDF) membrane and are then detected with MAb-CTX coating colored polystyrene beads. The intensity of the color on the membrane correlates to the concentration of toxin.

Preparation of Monoclonal Antibody to Purified Ciguatoxin

Highly purified ciguatoxin was obtained through the courtesy of Professor P.J. Scheuer of the University of Hawaii Department of Chemistry. The toxin was isolated from *Lycodontis* (*Gymnothorax*) *javanicus* (moray eel) livers and consisted of two interchangeable isomers (Nukina et al., 1984). The methods of Kohler and Milstein (1975) and presented by Schreier et al. (1980) were used in the hybridoma preparation.

Coupling of CTX1 to Human Serum Albumin

Purified ciguatoxin (1 μg) was coupled to HSA (1 mg) in 7.5 mL of 0.05-*M* phosphate-buffered saline (PBS) using the carbodiimide procedure (Hokama, 1985). Following exhaustive dialysis of the protein conjugate against saline at 4°C, the conjugate was precipitated with cold acetone in a ratio of acetone to conjugate of 4:1. The precipitate was centrifuged, rinsed twice with cold acetone, suspended in saline, and then used for the immunization of the BALB/c mice. After pervaporation, the acetone phase was analyzed for free ciguatoxin. These steps were critical for the immunization process (Hokama et al., 1989).

Immunization of BALB/c Mice

Three BALB/c mice, 10 weeks of age, were injected intraperitoneally once a week for 3 consecutive weeks with 0.1 mL of the CTX/HSA conjugate. A booster was given in the sixth week, 3 days prior to sacrificing the animals. Each mouse received a total of 80 to 100 ng CTX coupled with 80 to 100 μg HSA and 0.2 mL Freund's complete adjuvant (FCA) subcutaneously for each third injection of 0.1 mL of the conjugate.

Fusion Step

The non-immunoglobulin-synthesizing mouse myeloma cells selected for fusion were those previously reported by Kearney et al. (1978), designated PBX63-Ag8.656B. These cells were grown in Dulbecco's modified Eagle's medium (DMEM) supplemented with 10% fetal calf serum. Myeloma cells in the logarithmic growth phase were used for fusion.

The fusion of the sensitized cells from the BALB/c mice with the myeloma cells was done by the method of Kennet et al. (1980; see also Hokama et al., 1985, 1998a,b; Kearney et al., 1978). These procedures included hybridoma selection, media preparation, and limiting dilution methods. The original active hybridoma containing reactive anti-CTX was designated 5C8. Analysis of 5C8 with commercial immunofluorescence-labeled goat anti-mouse immunoglobulin isotypes (Sigma Chemical Co., St. Louis, MO) demonstrated the following hybrid cells: IgM, 85%; IgG$_1$, 55%; IgG$_{2a}$, 14%; IgG$_{2b}$, 3%; and possibly IgG$_3$. This suggested a mixture of clones, as the original myeloma produced no immunoglobulins. Nevertheless, 5C8 supernatants and ammonium sulfate fractions (50% precipitates) were used success-fully in numerous studies from 1987 through 1994 using a variety of test procedures (Hokama et al., 1987a,b, 1989, 1990a,b, 1993a,b, 1998a,b).

From 1987 to 1996, subculturing of 5C8 was shown to cause gradually dimin-ishing activity of the MAb-CTX; subsequent ELISA isotyping of different lots of 5C8 (50% ammonium sulfate fractions) showed the loss of the IgM, IgG_{2a}, and IgG_{2b} isotypes and the appearance of IgG_3. The first re-cloning of 5C8 resulted in six viable, moderately active clones out of 100 plated. The clone designated 2E6 was further cloned by limiting dilutions, resulting in 11 (6%) clones with good activity. All of the good and moderately active clones were frozen and stored at –80°C. One of the highly active clones designated 1C6 has been further cultured and used. Purification by gel affinity protein G column and isotyping in the ELISA procedure demonstrated equal amounts of IgG_1 and IgG_3 in the clone 1C6. The analyses for sensitivity and specificity were taken from Morgan et al. (1990):

$$\text{Sensitivity} = \frac{\text{Positive fish implicated in ciguatera detected by MIA} \times 100}{\text{Total number of positive fish implicated in ciguatera}}$$

$$\text{Sensitivity} = \frac{\text{Fish presumably without ciguatera toxins and negative in MIA} \times 100}{\text{Total number of fish tested presumed to be negative for ciguatera}}$$

Immunobead Preparation

The clone designated 1C6 was selected, and its cultured supernatants were collected and diluted 1:20 in saline in a final suspension of 0.1% colored polystyrene beads. The 1:20 dilution of antibody was selected as the optimal antibody concentration following titration of each batch of monoclone 1C6 cultured supernatants with the endpoint determined as approximately 1:100 dilution. The 1:20 dilution circumvents the "hook effect" (Morgan et al., 1990) and appears to be able to detect ciguatoxin at levels as low as 80 pg/g fish (80 ppt). Sensitivity can be enhanced by increasing the MAb-CTX concentration.

Polystyrene beads colored blue (0.314-μm diameter) and red (0.124-μm diam-eter) were used in a ratio of 3:1. These bead sizes were found to be satisfactory in suspension because larger sized beads (0.8-μm diameter and greater) tended to settle readily to the bottom of the vial. The use of a single color of beads was satisfactory, but the combination of two different colored beads gave a deeper hue.

Polyvinylidene fluoride membrane was laminated onto a plastic support stick (Figure 3.6). Other materials and chemicals used in the MIA included test tubes (8-mm I.D., 75-mm L.); a punch biopsy tool or sharp razor to cut fish samples; methanol for soaking fish samples; and a suspension of 0.1% colored microbeads (0.314 μm and 0.124 μm in diameter), coated with MAb-CTX. Standard control for positives consisted of pooled crude extracts of DOH-implicated fish from clin-ically diagnosed ciguatera poisonings. The presence of ciguatera in these crude extracts of Hawaiian reef fishes implicated in ciguatera poisoning was previously examined by Hokama et al. (1987) and Manger et al. (1995) using the neuroblas-toma cell bioassay. In addition, the presence of ciguatera was previously established

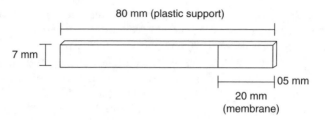

FIGURE 3.6 Membrane immunobead assay (MIA) procedure.

at 4 ng/12.5 mg of crude extract by immunoinhibition of the MAb-CTX with highly purified CTX1B (Khosravi, 1990).

Membrane Immunobead Procedure

The concept of the membrane immunobead assay (MIA) is similar to that of the solid-phase immunobead assay (SPIA): Colored immunobeads will adhere to cigua-toxin (antigen) on the membrane portion of a plastic stick previously exposed to the antigen; thus, positive samples will show visible color changes, while negative ones will not (Figure 3.7).

A fish tissue sample (approximately 5 ± 3 mg), cut with a punch biopsy tool or razor blade, was placed along with 0.5 mL methanol and a membrane stick into a test tube. After soaking for 20 minutes, the stick was removed from the test tube and thoroughly air dried for at least 20 minutes. The completely dried membrane stick was immersed into 0.5 mL of latex immunobead suspension, removed after 10 minutes, rinsed in saline or water, shaken to remove excess liquid, and air dried, after which the membrane was observed for color. The result was scored as negative for no distinct color on the membrane; weakly positive for a light blue-purple color on the membrane, with or without a darker band at the meniscus level; or strongly positive when membrane was colored and had more than one dark band at the meniscus level. All fish with results reading weakly positive and higher should not be eaten.

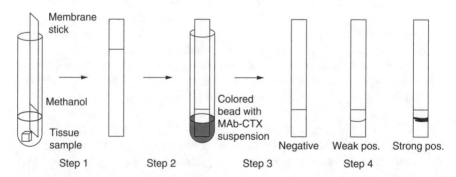

FIGURE 3.7 Membrane stick for membrane immunobead assay (MIA) with dimensions given. The membrane portion of the stick is directly laminated onto the longer plastic support.

TABLE 3.7
Membrane Immunobead Assay of Ciguatera-Implicated Fish Samples Reported by the Hawaii Department of Health

Species	Source	MIA Result	Remarks
Bodianus bilunulatus (a'awa)	Oahu	+	Cooked sample
Cephalopholis argus (roi)	Oahu	+	Cooked sample
Cephalopholis argus (roi)	Kauai	+	Cooked sample
Sphyraena barracuda (barracuda)	Big Island	$-^a$	Cooked sample
Mulloidichthys auriflamma (weke)	Oahu	+	Tissue
Unidentified	Kauai	+	Tissue
Unidentified	Kauai	+	Tissue
Kyphosus cinerascens (nenue)	Oahu	+	Cooked sample
Acanthurus dussumieri (palani)	Maui	+	Cooked sample
Snapper (sp. unidentified)	Barbados (via New Jersey)	±	Cooked sample
Redfish (sp. unidentified)	Texas Dept. of Health	+	Tissue
Barracuda (sp. unidentified)	Texas Dept. of Health	+	Tissue
Cephalopholis argus (roi)	Big Island	$\pm^b$	Cooked sample

[a] This sample was extracted and tested with the MIA; it reacted weakly at 7.0 mg/mL in methanol and was negative at 3.5 mg/mL. Mouse toxicity results (dead in 7 minutes after IP injection) suggest the presence of PTX- or MTX-like toxins. The guinea pig atrium analysis suggested the presence of low levels of CTX-like compounds in this sample (see Figure 3.7).

[b] One patient ate the same species for three consecutive meals; it is uncertain if the same or three different fishes were consumed. Three others ate only one meal of roi with no toxicity reported. A roi from the same catch was tested and found to be negative.

Note: +, positive; –, negative; ±, borderline.

Positive control samples at both high and low concentrations of toxins consisted of pooled extracts of implicated DOH ciguateric fish at 7.0 mg/mL and 3.0 mg/mL of methanol containing residual ciguatoxin of 2.24 ng and 0.96 ng ciguatoxin/mL of methanol, respectively. Negative controls were blank membranes used directly or soaked in methanol and dried thoroughly before immersing into the immunobead solution. The sequential steps of the MIA procedure are presented in Figure 3.6. During development of this method, several synthetic membranes were examined, and the hydrophobic membrane proved to be the best, as less than 3% of negative controls showed nonspecific binding of the immunobeads.

The data in Table 3.7 represent an assessment by MIA of fish involved in clinically documented ciguatera poisoning cases. Of the 13 fish samples examined, 10 were found to be positive and 2 borderline, containing approximately 60 to 160 pg ciguatoxin or related toxin per gram extract. This gave a sensitivity of 92.3%, with 7.7% false negatives. A *Sphyraena barracuda* sample from the Island of Hawaii gave an initial negative response in the MIA; however, further examination of the extract of this fish by mouse toxicity and guinea pig atrium analyses demonstrated it to contain a potent toxin unlike ciguatoxin. In comparison with a classical ciguatoxin pattern

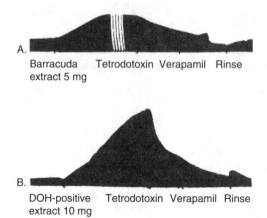

A.

Barracuda   Tetrodotoxin Verapamil   Rinse
extract 5 mg

B.

DOH-positive   Tetrodotoxin Verapamil   Rinse
extract 10 mg

FIGURE 3.8 Inotropic patterns from guinea pig atrium assays for (A) *S. barracuda* and (B) DOH-positive (containing CTX) extracts with addition of tetrodoxin (10^{-3} M, or 12.5 µL), verapamil (10^{-3} M, or 12.5 µL), and rinse. The difference in the TTX block is clearly demonstrated in the CTX-containing extract (B).

showing strong inhibition by tetrodotoxin (TTX), the *S. barracuda* pattern showed only a slight tetrodotoxin effect (Figure 3.8); nevertheless, the extract at 7.0 mg/mL showed a weak MIA response, and a 100-mg dose killed a mouse in 7 minutes. Still, the patient who consumed part of this fish demonstrated classical ciguatera symptoms (Hokama et al., 1996b). Taken together, these data suggested the presence of paly-toxin, maitotoxin, or as yet undetermined toxins in this barracuda, along with low levels of ciguatoxin-like compounds.

An analysis of various fish species by MIA is presented in Table 3.8. This table includes the species names, sources, total number of samples, and MIA results directly from fish tissues. *Caranx* (jack or papio) from Hawaii shows a higher percentage of borderline and positive results (23%) than those from Kwajalein and Kosrae (0% and 10%, respectively). In Hawaii, *Caranx* is a major target of sport fishermen and is the leading cause of ciguatera poisoning in nearly all of the islands in the state. Of the 154 samples tested by MIA, 132 (85.7%) were negative, 14 (9.1%) were borderline, and 8 (5.2%) were positive. The specificity (85.7%) shown is within acceptable levels for biological assays of this nature. All negative fishes were consumed without any reports of ciguatera poisoning; in other words, no false negatives were recorded.

Figure 3.9 illustrates titration of the standard pooled DOH positive extract in the MIA. The data show MIA results of the extracts tested at different concentrations and the approximate calculated ciguatoxin concentration. The minimal detection point was 0.08 ng or 80 pg (80 ppt) ciguatoxin in the crude DOH mixture.

This new MIA procedure was compared with previously developed immuno-logical test procedures that used correction-fluid-coated bamboo sticks (Hokama et al., 1984). The S-EIA uses bamboo skewers coated with correction fluid and MAb-CTX conjugated to horseradish peroxidase (HRP) with an appropriate substrate as

TABLE 3.8

Membrane Immunobead Assay of Routine Catches of Fish from the State of Hawaii and Other Pacific Islands

Species	Source	Total Number of Fish	MIA Results		
			Negative	Borderline	Positive
Caranx (papio/ulus)	Hawaii	26	20 (77.0%)	2 (7.6%)	4 (15.4%)
Caranx (papio)	Kwajalein	82	78 (95.0%)	4 (5.0%)	0
Caranx (papio)	Kosrae	20	18 (90.0%)	0	2 (10.0%)
Ctenochaetus trigosus (kole)	Midway	3	3	0	0
Mugil cephalus (mullet)	Hawaii	3	3	0	0
Mulloidichthys auriflamma (weke)	Hawaii	5	1	4	0
Seriola dumerili (kahala)	Hawaii	2	1	0	1
Aphareus furca (wahanui)	Hawaii	3	2	1	0
Mulloidichthys pflugeri (weke ula)	Hawaii	2	0	2	0
Bodianus bilinulatus (a'awa)	Hawaii	2	2	0	0
Aprion virescens (uku)	Maui	2	2	0	0
Cephalopholis argus (roi)	Oahu	1	0	0	1
Sphyraena helleri (barracuda)	Oahu	1	0	1	0
Priacanthus meeki (aweoweo)	Oahu	1	1	0	0
Acanthurus triostegus (manini)	Oahu	1	1	0	0
Total		154	132 (86.0%)	14 (9.0%)	8 (5.0%)

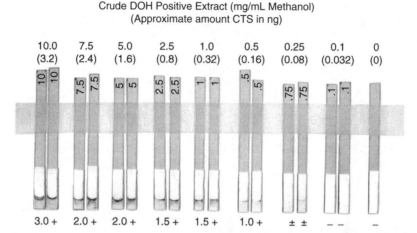

FIGURE 3.9 Examples of DOH mixed ciguateric fish extracts from 0.1 to 10.0 mg extract in 1 mL of methanol (in duplicate), tested by membrane immunobead assay (MIA). The numbers in the parentheses are calculated concentrations of CTX in the crude extracts. The −, ±, and + numbers represent relative degree of activity.

the detection system, while the SPIA uses a correction-fluid-coated bamboo paddle and MAb-CTX adhered to colored polystyrene beads to detect ciguatoxins. In contrast, the MIA system consists of a solid-phase hydrophobic synthetic membrane laminated onto a solid plastic support; the sensitized membrane is dipped into an aqueous suspension of mixed polystyrene beads of two different colors and diameters bound to MAb-CTX, and the intensity of the resulting color on the membrane is assessed.

This new procedure was used to assess clinically implicated DOH ciguatera fish samples, a variety of routine fish samples from endemic reef areas of Hawaii, and a number of *Caranx* species from Kwajalein and Kosrae. The results showed good detection of DOH ciguatera-implicated fish with one exception: Direct examination of the *S. barracuda* tissue showed no activity in the MIA, but the extract was highly toxic in the mouse toxicity assay and produced a response in the MIA at a higher dose or 7 mg. Analysis of the extract in the guinea pig assay suggested that its major toxic component was something other than ciguatoxin (Figure 3.8), as stated earlier.

Comparison of *Caranx* species from Hawaii, Kwajalein, and Kosrae showed that those from Hawaii had a higher toxicity level (23%) than the samples from Kwajalein (5%) and Kosrae (10%). In part, this may be attributed to the fact that the *Caranx* spp. from Hawaii were obtained from several areas on different islands, while the Kwajalein and Kosrae samples were from one area on a single island. Other groups of fish samples from Hawaii were too small to evaluate properly. Nonetheless, the overall sampling by MIA showed reasonable ciguatoxin detection levels with 86% negative, 9% borderline, and 5% positive. The variability due to nonspecific binding of the immunobeads to the membrane is minimized by the use of a hydrophobic membrane, with only 3% of 179 blank membranes tested showing a borderline reaction. The sensitivity achieved with the small number of DOH toxic samples was 92.3%, while the specificity indicated for unknown reef fish was 85.7%. These values were within the acceptable ranges for a biological test system.

The sensitivity of the older procedures (RIA, S-EIA, SPIA) ranged from 95.6 to 97.2%, but the specificity was close to 50%. This low specificity suggests non-specific binding of the antibody conjugate and the antibody bead to the correction fluid on the stick. In part, the antibody bead tended to bind to the bamboo paddles nonspecifically in 22 (10.6%) out of 207 blank sticks examined. As mentioned, the MIA blanks showed only 2.8% nonspecific binding. The low specificity with correction-fluid-coated bamboo paddles requires further study if these procedures are to be used for commercial ventures. However, the SPIA has been useful in preventing ciguatera for recreational fishermen in Hawaii (Hokama et al., 1990).

With the exception of okadaic acid, cross-reaction studies of the MAb-CTX with other polyethers are limited (Hokama et al., 1992, 1996b). As indicated by Land-steiner (1945), MAb-CTX was shown to react best with ciguatoxin, its homologous antigen (epitope), at the 1-ng level, while 5 ng of okadaic acid was necessary for comparable activity. Other related polyethers, including brevetoxin, palytoxin, mai-totoxin, and congeners of okadaic acid, require levels of 50 ng or greater to give comparable reactions with the MAb-CTX in the S-EIA.

In the development of the MIA, several factors critical to obtaining accurate and repeatable results were noted. First, the membrane portion of the membrane stick must not be touched, as this may cause false positive reactions. Second, the membrane stick must be soaked in the methanol/fish sample suspension for at least 20 minutes for optimal results. Third, both the stick and the test tube must be completely dried before adding the latex immunobead suspension to the test tube; failure to do so could also cause false positive reactions. Finally, to prevent false positive results, the membrane stick should not be soaked in the latex immunobead suspension for longer than 10 minutes. If these points are followed, the MIA procedure should prove to be simple and reliable for the detection of ciguatoxin and related polyethers in fish.

Preliminary studies suggested that the binding sites of ciguatoxin to sodium channel receptors and the monoclonal antibody to ciguatoxin were on opposite sites of ciguatoxin. Evidence for this interpretation was based on immunological analyses with epithelial extracts of pig small intestine (sodium channels) and MAb-CTX in the guinea pig atrium assay. Ciguatoxin added to the physiobath containing guinea pig atrium induces an inotropic (increase in the atrium contraction and thus amplitude of heartbeat) response. Pre-addition of varying concentrations of pig intestine extract or MAb-CTX into the physiobath inhibits the inotropic effect in the former (pig intestine extract) but not the latter (MAb-CTX). Further, immunological studies employing the stick-enzyme immunoassay demonstrated that the west sphere synthetic tricyclic rings A, B, and C did not react with the MAb-CTX, but the east sphere synthetic tetracyclic rings J, K, L, and M did react with the MAb-CTX (Sasaki et al., 1995). Furthermore, computer molecular modeling for ciguatoxin suggests that the reactive site of ciguatoxin on the fifth domain of the sodium channel is the west sphere, which is similar to brevetoxin in its reaction with the synaptosome of the rat brain tissue (Trainer et al., 1995).

Modified immunoassays for polyether toxins have been developed, including competitive binding radioimmunoassay for brevetoxin (Trainer et al., 1995); however, to date, no extensive testing or evaluation of this immunoassay has been conducted. This assay appears to show sensitivity, but specificity has not been evaluated, and the procedures generally are not applicable to the simple screening of toxic fish.

Summary

Various assays have been developed to identify the toxin of interest in natural marine products, in the purification processes, and for screening purposes to maintain wholesome and healthy products for consumption. The basic goals have been to achieve simplicity, sensitivity, and specificity in an assay system that is universally applicable for home, field, and laboratory use for detection of ciguatera fish poisoning. Most of the bioassays using animals or cell systems tend to be nonspecific; however, for ciguatoxin, use of sodium channel targets such as synaptosomes and cell bioassay with neuroblastoma suggest some level of specificity and sensitivity. The immunochemical assay appears to be the most promising for practical use commercially in the screening of toxic fish for ciguatera because of its simplicity, practicability, and, most of all, its specificity and sensitivity.

TISSUE AND BODY EFFECTS

Clinical

Acute-Phase Ciguatera

Consumption of toxic fish associated with ciguatera poisoning results in the appearance of clinical symptoms within 10 minutes to 12 hours and, on occasion, 24 hours after consumption (mean, 4 to 6 hours). The gastrointestinal symptoms are characteristic of many other food poisonings, but ciguatera poisoning can be differentiated by unique features affecting the neurological system. Table 3.1 summarized the many clinical symptoms associated with ciguatera poisoning (Bagnis, 1968; Russell, 1975). The major toxin implicated has been designated ciguatoxin (Scheuer et al., 1967), although the complex symptoms and peculiarities noted among patients from different tropical and subtropical areas (Caribbean vs. Pacific) suggest multiple toxins (Bagnis, 1968; Hokama and Miyahra, 1986). For example, Bagnis et al. (Bagnis and LeGrand, 1987; Bagnis et al., 1979) examined numerous cases from the South Pacific and found subtle differences in certain clinical symptoms between Melanesians and Polynesians. Pruritus, ataxia, abdominal pain, and weakness were more commonly reported by Melanesians than by Polynesians. Whether these differences were due to variability in toxins (source of fishes) or the susceptibility of different ethnicities to ciguatoxin remains unclear. Diagnosis was based on clinical presentation with paresthesia and dysethesia, considered clinical hallmarks of ciguatera poisoning, especially in the South Pacific. This clinical presentation essentially differentiates ciguatera from other forms of food poisoning or mild gastroenteritis (Palafox and Buenconsejo-Lum, 2001; Morris et al., 1982).

Chronic Ciguatera Poisoning

Chronic ciguatera poisoning symptoms initially resemble those defined in Table 3.1, but prolongation of the symptoms beyond 2 weeks is considered chronic ciguatera, which may persist for months and even years. Chronic ciguatera patients experience fatigue, lethargy, arthralgia, myalgia, and poor exercise tolerance and characteristically manifest with neurologic, joint, and muscle aches with constitutional symptoms (Palafox and Buenconsejo-Lum, 2001). Chronic ciguatera symptoms have been associated with chronic fatigue syndrome by some investigations in the clinical study of chronic ciguatera (Palafox and Buenconsejo-Lum, 2001; Racciatti et al., 2001; Pearn, 1997). Reports of ciguatera poisoning from the Caribbean (including Florida) and the Pacific (Hawaii, French Polynesia, American Samoa, and Australia) generally all show variations of the clinical symptoms included in Table 3.1. These variations can change from area to area. The neurological symptoms, especially dysethesia and paresthesia, are the major clinical diagnostic hallmarks of ciguatera poisoning following consumption of toxic fishes, although these symptoms can also occur in shellfish poisoning and tetrodotoxin intoxication (Yotsu et al., 1987; Noguchi et al., 1987).

Ciguatera poisoning caused by *Scarus gibbus* from the Gambier Islands showed initial clinical symptoms characteristic of the ciguatera syndrome; however, after 5 to 10 days, a second phase appeared, characterized by an ataxic gait, dysmetria, asthenia, loss of static and dynamic equilibrium, and muscle tremor, which was induced by an effect on the cerebellum. This second phase set in for about 7 days and required about 4 weeks for complete recovery (Bagnis, 1968).

Palytoxin was implicated by Japanese investigators (Noguchi et al., 1987) following consumption of a parrotfish (*Ypsiscarus ovifrons*) by a patient who died four days after consuming the fish and had symptoms not unlike ciguatera poisoning. Earlier, Yasumoto et al. (1983) reported the presence of palytoxin in two species of crabs (*Lophozozymus pictor* and *Demania alcalai*) associated with lethal poisoning of humans in the Philippines.

Palytoxin toxicity has also been reported in Hawaii from smoked *Decapterus macrosoma* imported from the Philippines (Kodama et al., 1989). In laboratory analysis of toxicity induced by several species, low levels of palytoxin were demonstrated in 4 of the total 14 fish examined (Hokama et al., 1996b). It seems that the term *ciguatera* encompasses fish poisoning associated with a group of lipid polyether compounds, of which ciguatoxin appears to be one of the most hazardous and probably the most prominent in carnivores (Scheuer et al., 1967).

A study of two outbreaks in Hawaii in 1985 involving a herbivore (*Ctenochaetus strigosus*) and a carnivore (*Seriola dumerili*) showed clinical similarities and differences (Hokama and Miyahara, 1986). *Ctenochaetus strigosus* induced only the gastrointestinal and neurological symptoms in all 16 patients with no hospitalization. Seven of the 14 patients who had eaten *S. dumerili* were hospitalized, and 7 had cardiovascular symptoms in addition to gastrointestinal and neurological problems. A similar observation was reported by Bagnis (1968) in Tahiti. This observation of ciguatera poisoning by two fish species of different eating habits suggests the following: (1) more than one toxin was involved, (2) changes in the toxin occurred during the passage from herbivore to carnivore, and (3) no differences existed between the toxins but poisoning was a dose–response effect because *C. strigosus* was small and the viscera (liver, roe, etc.) were not consumed.

Other Factors

Other factors in ciguatera poisoning worth noting include: (1) multiple poisonings of an individual causes an enhancement of clinical severity and greater sensitivity to the toxin in subsequent poisonings; (2) the poisoning is rarely lethal when the flesh is consumed (Cook et al., 1977; Engleberg et al., 1983; Quod 1992), but lethality (less than 1%) occurs when the most toxic part of fishes were eaten (liver, organs, roe, etc.); and (3) susceptibility to the toxin(s) may vary among individuals. Mammals susceptible to ciguatera fish poisoning include dogs, cats, dolphins, California sea lions, Hawaiian monk seals, and domestic pigs; therefore, care should be taken when feeding these animals fish from endemic areas.

Transmission of toxin via ciguateric mother's milk during breastfeeding has been demonstrated for ciguatera fish poisoning, along with placental transfer of the toxin, which has resulted in abortions during the first trimester of pregnancy (Bagnis and LeGrand, 1987). Also, sexual transmission via seminal fluid from an intoxicated husband to wife has also been reported (Lange et al., 1989). Thus, ciguatoxin and its congeners can be transmitted through breastfeeding, the placenta, and body fluids (seminal fluid) from a ciguateric patient to a healthy individual. This is probably made possible by the ability of ciguatera to bind to normal serum and tissue proteins, one of which may be albumin.

Table 3.4 summarizes the fish most commonly implicated in ciguatera poisoning in the Caribbean region, including Florida, and in the Pacific area (Hawaii, French Polynesia, American Samoa, and Australia). Most of the fishes listed in all of the areas are carnivores. Part of the variation in toxicity relative to fishes between areas may be attributed to ethnic variations in taste for various fish species; another contributing factor could be the variation due to the nature of secondary prevailing toxins. In all studies reported, the cyclic effect of a seasonal pattern of intoxication was inconsistent. In American Samoa, toxicity has occurred all year round. Toxicity in Florida occurs frequently in the spring and summer months. In Hawaii, no cyclic pattern of toxicity has been shown.

Hokama et al. (1996b) reported on their examination of 14 fish representing 8 species implicated in ciguatera fish poisoning in 1994 with respect to clinical symptoms, immunological tests of fish, and guinea pig atrium (sodium channel effect) and mouse bioassays. Based on a comparison of the clinical symptoms in the patients and analyses of the fish consumed using the immunological test and guinea pig atrium and mouse toxicity assays, they concluded that diverse toxins were present in the ciguateric fishes examined, and, potentially, in any given fish it was probable that more than one toxin caused the ciguatera symptoms. A diversity of toxins or congeners has been previously suggested by investigators in ciguatera fish poisoning studies (Hokama et al., 1996b; Kodama et al., 1989; Hokama and Miyahara, 1986; Morris et al., 1982; Bagnis et al., 1979; Bagnis, 1968).

Based on the mosquito, mouse, and membrane immunobead assays of consumed ciguateric fish, it has been estimated that illness occurs when humans consume at least 23 to 230 ng of ciguatoxin in a meal. This has been referred to as the pathogenic dose (PD) by Bagnis et al. (Bagnis and LeGrand 1987; Bagnis et al., 1985a,b). This wide range of toxicity suggests variability in individual susceptibility and the effect of previous exposures to very low concentrations of ciguatoxin or congeners (cumulative effect). Other researchers have indicated the minimal level of toxic fish consumption to be 50 to 100 pg/g fish (Labrousse et al., 1992).

PATHOLOGY

Human

Pathological findings in postmortem studies of humans following death from ciguatera poisoning are relatively scarce, in part due to the fact that deaths in ciguatera fish poisoning are very rare (less than 1% worldwide). Most deaths reported can probably be attributed to palytoxin, particularly due to intoxication from eating crustaceans. The crabs *Demania reynaudi*, *D. alcalai*, and *Lophozozymus pictor* from the Philippines and Singapore have been implicated in toxicities and death, but these involved palytoxin as the causative factor. Postmortem examinations of human tissues generally have shown little or no histological tissue changes with routine hematoxylin–eosin (H&E) staining.

Evidence of morphological tissue changes detectable either by light or electron microscopy in human deaths in ciguatera fish poisonings is very rare (Brusle, 1997); however, three reports in the literature demonstrated the following findings: (1) histological lesions in nerve fibers with striking edema in the vacuoles of Schwann cell cytoplasms and vesicular degeneration of myelin (Allsop et al., 1986); and (2) fiber-splitting degeneration and necrosis of the liver, revealed by muscle biopsy on a ciguatera fish poisoning victim (Bagnis and Rouanet 1970; Bagnis 1970). No electron microscopy findings have been reported in human fatalities as a consequence of ciguatera poisoning.

Animal Studies

Ciguatoxin and brevetoxin

Experimental animals administered whole fish tissues, crude organic solvent extracts, and purified ciguatoxin were presented with clinical symptoms characterized in human intoxication with ciguatera fish poisoning. Wild mongooses given toxic moray eel flesh were noted to have increases in ulcers of the stomach (Banner et al., 1960). In the natural state, however, the mongoose has been found to develop stomach ulcers due to stressful environments. Experimental mice models show little light microscope changes with routine H&E staining, but definite pathological changes can be seen with the electron microscope in target organs of mice administered pure ciguatoxin (Terao et al., 1992).

Repeated intraperitoneal and oral administrations of CTX1B, CTX4C, and brevetoxin PbTx-3 derived from *Lutjanus bohar* and CTX4C purified from *Gambierdiscus toxicus* to male ICR mice at a dose of 0.1 µg/kg for 15 days resulted in marked swelling of cardiac cells and endothelial lining cells of blood capillaries in the heart. A single dose showed no discernible pathological changes in the heart. Damage to the capillaries was followed by prominent effusion of serum and erythrocytes into the interstitial spaces of the myocardium. Swelling of the endothelial lining cells of the capillaries caused narrowing of the lumen and accumulation of blood platelets in the capillaries, which caused multiple necrosis of single cell cardiac muscle cells. Myocytes and capillaries appeared normal after 1 month of treatment with the toxins. The effusion in the interstitial spaces resulted in the formation of bundles of dense collagen, which persisted for 14 months. Diffuse interstitial fibrosis was prominent in the septum and ventricles, with bilateral ventricular hypertrophy. A single dose of 0.1 µg CTX1/kg IP resulted in severe acute heart injuries followed by diffuse myocardial fibrosis (Terao et al., 1992, 1995).

It is well established that the west sphere of ciguatoxin acts on the membrane of cells, with the receptor being the fifth domain of the sodium channel, similar in this respect to brevetoxin (Terao et al., 1994); however, ciguatoxin has been shown to have a greater affinity for the receptor than brevetoxin. Both compounds depolarize nerve terminals through their actions on sodium channels, which potentiate the membrane and cause the influx of sodium ions into the cells. It has been suggested that this increase in the sodium influx creates the pathological patterns of the targeted cells when examined by light or electron microscopy (Terao et al., 1992, 1995). Nevertheless, surprisingly, damage by acute levels of PbTx (200 µg/kg) showed less tissue pathology than CTX at a sample dose of CTX1 of 0.35 µg/kg. CTX1-treated animals showed marked edema in the heart muscles as well as the nerve tissues. Whether given in short-term successive or long-term intermittent doses, the effect of CTX1 on the heart muscles has been found to be similar to that of a single dose of 0.35 µg/kg.

Acute doses of brevetoxin cause tonic seizures by stimulation of the motor neurons and death with a short opisthotonos. Pathological changes in the heart, kidney, and liver by PbTx-3 were found to be less severe than those of ciguatoxicosis. Table 3.9 summarizes a comparison of the toxic effects of pure ciguatoxin and brevetoxin-3 in ICR mice (Terao et al., 1995). The effects of CTX1 (0.35 µg/kg) on the cardiac tissues at a lethal dose were much more severe than PbTx-3 at a larger lethal dose (200 µg/kg), although both toxins are sodium channel agonists. The affinity for the sodium channel, however, is much greater for CTX1 than PbTx-3. This physiological difference may account for the variance in the cardiac tissue pathology.

Mice given high (death in 65 minutes), moderate (death in 2 hours, 43 minutes), and low (death in 7 hours, 15 minutes) doses of ciguatoxin all demonstrated changes in the small and large intestines. Small intestines showed degeneration of nuclei and swelling (edema) of the lamina propia in the high-dose CTX1 administration, while mice given the moderate dose of CTX1 showed degeneration of the villi tips. Stripping of brush borders of the villi was observed in the small intestines with the low-dose CTX1 treatments. The low-dose CTX1 also caused epthelial surface degeneration, sloughing into the lumen, and increased mucin production. These findings were demonstrated by light microscopy (Bagnis, 1970).

TABLE 3.9

Comparison of Pure CTX1B and PbTx-3 Pathological Tissue Changes in ICR Mice

Category	Ciguatoxicosis	Brevetoxicosis
Lethal dose (LD)	1 mouse unit (0.35 µg/kg)	LD_{100} 200 µg/kg
Death	24 hours	0.5 hours
Clinical signs and symptoms	Paralysis, diarrhea, seizure, penile erection	Spasmodic seizures, opisthotonos, dyspnea
Major targeted organs	Heart, penis, unmyelinated nerves	Motor neurons (?)
Changes in the heart (relative intensity):		
Cardiac muscle cells	3+	+
Blood capillaries (endothelial lining cells)	3+	+
Thrombosis (heart, liver, penis)	3+	±
Cumulative effect in heart	2+	−

Note: Data from Bagnis (1970); Terao et al. (1992, 1994, 1995); Ito et al. (1996).

When 80% of a MU (mouse unit) of semipure ciguatoxin-1B from *Gymnothorax javanicus* was given per mouse, diarrhea resulted within 10 minutes after the IP injection and lasted for 30 minutes, with changes shown in the large intestines. CTX1B induced accelerated mucus secretion and peristalsis in the colon and stimulated defecation, resulting in prominent diarrhea. Large quantities of mucus were secreted in the colon from mature as well as immature goblet cells, and epithelial cell damages were observed in the upper portion of the large intestines but not the lower half. The morphological changes of the upper large intestine induced by CTX1B were similar to those seen with cholera toxin (Terao et al., 1991, 1995). Diarrhea appears to be induced in mice by CTX1B doses of 1 to 7 ng/mouse. Mice given less than 1 ng and greater than 7 ng IP injections showed no diarrhea. Mice given oral doses at any levels showed no diarrhea. It appears that variable patterns of diarrhea after IP injection of ciguatoxin crude extracts may be attributable to the CTX1B concentration in the crude extract.

The pathology induced after administration of ciguatoxin in experimental animals can be summarized as follows: (1) acute poisoning by CTX1B or CTX4C causes damage to the heart, medulla of the adrenal glands, autonomic nerves, penis, and small and large intestines (Terao et al., 1992, 1995); (2) atropine suppresses symptoms of diarrhea but has no effect on injury to cardiac muscle; (3) reserpine aggravates the clinical symptoms and pathological findings; and (4) guanethidine and 5-hydroxy dopamine and bilateral adrenalectomy have no significant effects on ciguatoxicosis. Table 3.10 presents the LD_{50} of mouse toxicity for various known pure marine toxins studied. The decreasing order of toxicity in mouse is as follows:

$$MTX > PTX > CTX > TTX > PbTx > OA > PbTx\text{-}B$$

TABLE 3.10
Comparative Potency of Marine Natural Toxins in Mice

Reference Toxin	LD$_{50}$ IP in Mice (μg/kg)	Molecular Weight (g/mol)	Source
Ciguatoxin-1B	0.35	1111	*Gymnothorax javanicus* (moray eel)
Maitotoxin	0.050	3422	*Gambierdiscus toxicus* (dinoflagellate)
Palytoxin	0.15	2677	*Palythoa* (soft coral)
Okadaic acid	192.0	786	*Prococentrum lima*
Brevetoxin A	95.0	900	*Ptychodiscus brevis* (dinoflagellate)
Brevetoxin B	500.0	885	*Ptychodiscus brevis* (dinoflagellate)
Tetrodotoxin	8.0	319	Tetraodontidae family (bacterial species *Shewanella alga*)

Note: LD$_{50}$ = lethal dose producing 50% mortality when injected intraperitoneally (IP) in a 20-g mouse.

Summary

The findings of studies in mice models with pure marine toxins carried out by Terao et al. (Terao et al., 1991, 1992, 1994, 1995, 1996; Ito et al., 1996) probably reflect the pathology in humans, for whom studies are very limited. The major target organs affected in humans by marine toxins are the gastrointestinal tract, nervous system, and muscles, thus explaining the symptomology seen for ciguatera fish poisoning (Table 3.1).

THERAPY

Earlier Treatment

Treatment of ciguatera poisoning can be separated into two periods. In the first period, limited information was available with regard to the mode of action, chemistry of the toxins, and definite patterns of symptoms for ciguatera fish poisoning. A thesis by Chanfour (1988) described a treatment for ciguatera poisoning in French Polynesia which was quite similar to the therapy devised by Russell (1975). Essentially, treatment was based on the action of the drugs on the symptoms observed; thus, in humans, drips of atropine at 0.5 mg were administered every 4 hours in a continuous, multiple electrolyte solution (Russell, 1975). Atropine appeared to have an effect on the gastrointestinal and cardiovascular symptoms and signs; however, it had no significant effect on the skeletal muscle symptoms and showed only a slight improvement in the neurological findings following injection of atropine. Cyanotic and respiratory diseased patients were placed on oxygen. Patients were maintained on high electrolyte solutions and daily intravenous doses of calcium gluconate, a vitamin B complex, vitamin C, and time-release capsules that included phenobarbital, hyoscyamine sulfate, atropine sulfate, and hyoscine hydrobromide. Use of these drugs was an attempt to control the presumed pharmacological action of the fish poisoning toxins. These treatments were confined to patients seen within 48 hours of the fish poisoning (Russell, 1975). In cases seen 3 to 14 days after poisoning, the most severe complaints reported were sensory disturbances. Atropine had no effect on these patients; that is, no demonstrable improvements were seen. These patients did best with a high-protein diet and administration of intravenous vitamin B complex, calcium gluconate, and oral vitamin C. Extremes in temperature were avoided, as they caused recurrence of painful pruritus, paresthesia, and nausea (Russell, 1975). The use of pyridine-2-aldoxime methiodide (2-PAM) based on the anticholinesterase concept of ciguatoxin action could provide no improvement in a patient's condition, as was demonstrated in earlier reports (Okihiro et al., 1965).

In 1975, one of the best courses of treatment for ciguatoxin was recommended by Russell (1975): (1) atropine to control the gastrointestinal complaints and cardiovascular disturbances in the early phases of ciguatera poisoning; and (2) intravenous high electrolytes, calcium gluconate, and vitamin B complex, coupled with a high-protein diet and vitamin C, which appeared to give the most satisfactory results following the acute period and shortened the duration of illness. For pruritus, analgesic cream was used as steroid creams were of no value. For insomnia, diazepam (10 mg) was recommended because, again, steroids were ineffective.

Recent Treatment

Tocainide has been used with some success in three patients with long-term, chronic ciguatera, in which neurological symptoms seem to persist over several years (Lange et al., 1988). Amitriptyline was also given to these same patients prior to tocainide with no effect (Bowman, 1984). To date, no significant large-scale studies on the treatment of ciguatera fish poisoning with tocainide or amitriptyline have been reported, in part due to the fact that studies of chronic ciguatera poisoning are limited in the United States because of an insufficient patient population. A more recent preliminary study suggested the use of long-term antioxidant therapy for chronic ciguatera poisoning (Lange et al., 1994). Vitamin E has been shown to provide protection from various chemicals thought to initiate free-radical-induced injury by blocking the deleterious effect of free radicals in the cellular membrane (Lange et al., 1994). A suggested therapy for chronic ciguatera poisoning is vitamin E at 1000 IU/day for 1 week, followed by vitamin E at 2000 IU/day for 2 to 8 weeks, in addition to vitamin C at 500 mg/day and beta-carotene at 100 mg/day.

Amitriptyline (an antisuppressant drug) given at a low dose of 25 mg to an individual with ciguatera poisoning resulted in improvement and eventual recovery after several weeks (Bowman, 1984); however, amitriptyline was not shown to have a significant effect in studies carried out on the Marshall Islands (Palafox et al., 1988).

In the Western Pacific, traditional remedies prepared from numerous plants have been used as both oral treatments and topical applications for rashes, pruritus, and other skin ailments associated with ciguatera fish poisoning. Extracts of leaves, bark, roots, and fruits of various plants have been traditionally used for fish poisoning. Although some plant extracts alleviate some of the symptoms of ciguatera poisoning, none of the hundreds of plants examined has been specific for the treatment of ciguatera fish poisoning.

The most significant clinical discovery in the treatment of ciguatera fish poisoning occurred serendipitously, when two coma patients suspected of ciguatera fish poisoning in the Marshall Islands (Jaluit Atoll) were treated with mannitol for edema of the brain. A few minutes after intravenous infusion of mannitol, both patients remarkably awoke from their state of coma (Palafox et al., 1988). Subsequently, all patients with severe ciguatera fish poisoning have been routinely treated with intravenous infusion of mannitol at the Majuro Hospital in the Marshall Islands.

In the report by Palafox et al. (1988), 24 patients with acute ciguatera fish poisoning were treated with intravenous mannitol, and each patient's condition improved dramatically. All of the patients exhibited marked lessening of the neurological and muscular dysfunction within minutes of the mannitol infusion. Relief from gastrointestinal symptoms took longer. Two patients in coma and one in shock responded within minutes with full recovery after mannitol infusion. These observations were empirical and uncontrolled; nevertheless, later studies in Australia and the United States have verified and repeated the results reported by Palafox et al. (1988).

Mannitol is currently used in severe ciguatera poisoning in most emergency units located where ciguatera poisoning occurs (Hawaii, Florida, Puerto Rico, Australia). Mannitol treatment is most effective when given within the first 24 to 72 hours after exposure to ciguatera poisoning; after 4 weeks following intoxication, mannitol may be of no help (Blythe et al., 1992; Pearn et al., 1989; Palafox et al., 1988). The exact mode of mannitol action in acute ciguatera fish poisoning is not clear, but it may be attributable to its pharmacological actions. In addition to being a potent diuretic, mannitol can cause decreasing cellular edema, re-establishing ionic balance and decreasing plasma pH; also, mannitol is a scavenger of selected chemical structures, including hydroxyl group and free radicals (Huang and Huang, 1990). A major effect may be the interference or removal of bound ciguatoxin at the receptor sites of sodium channels of the nerve and muscle tissues (Hokama and Miyahara, 1994). Thus, mannitol is most effective during the initial period of acute ciguatoxin poisoning.

Summary

As can be seen by these recent approaches to treatment, nontoxic drugs that could have a protective effect on the sodium channel of the nerves and muscles would probably be the choice to alleviate the clinical symptoms associated with ciguatera fish poisoning.

ACKNOWLEDGMENT

The author wishes to thank Lisa Whang for her excellent work of word processing and editing of the chapter.

REFERENCES

Adachi, R. and Fukuyo, Y. (1979) The thecal structure of a marine toxic dinoflagellate *Gambierdiscus toxicus* gen. et sp. nov. collected in a ciguatera-endemic area, *Bull. Jpn. Soc. Sci. Fish*, 45: 67–71.

Allsop, J.L., Martini, L., Lebrus, H., Pollard, J., Walsh, J., and Hodgkin, S.M.S. (1986) Les manifestations neurologiques de la ciguatera, *Rev. Neurol.*, 142: 590.

Amade, P., Gonzalez, G., Rogeau, D., and Puel, D. (1990) Intoxication experimentale de *Serranus cabrilla* (Teleosteen, Serrinidae) par *Gambierdiscus toxicus* (dinoflagellate), *Bull. Soc. Zool. Fr.*, 115: 183.

Bagnis, R.A. (1968) Clinical aspects of ciguatera (fish poisoning) in French Polynesia *Haw. Med. J.*, 20: 25–28.

Bagnis, R.A. (1970) Concerning a fatal case of ciguatera poisoning in the Tuamotu Islands, *Clin. Toxicaol.*, 3: 579.

Bagnis, R.A. and LeGrand, A.M. (1987) Clinical features in 12,890 cases of ciguatera fish poisoning in French Polynesia, in *Progress in Venom and Toxin Research*, Gopolakrisnakove, P. and Tan, C.K., Eds., National University of Singapore, Singapore, p. 372.

Bagnis, R.A. and Rouanet, M. (1970) A propos dun cas mortulde ciguatera dans les ides Tuamo Fr., *Rev. Med. Vet.*, 121: 459.

Bagnis, R.A., Kuberski, T., and Langier, S. (1979) Clinical observations on 3009 cases of ciguatera (fish poisoning) in the South Pacific, *Am. J. Trop. Med. Hyg.*, 28: 1067.

Bagnis, R.A., Benett, J., Barsinas, M., Chebret, M., Jacquet, G., Lechat, I., Mitermite, Y., Perolat, P.H., and Rongeras, S. (1985a) Epidemiology of ciguatera in French Polynesia from 1964–1984, *Proc. 5th Int. Coral Reel Congress*, Tahiti, p. 475.

Bagnis, R.A., Chanteau, S., Chungue, E., Droillet, J.H., Lechat, I., LeGrand, A.M., Pompon, A., Prieur, C., Roux, U., and Tetaria, C. (1985b) Comparison of the cat bioassay, the mouse bioassay, and the mosquito bioassay to detect ciguatoxicity in fish, in *Proc. 5th Int. Coral Reef Congress*, Tahiti, p. 491.

Bagnis, R.A., Barsinas, M., Prieur, C., Pompon, A., Chungue, E., and LeGrand, A.M. (1987) The use of the mosquito bioassay for determining the toxicity to man of ciguateric fish, *Biol. Bull.*, 172: 137.

Banner, A.H. (1974) The biological origin and transmission of ciguatoxin, in *Bioactive Products from the Sea*, Hum, H.J. and Lance, C.E., Eds., Marcel Dekker, New York, pp. 15–36.

Banner, A.H., Scheuer, P.J., Sasaki, S., Helfrich, P., and Alender, C.B. (1960) Observations on ciguatera type toxin in fish, *Ann. N.Y. Acad. Sci.*, 90: 770–787.

Banner, A., Helfrich, H.P., and Piyakarnchana, T. (1966) Retention of ciguatera toxin by the red snapper *Lutjanus bohar*, *Copeia*, 2: 297.

Bieri, J.G., Corash, L., and Hubbard, U.S. (1993) Medical use of vitamin E, *New Engl. J. Med.*, 308: 1063.

Blythe, D.G., DeSylva, D.P., Fleming, L.E., Ayyar, R.A., Baden, D.G., and Shrank, K. (1992) Clinical experience with IV mannitol in the treatment of ciguatoxin, *Bull. Soc. Pathol. Exot.*, 85: 425.

Boisier, P., Ranaivoson, G., Rasolofonirina, N., Andriamahefazafy, B., Roux, J., Chantau, S., Satake, M., and Yasumoto, T. (1995) Fatal mass poisoning in Madagascar following ingestion of shark (*Carcharhimus leucas*): clinical and epidemiological aspects and isolation of toxins, *Toxicon*, 33: 1359.

Bourdeau, P. (1986) Epidemiologie de la ciguatera aux antilles: plateau de Saint-Barthemlemy, Saint-Martin et Anguilla, Etude in 1985 et 1986, *Rapport IFREMER-EVAN*, 84: 3303–3304.

Bowman, P.B. (1984) Amitriptyline, and ciguatera, *Med. J. Aust.*, 40: 802.

Brusle, I. (1997) *Ciguatera Fish Poisoning: A Review—Sanitary, and Economic Aspects*, INSERM, Paris.

Cameron, J., Flowers, A.E., and Capra, M.F. (1991a) Effects of ciguatoxin on nerve excitability in rats, Part I, *J. Neurol. Sci.*, 101: 87.

Cameron, J., Flowers, A.E., and Capra, M.F. (1991b) Electrophysiological studies on ciguatera poisoning in men, Part II, *J. Neurol. Sci.*, 101: 93.

Campbell, B., Nakagawa, K.M., Kobayashi, N., and Hokama, Y. (1987) *Gambierdiscus toxicus* in gut content of the surgeon fish *Ctenochaetus strigosus* (herbivore) and its relationship to toxicity, *Toxicon*, 25: 1125–1127.

Catterall, W.A. (1992) Molecular properties of the voltage-sensitive Na^+ channel: a receptor for multiple toxins, in *Proc. of the 4th Int. Conf. on Ciguatera Fish Poisoning*, Tahiti, p. 28.

Chanfour, B. (1988) Lintoxication Ciguaterique en Polynesie Francaise, Doctorat en Medicine Diplome DETAT, Universite Louis Pasteur, Strasbourg, France.

Cheng, K.K., Li, K.M., and Quinctillis, Y.H.M. (1969) The mechanism of respiratory failure in ciguatera poisoning, *J. Pathol.*, 97: 89.

Cook, J., Gurneaux, T., and Hodoes, W., Eds. (1977) *A Voyage Towards the South Pole and Around the World*, 3rd ed., W. Strahan and T. Cadell, London.

Danielson, M.T. and Danielson, B. (1985) The Mangaravea story: Greenpeace v. *Gambierdiscus*, *Pacific Isl. Monthly*, 1: 29–30.

Demotta, E., Feliu, G., and Izquierdo, A. (1996) Identification, and epidemiological analysis of ciguatera cases in Puerto Rico, *Marine Fish Rev.*, 48: 14.

Engleberg, N.C., Morris, J.G., Lewis, J., McMillan, J.P., Pollard, R.A., and Blake, P.A. (1983) Ciguatera fish poisoning: a major common-source outbreak in the U.S. Virgin Islands, *Ann. Int. Med.*, 98: 336–338.

Fuhrman, F.A. (1986) Tetrodotoxin, tarichatoxin, and chiriquitoxin: historical perspectives, *Ann. N. Y. Acad. Sci.*, 479: 1–14.

Fukuyo, Y., Takano, H., Chihara, M., and Matsuoka, K., Eds. (1990) *Red Tide Organisms in Japan: An Illustrated Taxonomic Guide*, Rokakuho, Japan, pp. 114–115.

Ganal, C.A., Asahina, A.Y., Hokama, Y., and Miyahara, J.T. (1993) Characterization of toxin(s) in *Myripristis* sp. by immunological, mouse toxicity, and guinea pig assays, *J. Clin. Lab. Anal.*, 7: 41.

Granade, H.R., Cheng, P.C., and Doorenbos, N.C. (1976) Ciguatera. 1. Brine shrimp (*Artemia salina L.*) larval assay for ciguatera toxins, *J. Pharmaceut. Sci.*, 65: 1414.

Habermehl, G.G., Krebs, H.C., Rasoanaivo, P., and Ramialihariso, A. (1994) Severe ciguatera poisoning in Madagascar: a case report, *Toxicon*, 32: 1539.

Halstead, B.W. (1988) *Poisonous and Venomous Marine Animals of the World*, 2nd ed., Darwin Press, Princeton, NJ, p. 1006.

Hashimoto, Y. (1979) Ciguatera, in *Marine Toxins, and Other Bioactive Marine Metabolites*, Konosu, S., Hashimoto, K., Onoue, Y., and Fusetani, N., Eds., Japan Scientific Societies Press, Tokyo, p. 91.

Helfrich, P. (1964) Fish poisoning in Hawaii, *Haw. Med. J.*, 22: 361–372.

Hessel, D.W. (1960) Marine biotoxins. 1. Ciguatera poison: some biological, and chemical aspects, *Ann. N.Y. Acad. Sci.*, 90: 788.

Hirama, M., Oishi, T., Vekara, H., Inuoe, M., Murayama, M., Oguri, H., and Satake, M. (2001) Total synthesis of ciguatoxin CTX3C, *Science*, 294: 1904–1907.

Hokama, Y. (1985a) A rapid simplified enzyme immunoassay stick test for the detection of ciguatoxin and related polyether from fish tissues, *Toxicon*, 23: 939.

Hokama, Y. (1985b) Immunological approaches to understanding marine toxins, in *Aquaculture*, 2nd ed., Kimble, C.E., Ed., Zarcon Press, Silver Springs, MD, p. 80.

Hokama, Y. (1990) Simplified solid-phase immunobead assay for detection of ciguatoxin, and related polyethers, *J. Clin. Lab. Anal.*, 4: 213.

Hokama, Y. and Miyahara, J.T. (1986) Ciguatera poisoning: clinical, and immunological aspects, *J. Toxicol. Toxin Rev.*, 5: 25.

Hokama, Y. and Miyahara, J.T. (1994) *In vitro* effect of 6-carbon monosaccharides on the sodium channel response to crude fish extracts containing ciguatoxin, *J. Natural Toxin*, 3: 35.

Hokama, Y. and Yoshikawa-Ebesu, J. (2001) Ciguatera fish poisoning: a foodbourne disease, *J. Toxicol. Toxin Rev.*, 20(2): 85–139.

Hokama, Y., Banner, A.H., and Boyland, D. (1977) A radioimmunoassay for the detection of ciguatoxin, *Toxicon*, 15: 317–325.

Hokama, Y., Kimura, L.H., Abad, M.A., Yokochi, L., Scheuer, P.J., Nukima, M., Yasumoto, T., Baden, D.G., and Shimizu, Y. (1984) *An* enzyme immunoassay for the detection of ciguatoxin and competitive inhibition by related natural polyether toxins, in *Seafood Toxin*, Ragelis, E.P., Ed., American Chemical Society, Washington, D.C., p. 307.

Hokama, Y., Osugi, A.M., Honda, S.A.A., and Matsuo, M.K. (1985) Monoclonal antibodies in the detection of ciguatoxin and other toxic polyethers in fish tissue by rapid poke stick tests, in *Proc. 5th Int. Coral Reef Cong.*, Antenne Museum-Ephe, Morea, French Polynesia, p. 449.

Hokama, Y., Honda, S.A.A., Kobayashi, M.N., Nakagawa, L.K., Kurihara, J., and Miyahara, J.T. (1987a) The similarity between cultured *Gambierdiscus toxicus* (T39) and fish extracts of *Ctenochaetus strigosus* (herbivore), in *Progress in Venom, and Toxin Research*, Gopatakrisnakone, P. and Tan, C.K., Eds., National University of Singapore, Kent Ridge, Singapore, p. 356.

Hokama, Y., Shirai, L.K., Iwamoto, L., Kobayashi, M.K., Goto, C.S., and Nakagawa, L.K. (1987b) Assessment of a rapid enzyme immunoassay stick test for the detection of ciguatoxin and related polyether toxins in fish tissues, *Biol. Bull.*, 172: 144.

Hokama, Y., Honda, S.A.A., Kobayashi, M.N., Nakagawa, L.K., Asahina, A.Y., and Miyahara, J.T. (1989) Monoclonal antibody (MAb) in detection of ciguatoxin (CTX) and related polyethers by the stick enzyme immunoassay (S-EIA) in fish tissues associated with ciguatera poisoning, in *Mycotoxins and Phycotoxins*, Natori, S., Hashimoto, K., and Ueno, Y., Eds., Elsevier, Amsterdam, p. 399.

Hokama, Y., Asahina, A.Y., Hong, T.W.P., Shang, E.S., and Miyahara, J.T. (1990) Evaluation of the stick enzyme immunoassay in *Caranx* sp. and *Seriola dumerili* associated with ciguatera, *J. Clin. Lab. Anal.*, 4: 363.

Hokama, Y., Hong, T.W.P., Isobe, M., Ichikawa, Y., and Yasumoto, T. (1992) Cross reactivity of highly purified okadaic acid (OA) synthetic spirochetal east sphere of OA and ciguatoxin, *J. Clin. Lab. Anal.*, 6: 54.

Hokama, Y., Asahina, A.Y., Shang, E.S., Hong, T.W.P., and Shirai, J.L.R. (1993) Evaluation of the Hawaiian reef fishes with solid-phase immunobead assay, *J. Clin. Lab. Analy.*, 7: 26.

Hokama, Y., Ebesu, J.S.M., Ascunsion, D.A., and Nagai, H. (1996a) Growth, and cyclic studies of *Gambierdiscus toxicus* in the natural environment and in culture, in *Harmful and Toxic Algal Blooms*, Yasumoto, T., Oshima, Y., and Fukuyo, Y., Eds., Intergovernmental Oceanographic Commission of UNESCO, Paris, p. 313.

Hokama, Y., Ebesu, J.S.M., Nishimura, K., Oishi, S., Mizuo, B., Stiles, M., Sakamoto, B., Takenaka, W., and Nagai, H. (1996b) Human intoxication from Hawaiian reef fishes associated with diverse marine toxins, *J. Nat. Toxin*, 5: 235.

Hokama, Y., Ebesu, J.S.M., Takenaka, W., Nishimura, K.L., Bourke, R., and Sullivan, P.K. (1998a) A simple membrane immunobead assay (MIA) for detection of ciguatoxin and related polyethers from ciguatera intoxication and natural reef fish, *J. AOAC Int.*, 88(4): 727–735.

Hokama, Y., Nishimura, K.L., Takenaka, W., and Ebesu, J.S.M. (1998b) Simplified solid-phase membrane immunobead assay (MIA) with monoclonal anti-ciguatoxin antibody (MAb-CTX) for detection of ciguatoxin, *J. Nat. Toxin*, 7: 1.

Huang, T.F. and Huang, L.L. (1990) Effect of mannitol, N-2-mercaptopropionyl glycerine, and sodium nitropriusside in EEG recovery following cerebral ischemia and reperfusion in rat, *Clin. J. Physiol.*, 33: 121.

Ichinotsubo, D., Asahina, A.Y., Titus, E., Chun, S., Hong, T.L.W.P., Shirai, J.L., and Hokama, Y. (1994) Survey of ciguatera fish poisoning in West Hawaii, *Mem. Queensl. Mus.*, 34: 513–522.

Ito, E., Yasumoto, T., and Terao, K. (1996) Morphological observations of diarrhea in mice caused by experimental ciguatoxicosis, *Toxicon*, 34: 111.

Kearney, J.F., Radbrush, A., Liesegang, B., and Rajewsky, K. (1978) A new marine myeloma cell line that has lost immunoglobulin expression but permits the construction of antibody-secreting hybrid cell lines, *J. Immunol.*, 123: 1548.

Kennet, R.H., McKearn, T.J., and Bechtol, K.B., Eds. (1980) *Monoclonal Antibodies*, Plenum Press, New York.

Khosravi, M.J. (1990) Shifting the "hook effect" in one-step immunometric assays, *Clin. Chem.*, 36: 169.

Kimura, L.H., Abad, M.A., and Hokama, Y. (1982a) Evaluation of the radioimmunoassay (RIA) for detection of ciguatoxin (CTX) in fish tissue, *J. Fish Biol.*, 21: 671.

Kimura, L.H., Hokama, Y., Abad, M.A., Oyama, M., and Miyahara, J.T. (1982b) Comparison of the different assays for the assessment of ciguatoxin in fish tissue: radioimmunoassay, mouse bioassay, and *in vitro* guinea pig atrium assay, *Toxicon*, 20: 907–912.

Kodama, A., Hokama, Y., Yasumoto, T., Fukui, M., Maneaand, S.J., and Sutherland, N. (1989) Clinical and laboratory findings implicating palytoxin as a cause of ciguatera poisoning due to *Decapterus mucrosoma* (mackerel), *Toxicon*, 27: 1051.

Kohler, G. and Milstein, C. (1975) Continuous cultures of fused cells secreting antibody of predefined specificity, *Nature*, 256: 494.

Kosaki T.I. and Anderson, H.H. (1968) Marine toxins from the Pacific. IV. Pharmacology of ciguatoxin(s), *Toxicon*, 6: 55.

Labrousse, H., Pauillac, S., Jehl-Martinez, E., LeGrand, A.M., and Avrameas, S. (1992) Techniques de detection de la ciguatoxine *in vivo* el *in vitro*, *Oceanis*, 18: 189.

Landsteiner, K., Ed. (1945) *The Specificity of Serological Reactions*, Harvard University Press, Cambridge, MA.

Lange, W.R., Kreider, S.D., Hattwick, M.M.D., and Hobbs, J. (1988) Potential benefit of tocainide in the treatment of ciguatera: report in three cases, *Am. J. Med.*, 84: 1087.

Lange, W.R., Lipkin, K.M., and Yang, G.C. (1989) Can ciguatera be a sexually transmitted disease?, *J. Toxicol. Clin. Toxicol.*, 27: 193.

Lange, W.R., Contoreggi, C.S., Herring, R.I., and Cardent, J.L. (1994) *Proc. of the Int. Symp. on Ciguatera and Marine Natural Products*, Asian Pacific Research Foundation, Honolulu, p. 273.

LeGrand, A.M., Galonnier, M., and Bagnis, R.A. (1982) Studies on the mode of ciguatera toxins, *Toxicon*, 20: 311.

LeGrand, A.M., Fukui, M., Cruchet, P., Ishibashi, Y., and Yasumoto, T. (1992) Characterization of ciguatoxins from different fish species and wild *Gambierdiscus toxicus*, in *Proc. of the 3rd Int. Conf. on Ciguatera Fish Poisoning*, Toteson, T.R., Ed., San Juan, PR, pp. 25–32.

Lewis, J.N., Caines, O., Christian, C.L.E., and Schneider, R. (1981) Ciguatera fish poisoning: St. Croix, Virgin Islands of the United States, *MMWR*, 30: 138.

Lewis, N.D. (1986) Epidemiology and impact of ciguatera in the Pacific: a review, *Mar. Fish. Rev.*, 48: 6.

Lewis, R.J., Sellin, M., Poll, M.A., Norton, R.S., Macleod, J.K., and Shell, M.M. (1991) Purification, and characterization of ciguatoxins from moray eel (*Lycodontis javanicus*, Muraenidae), *Toxicon*, 29: 1115.

Li, K.M. (1965a) A note on ciguatera fish poisoning and action of its proposed antidotes, *Haw. Med. J.*, 24: 358.

Li, K.M. (1965b) Ciguatera fish poison: a cholinesterase inhibitor, *Science*, 147: 1580.

Lin, Y.Y., Rish, M., Ray, S.M., Van Engen, D., Clardy, J., Golik, J., James, J.C., Lombert, A., Bidard, J.N., and Lazdunski, M. (1987a) Ciguatoxin and brevetoxins share a common receptor site on the neuronal voltage-dependent Na+ channel, *FEBS Lett.*, 219: 355.

Lin, Y.Y., Rish, M., Ray, S.M., Van Engen, D., Clardy, J., Golik, J., James, J.C., Nakanishi, K. (1987b) Isolation and structure of brevetoxin B from the "red tide" dinoflagellate *Ptychodiscus brevis* (*Gymnodinium breve*), *J. Am. Chem. Soc.*, 103: 6773–6775.

Lombert, A., Bidard, J.N., and Lazdunski, M. (1987) Ciguatoxin and brevetoxins share a common receptor site on the neuronal voltage-dependent Na+ channel, *FEBS Lett.*, 219: 355.

Manger, R., Leja, L.S., Lee, S.Y., Hungerford, J.M., Hokama, Y., Dickey, R.W., Granade, H.R., Lewis, R., Yasumoto, T., and Wekell, M.M. (1995) Detection of sodium channel toxins: directed cytotoxicity assays of purified ciguatoxins, brevetoxins, saxitoxins, and seafood extracts, *J. AOAC Int.*, 78: 521.

Miyahara, J.T., Oyama, M.M., and Hokama, Y. (1985) The mechanism of cardiotonic action of ciguatoxin, *5th Int. Coral Reef Cong.*, 4: 449.

Moore, R.E. and Scheuer, P.J. (1971) Palytoxin: a new marine toxin from coelenterate, *Science*, 172: 495.

Morgan, R.F., Hebel, J.R., and McCarter, R.J. (1990) *A Study Guide to Epidemiology and Biostatistics*, 3rd ed., Aspen Publications, Gaithersburg, MD.

Morris, J.G., Lewin, P., Hargrett, N.T., Smith, C.W., Blake, P.A., and Schneider, R. (1982) Ciguatera fish poisoning: epidemiology of the disease on St. Thomas, U.S. Virgin Islands, *Am. J. Trop. Med. Hyg.*, 31: 574.

Murakami, Y., Oshima, Y., and Yasumoto, T. (1982) Identification of okadaic acid as a toxic component of a marine dinoflagellate *Prorocentrum lima*, *Bull. Jpn. Soc. Fish.*, 48: 69–72.

Murata, M., LeGrand, A.M., Ishibashi, Y., Fukui, M., and Yasumoto, T. (1990) Structures, and configurations of ciguatoxin from the moray eel *Gymnothorax javanicus* and its likely precursor from the dinoflagellate *Gambierdiscus toxicus*, *J. Am. Chem. Soc.*, 112: 4380.

Nagai, H., Mikami, Y., Yazawa, K., Gonoi, T., and Yasumoto, T. (1993) Biological activities of novel polyether antifungals, gambieric acids A and B, from a marine dinoflagellate *Gambierdiscus toxicus*, *J. Antibiotics*, 46: 520.

Nagumo, Y., Oguri, H., Shindo, Y., Sasaki, S., Oishsi, T., Hirama, M., Tomioka, Y., Mizugaki, M., and Tsumuraya, T. (2001) Concise synthesis of ciguatoxin ABC-ring fragments and surface plasmon resonance study of the interaction of their BSA conjugates with monoclonal antibodies, *Bioorg. Med. Lett.*, 11: 2037–2040.

Nakanishi, K. (1981) Isolation, and structure of brevetoxin B from the "red tide" dinoflagellate *Ptychodiscus brevis (Gymnodinium breve), J. Am. Chem. Soc.*, 103: 6773

Noguchi, T., Hwang, D.F., Arakawa, O., Daigo, K., Sato, S., Ozaki, H., Kawai, N., Ito, M., and Hashimoto, K. (1987) Palytoxin as the causative agent in parrotfish poisoning, in *Progress in Venom and Toxin Research*, Gopalakrishnakone, P. and Tan, C.K., Eds., National University of Singapore, Kent Ridge, Singapore, p. 325.

Nukina, M., Koyanagi, I.M., and Scheuer, P.J. (1984) Two interchangeable forms of ciguatoxin, *Toxicon*, 22: 169–176.

Nukina, M., Tachibana, K., and Scheuer, P.J. (1986) Recent developments in ciguatera research, in *Natural Toxins: Animal, Plant, and Microbial*, Harris, J.B., Ed., Clarendon Press, Oxford, p. 46.

Ohizumi, Y., Shibata, S., and Tachibana, K. (1981) Mode of the excitatory and inhibiting actions of ciguatoxin in the guinea pig vas deferens, *J. Pharmacol. Exp. Ther.*, 217: 474.

Okihiro, M.M., Keenan, J.P., and Ivy, A.C., Jr. (1965) Ciguatera poisoning with cholinesterase inhibition, *Haw. Med. J.*, 24: 354.

Oshima, Y., Buckely, L.J., Alam, M., and Shimizu, Y. (1977) Heterogeneity of paralytic shellfish poisons: three new toxins from cultured *Gonyaulax tumerensis* cells, *Mya arenaria*, and *Saxidomus giganteus, Comp. Biochem. Physiol.*, 57: 31–34.

Palafox, N.A. and Buenconsejo-Lum, L.E. (2001) Ciguatera fish poisoning: review of clinical manifestation, *J. Toxicol. Toxin Rev.*, 20(2): 141–160.

Palafox, N.A., Jain, L., Pinano, A., Gulick, T., Williams, R., and Schatz, I. (1988) Successful treatment of ciguatera fish poisoning with intravenous mannitol, *JAMA*, 250: 2740.

Pauillac, S., Sasaki, M., Inuoe, M., Naar, J., Brahaa, P., Chinain, M., Tachibana, K., and LeGrande, A.M. (2000) Characterization of mice antisera elicited with a ciguatoxin tetracyclic synthetic ring fragment (JKLM) conjugated to carrier proteins, *Toxicon*, 38, 669–685.

Pearn, J.H. (1997) Chronic fatigue syndrome: chronic ciguatera poisoning as differential diagnosis, *Med. J. Austr.*, 166: 309–310.

Pearn, J.H., Lewis, R., Ruff, T., Tait, M., Quinn, J., and Gillespie, N. (1989) Ciguatera, and mannitol: experience with a new treatment regimen, *Med. J. Austr.*, 151: 77.

Perl, T.M., Bedard, L., Kosatsky, T., Hockin, J.C., Todd, E.C.D., and Remis, R.S. (1990) An outbreak of toxic encephalopathy caused by eating mussels contaminated with domoic acid, *New. Engl. J. Med.*, 322: 1775–1780.

Quod, J.P. (1992) Ciguatera in the Indian Ocean: an overview, in *Proc. of the 4th Int. Conf. on Ciguatera Fish Poisoning*, Tahiti, p. 37.

Racciatti, D., Vecchiet, J., Ceccomancini, A., Ricci, F., and Pizzigallo, E. (2001) Chronic fatigue syndrome following toxic exposure, *Sci. Total Environ.*, 270: 27–31.

Randall, J.E. (1958) A review of ciguatera tropical fish poisoning with a tentative exploration of its cause, *Bull. Mar. Sci. Gulf Carib.*, 8: 236–237.

Randall, J.E. (1980) A survey of ciguatera at Enewetak, and Bikini Marshall Islands, with notes on the systemic and food habits of ciguatoxic fishes, *Fish Bull. U.S.*, 78: 201.

Rayner, M.D. (1972) Mode of action of ciguatoxin, *Fed. Proc.*, 31: 1139.

Rigby, G. and Hallegraff, G.A. (1996) Ballast water controls to minimize translocation: what progress have we made and where are we going?, in *Harmful Toxic Algal Blooms*, Yasumoto, T., Oshima, Y., and Fubuyo, Y., Eds., Intergovernmental Oceanographic Commission of UNESCO, Paris, p. 201.

Russell, F.E. (1975) Ciguatera poisoning: a report of 35 cases, *Toxicon*, 13: 383–385.

Satake, M., Murata, M., and Yasumoto, T. (1993) The structure of CTX3C, a ciguatoxin congener isolated from cultured *Gambierdiscus toxicus, Tetrahedron Lett.*, 34: 1975.

Sasaki, M., Inoue, M., Murata, M., and Tachibana, K. (1995) Synthesis of a tetracyclic fragment of ciguatoxin toward preparation of an artificial antigen for ciguatoxin immunoassay, in *Proc. of the Int. Symp. on Ciguatera and Marine Natural Products*, Hokama, Y., Scheuer, P.J., and Yasumoto, T., Eds., Asian Pacific Research Foundation, Honolulu, p. 229.

Satake, M., Fukui, M., LeGrand, A.M., Cruchet, P., and Yasumoto, T. (1998) Isolation and structures of new ciguatoxin analogs, 2,3-dihydroxy CTX3C and 51-hydroxy CTX3C, accumulated in tropical reef fish, *Tetrahedron Lett.*, 39: 1197.

Scheuer, P.J., Takahashi, W., Tsutsumi, J., and Yoshida, T. (1967) Ciguatoxin: isolation and chemical nature, *Science*, 155: 1267–1268.

Schreier, M., Kohler, G., Heingartner, H., Berek, C., Trucco, M., and Forni, L. (1980) *Hybridoma Techniques*, Cold Spring Harbor Laboratory Press, Cold Spring Harbor, NY.

Shimizu, Y. (1982) Shellfish aquaculture and paralytic shellfish poisoning, in *Aquaculture: Public Health Regulatory and Management Aspects, Proc. of the 6th U.S. Food, and Drug Administration Science Symp. on Aquaculture*, Sea Grant College Program, Texas A&M University, College Station, pp. 38–46.

Shimizu, Y., Shimizu, H., Scheuer, P.J., Hokama, Y., Oyama, M., and Miyahara, J.J. (1982) *Gambierdiscus toxicus:* a ciguatera-causing dinoflagellate from Hawaii, *Bull. Jpn. Soc. Sci. Fish*, 48: 811–813.

SPC. (1990) *Coordination of SPC Work in Ciguatera*, SPC/WP29, South Pacific Commission, Canberra, Australia, p. 3.

Tachibana, K., Scheuer, P.J., Tsukitani, Y., Kikuchi, H., Van Engen, D., Clardy, J., Gopichand, Y., and Shimtz, F. (1981) Okadaic acid: a cytotoxic polyether from two marine sponges of the genus *Halichondria*, *J. Am. Chem. Soc.*, 103: 2469–2471.

Tachibana, K., Nukina, M., John, Y.G., and Scheuer, P.J. (1987) Recent developments in the molecular structure of ciguatoxin, *Biol. Bull.*, 172: 122.

Taylor, S.L., Hui, J.Y., and Lyons, D.E. (1984) Toxicology of scombroid poisoning, in *Seafood Toxins*, Ragelis, E.P., Ed., American Chemical Society, Washington, D.C., pp. 417–430.

Terao, K., Ito, E., Oarada, M., Ishibashi, Y., LeGrand, A.M., and Yasumoto, T. (1991) Light and electron microscopic studies of pathological changes induced in mice by ciguatoxin poisoning, *Toxicon*, 29: 633.

Terao, K., Ito, E., and Yasumoto, T. (1992) Light, and electron microscopic studies of the murine heart after repeated administrations of ciguatoxin or ciguatoxin-4C, *Nat. Toxins*, 1: 19.

Terao, K., Ito, E., Ohkusu, M., and Yasumoto, T. (1994) Pathological changes in murine hearts induced by intermittent administration of ciguatoxin to ICR mice (Charles River, Japan), *Mem. Queensl. Mus.*, 34: 621.

Terao, K., Ito, E., Ohkusu, M., and Yasumoto, T. (1995) Pathomorphological aspects of poisonings induced by marine toxins acting on the sodium channel in mice, in *Proc. of the Int. Symp. Ciguatera and Marine Natural Products*, Hokama, Y., Scheuer, P.J., and Yasumoto, T., Eds., Asian Pacific Research Foundation, Honolulu, p. 263.

Trainer, V.L., Baden, D.G., and Catterall, W.A. (1995) Detection of marine toxins using reconstituted sodium channels, *J. AOAC Int.*, 78: 570.

Usami, M., Satake, M., Ishida, M., Inoue, A., Kan, Y., and Yasumoto, T. (1995) Palytoxin analogs from the dinoflagellate *Ostreopsis siamensis*, *J. Am. Chem. Soc.*, 117: 5389.

Vernoux, J.P. and Lewis, R.J. (1997) Isolation, and characterization of Caribbean ciguatoxins from the horse-eye jack (*Caranx latus*), *Toxicon*, 35: 889.

Vijverberg, J.N., Frenlin, C., Chungue, E., LeGrand, A.M., Bagnis, R., and Lazocunski, M. (1984) Ciguatoxin is a novel type of Na+ channel toxin, *J. Biol. Chem.*, 259: 8353.

Yasumoto, T. and Murata, M. (1993) Marine toxins, *Chem. Rev.*, 93: 1897–1909.

Yasumoto, T., Bagnis, R., and Vernoux, J.P. (1976) Toxicity of surgeonfishes. II. Properties of the principle water-soluble toxin, *Bull. Jpn. Soc. Sci. Fish*, 42: 359–365.

Yasumoto, T., Nakajima, I., Bagnis, R., and Adachi, R. (1977) Finding of a dinoflagellate as a likely culprit of ciguatera, *Bull. Jpn. Soc. Sci. Fish.*, 43, 1977, 1021–1026.

Yasumoto, T., Inoue, A., and Bagnis, R. (1979) Ecological survey of a toxic dinoflagellate associated with ciguatera, in *Toxic Dinoflagellate Blooms*, Taylor, D. L. and Seliger, H. H., Eds., Elsevier, New York, p. 221.

Yasumoto, T., Fujimoto, K., Oshima, Y., Inoue, A., Ochi, T., Adachi, R., and Fukuyo, Y. (1980a) *Ecological Distributional Studies on a Toxic Dinoflagellate Responsible for Ciguatera*, a report to the Ministry of Education, Tokyo, Japan, p. 1.

Yasumoto, T., Oshima, Y., Murakami, Y., Nakajima, I., Bagnis, R., and Fukuyo, Y. (1980b) Toxicity of benthic dinoflagellates, *Bull. Jpn. Soc. Fish*, 46: 327–331.

Yasumoto, T., Yamamura, D., Ohizumi, Y., Takahashi, M., Alcala, A.C., and Alcala, L.C. (1983) Palytoxin in two species of Philippine crabs, in *Studies on Tropical Fish and Shellfish Infected by Dinoflagellates*, Yasumoto, T., Ed., Tohoku University, Japan, p. 45.

Yasumoto, T., Raj, U., and Bagnis, R. (1984) *Seafood Poisoning in Tropical Regions*, Faculty of Agriculture, Tohoku University, Japan, pp. 1–74.

Yasumoto, T., Seino, N., Murakami, Y., and Murata, M. (1987) Toxins produced by benthic dinoflagellates, *Biol. Bull.*, 172: 128–131.

Yasumoto, T., Fukui, M., Sasaki, K., and Sugiyama, K. (1995) Determinations of marine toxins in food, *J. AOAC Int.*, 78: 514.

Yotsu, M., Yamazaki, T., Meguro, Y., Endo, A., Murata, M., Naoki, H., and Yasumoto, T. (1987) Production of tetrodotoxin and its derivatives by *Pseudomonas* sp. isolated from the skin of pufferfish, *Toxicon*, 25: 225–228.

4 Hepatitis A: Sources in Food and Risk for Health

Michele Quarto and Maria Chironna

CONTENTS

Abstract   Hepatitis A is the prevalent form of acute viral hepatitis, which represents an important public health problem in many countries. Hepatitis A virus (HAV) is resistant in the environment, and the infection is mainly transmitted by the fecal–oral route, either through contaminated food and water or through direct contact with an infected person. HAV is present worldwide, although the risk of transmission depends upon the socioeconomic conditions of populations. In much of the developing world, HAV infection is hyperendemic, and the majority of persons are infected in early childhood. Outbreaks are rare because most infections occur among young children who generally remain asymptomatic. In such countries, hepatitis A does not represent a significant healthcare problem. In many developed countries, the progressive improvement of hygienic conditions and environmental sanitation has led to a much-reduced risk of acquiring the infection during infancy, when most cases are asymptomatic. The creation of large cohorts of susceptibles allows the occurrence of epidemics, sometimes with a large number of subjects involved, including adults in whom the infection is almost always clinically overt and may be particularly serious. The role of HAV as a cause of foodborne disease is widely recognized, and it is likely to appear among the most frequent causes of viral foodborne diseases. Outbreaks of hepatitis A occur periodically throughout the world, and fecally contaminated water and food are the main vehicles. The main food type associated with recent hepatitis A outbreaks is molluscan shellfish. Nevertheless, current regulations regarding the commercialization of shellfish are unable to guarantee the protection of consumers, as sanitary controls for bivalve shellfish rely on microbiological criteria to define the suitability of these products, and no specific microbiological criteria concerning the presence of enteric virus have been established. Depuration is the current method used to obtain marketable shellfish. This method is inadequate for complete virus elimination, even if performed with advanced systems; therefore, the problem of sanitary control of shellfish commercialized for human consumption remains an important issue.

Contamination of food by infected foodhandlers is probably the most common cause of viral foodborne illness. Food items such as salads and desserts that receive considerable handling during preparation are often implicated in foodborne outbreaks. Many reports confirm the role of foodhandlers in spreading foodborne diseases and underline the need for appropriate training in safe food-handling practices.

The strategy to control hepatitis A varies in different areas and population groups. Among the measures, improving sanitation and hygienic standards is the primary and permanent goal. In addition, the HAV vaccine represents the most promising measure to control the disease. A suitable knowledge of the size and epidemiologic characteristics of the disease should be the first step in developing an appropriate strategy.

Because there are several steps at which the food can be contaminated, a hazard analysis and critical-control points (HACCP) program or other systematic quality-control programs are needed to prevent HAV contamination. Food safety is one of the World Health Organization's top eleven priorities, and the member states have adopted a strongly worded resolution that recognizes food safety as an essential public health function.

INTRODUCTION

Acute viral hepatitis is one of the most prevalent infectious diseases in the world. Hepatitis A virus (HAV) is responsible for the most common form of acute viral hepatitis, which represents a significant public health problem in many countries. The disease was previously referred to as "infectious hepatitis" because it was known that the infection was orally transmitted, contrary to the other type of hepatitis, which is transmitted by blood and therefore is referred to as "serum hepatitis." Under the impression that there were only two forms of hepatitis, it seemed logical at the time to label them with the first letters of the alphabet: A and B.

It has been stressed that the morbidity of hepatitis A is often underestimated. Because it does not cause chronic infection, a common misperception regarding hepatitis A is that it is not a serious disease (Van Damme and Bell, 2001). In fact, hepatitis A is a cause of substantial morbidity, with approximately 1.4 million cases reported worldwide each year, but this figure is regarded as an underestimate, with the true incidence being three to ten times higher. Although a viral etiology for this disease was already predicted in 1908 and was confirmed to be different from hepatitis B during World War II, HAV was identified by immune electron microscopy for the first time in 1973 (Feinstone et al., 1973).

Hepatitis A virus, lacking a lipid envelope, is resistant to the action of chemical and physical agents in the environment, and the infection is primarily transmitted by the fecal–oral route, either through contaminated food and water or through direct contact with an infected person. HAV is present worldwide, although the risk of transmission depends upon the socioeconomic conditions of populations. In the past, poor environmental and sanitary conditions made contact with fecal-infected material extremely frequent and most children were infected with HAV, although the disease was clinically evident only in a few cases. In many developed countries, the progressive improvement of hygienic conditions and environmental sanitation has led to a much-reduced risk of acquiring the infection during infancy, when most cases are asymptomatic. The creation of large cohorts of susceptibles allows the occurrence of epidemics, sometimes with a large number of subjects involved, including adults, in whom the infection is almost always clinically overt and may be particularly serious. The change in epidemiological features of HAV infection depends on modes of transmission.

Until very recently, in countries with high social and healthcare standards, hepatitis A was seen as an infection typical of tourists traveling to highly endemic areas (Franco and Vitiello, 2003), even though several outbreaks of hepatitis A occur periodically throughout the world, and fecally contaminated foods are the main vehicle.

In the United States, 25,000 to 30,000 cases are reported each year, of which approximately 12 to 25% can be attributed to household or sexual contact with a case (Koopmans et al., 2002). Other identified potential sources of HAV infection include an association with childcare centers (11 to 16%) and international travel (4 to 6%). Although several water- and foodborne outbreaks of hepatitis A have been described in the United States, surveillance data suggest that water- or food-borne outbreaks account for less than 5% of reported cases of the disease (Mead et al., 1999); however, approximately 50% of reported cases do not have a recognized source of infection (Koopmans et al., 2002). Some of these cases may be caused by the ingestion of contaminated food, but small clusters of foodborne disease are unlikely to be recognized with current methods of investigation (Hutin et al., 1999). In addition, the hepatitis A outbreaks are less frequently reported than foodborne outbreaks with other clinical presentations, particularly gastroenteritis (Lees, 2000).

It is also notable that many of the reported hepatitis A outbreaks involve large numbers of cases. The fairly protracted incubation period of HAV infection (mean duration, 4 weeks) makes association with a particular food vehicle in individual or sporadic cases very difficult; normally, the food is not available for testing at the time of diagnosis, and consumption histories are inconclusive (Lees, 2000). Moreover, substantial costs are incurred by both society and the food industry as a result of foodborne outbreaks of hepatitis A in the United States (Dalton et al., 1996).

In Europe, in a "dining out" society, the preference for exotic and fast food has increased the exposure to a far wider range of food (Van Damme and Bell, 2001).

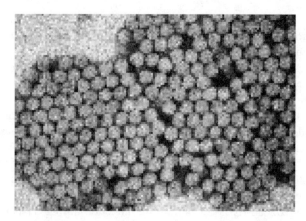

FIGURE 4.1 Electron microscopy picture of hepatitis A virus. (Courtesy of the Centers for Disease Control and Prevention, Atlanta, GA.)

Currently, HAV is often spread through contaminated food coming from highly endemic countries, where the food might not have been prepared and/or controlled according to the provisions of European legislation (Franco and Vitiello, 2003).

As a consequence of globalization, multistate and transnational foodborne outbreaks of hepatitis A are being reported with increasing frequency (Rosenblum et al., 1990; Desenclos et al., 1991; Niu et al., 1992; Hutin et al., 1999; Sànchez et al., 2002). Foodborne diseases are among the most widespread health problems in the world and have implications on both the health of individuals and the development of societies (Schlundt, 2002). Many countries now realize that foodborne disease continues to be a major public health issue. Today, food safety is an essential public health function and is one of the World Health Organization's top 11 priorities (WHO, 2000). WHO has called for more systematic and aggressive steps to be taken to significantly reduce the risk of microbiological foodborne diseases.

HEPATITIS A VIRUS

Hepatitis A is one of the smallest and structurally simplest of the RNA animal viruses. The virion is small, 27 to 32 nm in diameter, and is classified within the picornavirus family (Lemon and Robertson, 1993). It is spherical with a protein shell that encapsulates a single-stranded RNA of approximately 7500 bases. The structure is icosohedral, and HAV particles are indistinguishable from other picornaviruses (Figure 4.1). HAV was originally thought to be an enterovirus but, because of several differences from enteroviruses, it has been assigned to a separate genus, that of *Hepatovirus* (Minor, 1991). The viral proteins (VPs) are conformational (i.e., individual capsid proteins have to be assembled for the expression of significant antigenic activity) and therefore do not raise antibodies; on the other hand, the intact viral particle is very immunogenic.

The hepatitis A genome (Figure 4.2) consists of a linear, single-stranded, positive sense RNA and is organized to include a relatively lengthy 5′ non-translated

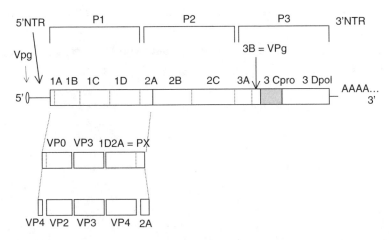

FIGURE 4.2 Organization of the HAV genome. (Adapted from Lemon, S.M., in *Viral Hepatitis and Liver Disease*, Rizzetto, M. et al., Eds., Minerva Medica, Turin, 1997, pp. 559–561.)

RNA segment (5′NTR) followed by a single, long, open reading frame encoding a polyprotein of about 2200 amino acids, as well as a short non-translated RNA segment (Najarian et al., 1985; Cohen et al., 1987). The 5′ terminus of the positive-stranded RNA genome is covalently linked to a small viral protein, VPg (Weitz et al., 1986), while the 3′ end terminates in a poly-A segment.

The polyprotein of HAV undergoes multiple proteolytic cleavages under direction of a virally encoded protease (3C^{pro}) (Schultheiss et al., 1994) and is generally considered to be organized into three functionally separate domains. The primary cleavage of the HAV polyprotein appears to occur at the junction of 2A and 2B. The P1 domain is located at the amino end of the polyprotein and includes the major capsid polypeptides, VP2, VP3, and VP1. A fourth, very small polypeptide, VP4, is located at the extreme amino terminus of the polyprotein; it may also be present within the HAV capsid, but this has never been demonstrated (Lemon and Robertson, 1993). Early capsid assembly intermediates also appear to contain an incompletely processed VP1 capsid polypeptide precursor with a carboxy terminal (the so-called PX protein) (Anderson and Ross, 1990). The 2A protein originates from PX cleavage.

The P2 and P3 segments of the polyprotein are comprised of at least six proteins involved in the synthesis of new viral RNAs. These include the 2B and 2C (helicase) proteins, as well as 3A, 3B (VPg), 3C^{pro} (which is also the viral protease), and 3D^{pol} (an RNA-dependent RNA polymerase).

After entry into the host cell, the virus loses the capsid, and the uncoated RNA induces the host cell to produce the viral polyprotein without shutting off protein synthesis of the cell. Slow growth, accompanied by low viral yields, absence of cytopathic effects, and rapid establishment of persistent and non-lytic infection, has characterized the propagation of HAV in cell lines originating from non-human primates or human beings. Attenuated HAV strains adapted to cell culture have been used to develop vaccines.

TABLE 4.1

Classification of HAV Genotypes and Subgenotypes, Source, and Country of Recovery

Genotype	Subgenotype	Representative Strain	Source	Location
I	IA	GA90	Human	United States
	IB	HM-175	Human	Australia
II	—	CF-53	Human	France
III	IIIA	H-141	Human	Sweden
	IIIB	A-229	Human	Japan
IV	—	Cy 145	Monkey	Philippines
V	—	AGM27	Monkey	Kenya
VI	—	JM55	Monkey	Indonesia
VII	—	SLF88	Human	Sierra Leone

Because HAV has no lipid envelope, it is stable and is not inactivated in the gastrointestinal tract. In addition, it has been found to survive in experimentally contaminated freshwater, seawater, wastewater, soils, marine sediments, shellfish, and food. It is resistant to thermal denaturation, acid treatment, and detergent inactivation; when stored at −20°C, it is resistant for years. HAV is inactivated only by heating to 85°C for a few minutes, after sterilization (121°C for 20 minutes), or by ultraviolet and other chemical treatments (e.g., iodine, chlorine-containing compounds) at particular concentrations. It should be emphasized that shellfish from contaminated areas should be heated to 90°C for at least 4 minutes or steamed for 90 seconds to inactivate the virus.

GENOTYPIC CLASSIFICATION AND MOLECULAR EPIDEMIOLOGY OF HEPATIS A VIRUS

All strains of HAV, irrespective of their genotype, have a single, conserved, immunodominant epitope that is responsible for generating neutralizing antibodies; however, a comparison of sequences of the capsid regions of strains from different sources has revealed that selected regions of the capsid vary between groups of viruses (Robertson and Nainan, 1997).

The most variable regions include the VP3 C terminus, the VP1 amino terminus, and the VP1/P2A junction. In particular, the putative VP1/P2A junction contains more informative variable positions between strains. Studies on the nucleic acid heterogeneity of HAV isolates and, in particular, of the VP1/2A junction have allowed the characterization of strains and grouping into various genotypes (I to VII; see Table 4.1) and subgenotypes (IA, IB, IIIA, and IIIB) (Nainan et al., 1991; Robertson et al., 1992). Genotypes distinguish from 15 to 25% sequence diversity whereas subgenotypes, within each genotype, differ in about 7.5% of base positions. Viruses from four of the genotypes (I, II, III, and VII) were recovered from cases of hepatitis A in humans, whereas viruses from the other three genotypes (IV, V, and VI) were isolated from simian species (Robertson et al., 1992). Genotype I includes about 80% of the human strains and is the most widespread. It is particularly prevalent in North and South America, Japan, North Africa, Australia, and Europe. In addition, subgenotype IA includes the majority of human isolates.

Most of the remaining human HAV strains segregate into a single genotype that can also be divided into two subgenotypes, IIIA and IIIB. Human genotypes II and VII are quite rare, while genotypes IV (isolate Cy145), V (isolate AGM27), and VI (isolate JM55) are each represented by a unique virus strain recovered from monkey species, as reported by Robertson et al. (1992).

The ability to characterize HAV strains during epidemic or endemic periods offers the potential to clarify some important aspects of HAV infection and transmission at a molecular level. Recently, new insights into the molecular epidemiology of HAV have been provided throughout the world.

Analysis of HAV sequences of clinical and environmental wild-type isolates from South Africa showed the presence of solely genotype I with the majority of strains (>80%) clustering within subgenotype IB (Taylor, 1997). In contrast, the most prevalent subgenotype within North America is IA (Robertson et al., 1992, 2000; Hutin et al., 1999). In addition, a limited number of isolates circulate in this area, even during outbreaks, suggesting that these strains probably represent circulating endogenous strains. Also, the genetic relatedness of Cuban HAV wild-type isolates showed the presence of only subgenotype IA and a new subgenotype IA variant (Diaz et al., 2001).

Latest data from South America reported the circulation of a single subgenotype (IA) in Argentina, although it has a high genetic diversity, whereas in Rio de Janeiro, Brazil, the concomitant circulation of isolates from subgenotypes IA and IB, with a wide prevalence of IB, are observed (Mbayed et al., 2002; de Paula et al., 2002). Data from China show that epidemic or sporadic strains may belong to HAV genotype IA or IB (Chen et al., 2001), while findings from Korea show about 95% identity, clustering within genotype IA (Byun et al., 2001).

The molecular characterization of HAV strains from Western Europe seems to confirm the wide difference among genotypes due to little endemic transmission of HAV in this geographical region (Bruisten et al., 2001; Costa-Mattioli et al., 2002; Chironna et al., 2003b). Also, the presence of a IIIA subgenotype in a Mediterranean country has been reported for the first time (Costa-Mattioli et al., 2001). An extensive heterogeneity of HAV strains was evident among strains recovered from patients with acute viral hepatitis and from environments in Spain (Pina et al., 2001). Sequence analysis of strains from France showed the contemporary presence of various subgenotypes (Apaire-Marchais et al., 1995). Moreover, a new HAV genotype IB variant has been recently characterized in Italy (Chironna et al., 2004).

The peculiarity of HAV epidemiology in Western Europe, particularly Spain, Italy, and France, and the role of raw seafood as a main risk factor for hepatitis A cases seem to support the hypothesis that shellfish could be a reservoir of various HAV genotypes circulating in a limited period. Such an assumption has been hypothesized by Costa-Mattioli et al. (2001), who analyzed the molecular characteristics of the strains isolated during an outbreak that occurred in North Bretagne,

France, due to the consumption of raw shellfish; the co-circulation of IA and IB subgenotypes and the presence of IIIA subgenotype were observed among cases. The heterogeneity of strains isolated from shellfish has been further confirmed by other authors (Romalde et al., 2001; Sanchez et al., 2002; Bosh et al., 2001). More wide-ranging studies on such a vehicle of infection (e.g., sequence analysis) could help to clarify this issue.

Currently, data available on HAV genotypes from environmental samples, although scarce (Morace et al., 2002; Pina et al., 2001), also show the circulation of different genotypes. Based on data from the latest studies, a higher degree of heterogeneity than expected in different areas of the world is being hypothesized. Further studies would help to better define the molecular epidemiology of HAV.

The molecular characterization of HAV has become an important tool during outbreak investigation to identify the sources of infections and to complement the classical epidemiological methods. Recently, different outbreaks of hepatitis A have been investigated by molecular techniques and additional sequencing (De Serres et al., 1999; Hutin et al., 1999; Arauz-Ruiz et al., 2001; Dentiger et al., 2001; Sànchez et al., 2002; Stene-Johansen et al., 2002; Chironna et al., 2004), which has helped to clarify some important epidemiological features of HAV infection.

NATURAL HISTORY AND CLINICAL PICTURE

Viral hepatitis A is a systemic infection in which the liver is the major target organ. Over 95% of HAV infections are transmitted by the fecal–oral route. The precise oral infective dose of HAV in human beings is not well defined. After oral inoculation, HAV is thought to be transported across the intestinal epithelium by a vectorial transport process and is taken up by hepatocytes. The liver is the only target organ of injury, and HAV genomic replication occurs exclusively in the cytoplasm of the infected hepatocytes by a mechanism involving an RNA-dependent RNA polymerase. From the liver, HAV is transported through the biliary tree to the intestine. Its resistance to inactivation by bile and intestinal proteolytic enzymes allows it to be shed in the feces and facilitates fecal–oral transmission. The disease is expressed in two major forms, symptomatic and asymptomatic, representing a broad spectrum of infection. The likelihood of showing symptoms associated with HAV infection is related to the age of the patient. Most infections in children less than 6 years old are asymptomatic, whereas those in older children and adults are usually symptomatic, with jaundice occurring in more than 70% of patients. Asymptomatic infection can be classified into two categories: subclinical and unapparent. In subclinical infections, only the biochemical features of hepatitis can be detected; unapparent infection can be identified only by serological studies. The acute illness can be divided into four phases: (1) incubation period, (2) prodromal symptoms, (3) acute hepatitis, and (4) protracted hepatitis (Table 4.2).

The incubation period lasts about 15 to 50 days (mean, 30 days). HAV is already present in feces, bile fluid, blood, and liver from the late incubation period. Also, immunoglobulin M (IgM) anti-HAV antibodies may already be detectable. In most people, IgM anti-HAV, which is the main serological marker for diagnosis, becomes

TABLE 4.2
Clinical Phases of Hepatitis A

Phase	Duration	Symptoms	Laboratory Features
Incubation	15 to 50 days (mean, 30 days)	None	HAV–IgM positive; HAV in feces
Prodromal symptoms	1 to 2 weeks	Lack of appetite, nausea, vomiting, aching joints	IgM positive and IgG positive; HAV in feces
Acute hepatitis	3 months	Jaundice, dark urine, pale stools	High levels of serum ALT, AST, γGT, and bilirubin; HAV–IgM and HAV–IgG positive; HAV in feces
Protracted hepatitis	6 months	Persisting jaundice, dark urine, pale stools	Persisting high levels of ALT and AST; HAV replicating and shedding in feces

Note: ALT = alanine aminotransferase; AST = aspartate aminotransferase; γGT = gamma-glutamyl transferase; HAV = hepatitis A virus; IgG = immunoglobulin G; IgM = immunoglobulin M.

detectable 5 to 10 days after exposure and can persist for up 6 months after infection. Although IgG anti-HAV also begins to appear early in infection, it is always accompanied by IgM after acute HAV infection and reflects recovery and lifelong protection against reinfection. Obviously, the still healthy-feeling patients are very contagious in this phase of the disease. The prodromal symptoms of acute viral hepatitis usually last 1 to 2 weeks and include, for example, lack of appetite, nausea and vomiting, tiredness, aching joints and muscles, headache, sore throat, coughing, and subfebrile temperature. Especially in young children, the clinical course of the disease may be restricted to these symptoms or give no symptoms at all. Prodromal symptoms tend to abate with the onset of jaundice, although the anorexia, malaise, and weakness may persist or increase transiently. The specific signs of clinical overt acute hepatitis are dark urine and pale stools, which precede jaundice for some days. The most prominent biochemical feature during symptomatic HAV infection is the very high concentrations of serum aminotransferases, which may reach a maximum of 500 to 5000 U/L. In those patients who develop jaundice, serum bilirubin concentrations are rarely higher than 171 µmol/L, except in acute liver failure and cholestatic hepatitis A. The total duration of symptomatic disease usually is about 3 months, sometimes 6 months. After the acute illness, a state of persistent immunity remains, probably lifelong, regardless of the former clinical course of acute disease. Protracted hepatitis A may last for 6 months, during which period the viral antigens and HAV RNA are detected in blood, stool samples, or liver biopsies (Yotsuyanagi et al., 1996).

Several unusual clinical manifestations of hepatitis A are worth noting, including relapsing hepatitis, cholestatic hepatitis, and fulminant and subfulminant hepatitis. Relapsing hepatitis is characterized by a second appearance of signs and symptoms, usually 2 to 3 months after the initial presentation. It has been reported in 3 to 20%

of children. Patients with this clinical form of infection may be host to replicating virus, and shedding of HAV may be detectable (Ciocca, 2000). Despite the protracted course characteristic of this variant, the prognosis is excellent for complete recovery. Cholestatic hepatitis is characterized by persistent jaundice, intense pruritus, and biochemical evidence of intrahepatic cholestasis. Despite their long-lasting jaundice, such patients typically feel quite well and the prognosis is good. Fulminant hepatitis is defined as the consequence of severe liver injury complicated by the development of hepatic encephalopathy within 8 weeks of the onset of the jaundice.

In the subfulminant form, encephalopathy occurs after 8 weeks but before 6 months after the onset symptoms. Characteristics include the presence of anorexia, hepatic encephalopathy, increasing jaundice, and decreasing liver function. The presence of complications (e.g., bacterial or fungal infection, renal failure, pulmonary failure, and other electrolytic complications) worsens the prognosis. Fulminant hepatitis resulting from acute hepatitis A is relatively rare, occurring in about 0.008% of cases. The frequency of fulminant hepatitis A is strongly age dependent and is an increasing problem in Western countries. Increased risk for fulminant hepatitis was described in patients with chronic hepatitis C, regardless of whether they had liver cirrhosis (Vento et al., 1998). An autoimmune phenomenon is probably involved here. In general, acute hepatitis A superinfection on top of severe chronic liver disease of another origin may be fatal. The case fatality rate of fulminant hepatitis is about 80% and has changed little even with modern management in intensive-care units.

EPIDEMIOLOGY

Worldwide, different patterns of the endemicity of HAV infection can be identified, each characterized by distinct prevalence rates of anti-HAV antibodies and hepatitis A incidence and associated with different levels of prevailing environmental (sanitary and hygienic) and socioeconomic conditions (Koopmans et al., 2002). The global pattern of hepatitis A virus transmission can be represented by four different levels of endemicity: high, moderate, low, and very low (Table 4.3). In much of the developing world, HAV infection is hyperendemic, and the majority of persons are infected in early childhood; virtually all adults are immune. In these areas, HAV transmission is primarily from person to person. Outbreaks are rare because most infections occur among young children, who generally remain asymptomatic. In such countries, hepatitis A does not represent a primary health care problem at the present time. Paradoxically, as socioeconomic and environmental conditions improve and HAV infection decreases in endemicity, the overall incidence and average age of reported cases often increase because older individuals are susceptible and develop symptoms with infection.

In the United States, about 33% of the population has serological evidence of previous HAV infection (Koff, 1998), and approximately 50% of clinically apparent acute viral hepatitis has been attributable to hepatitis A (Alter et al., 1997). Approximately 25,000 to 83,000 cases of hepatitis A are reported each year (Mead et al., 1999; Koopmans et al., 2002), and costs associated with the disease were recently calculated to be $332 million to $580 million annually in the United States (Berge et al., 2000). Currently, outbreaks across a community are thought to be the main

TABLE 4.3
Patterns of Hepatitis A Virus Transmission in the World

Endemicity Level	Disease Rate	Peak Age of Infection	Transmission Patterns
High	Low to high	Early childhood	Person to person; outbreaks uncommon
Intermediate	High	Late childhood/ young adults	Person to person; food and waterborne outbreaks
Low	Low	Young adults	Person to person; food and waterborne outbreaks
Very low	Very low	Adults	Travelers; outbreaks uncommon

source of HAV infection, affecting schoolchildren, adolescents, and young adults (Koff, 1998). Large families, household crowding, poor education, inadequate human-waste disposal systems, and mixing with other children in daycare centers are all factors linked to HAV endemicity and outbreaks (Redlinger et al., 1997). Occasionally, widespread foodborne outbreaks are associated with uncooked or fresh food contaminated before distribution, including shellfish, lettuce, and frozen raspberries and strawberries (Cuthbert, 2001).

Canada continues to record over 1000 hepatitis A case reports annually, although the true number is much larger due to underreporting and nonrecognition of milder cases, especially among young children (Wu et al., 2001). In the past, Latin America was considered to be an area of high endemicity for HAV infection, with most people being infected in early childhood. Several serological studies were recently undertaken to determine whether this pattern has changed. In Mexico, Argentina, and Brazil, anti-HAV seroprevalence was significantly higher in low socioeconomic groups than in middle and high socioeconomic groups. These results indicate a shift from high to medium endemicity of HAV infection throughout Latin America, which may result in more clinical cases in adolescents and adults and a greater potential of outbreaks (Tanaka, 2000).

A review of the epidemiology of HAV infection over the last 20 years shows shifting patterns in the prevalence of anti-HAV antibodies throughout Southeast Asia and China. A number of countries have shifted from high to moderate and from moderate to low endemicity, with a corresponding increase in the age of exposure from childhood to early adulthood. The changes have resulted from improvements in hygiene, sanitation, and the quality of drinking water, reflecting improvements in living standards and socioeconomic progress. As noted earlier, exposure to HAV at a later age may be associated with an increase in hepatitis A morbidity and a greater propensity for outbreaks (Barzaga, 2000).

Data on the endemicity level of HAV infection in Africa and the Middle East are scant, but most of Africa appears to remain a high endemicity region, with the exception of subpopulations in some areas, such as Caucasians in South Africa. Saudi Arabia is a model for the Middle East, and it is a country in which shifting HAV epidemiology has been documented in recent years, concurrent with the social and economic development that has occurred over the last two decades. Here, again, the seroprevalence for anti-HAV is related to socioeconomic status, being highest in the lowest groups. Similar findings have been reported from other countries in the Middle East. The existence of pockets of high endemicity for HAV infection with surrounding areas shifting toward intermediate endemicity may lead to outbreaks (Tufenkeji, 2000).

Data from the World Health Organization indicate, in general, a decline of hepatitis A in Eastern European countries. The countries can be divided into two groups on the basis of the morbidity data. One group consists of countries that have been intermediate endemicity areas for many years, whereas the second group is comprised of Lithuania, Latvia, Russia, and Romania, which are in a period of transition toward intermediate endemicity. The shift from high to intermediate endemicity in these countries has led to a lower level of HAV circulation in the population, to fewer cases of hepatitis A in children, and to fewer people becoming immune in childhood. An increased potential risk for HAV infection in adults can then be expected, with the possibility of large outbreaks (Cianciara, 2000).

Over the last several decades, the morbidity of hepatitis A in northern Europe has been low (Nordenfelt, 1997). The incidence of the disease in Nordic countries is low, the mean incidence varying between the lowest in Finland (1.8 cases per 100,000 inhabitants) and the highest in Denmark and Sweden (3.8 cases per 100,000). Iceland and Norway have had a mean incidence of 2.5 and 3.4, respectively. In Ireland, England, and Germany, the reported incidence is slightly higher. This continuous decline of the incidence of hepatitis A has also been confirmed by serologic study. The explanation for this decline, again, is the improved socioeconomic conditions, which have allowed better housing accompanied by less crowded living, improved sewage systems, and easy access to running water, all of which can contribute to better standards of hygiene.

Even in low endemicity areas such as northern Europe, however, community-wide outbreaks continue to occur, and an important risk group for HAV infection is travelers who have visited hyperendemic areas. In areas of very low endemicity, such as Scandinavia, international travel accounts for the majority of reported cases. In Sweden, up to 60% of the registered cases have been associated with travel to high-risk areas (Nordenfelt, 1992). Up to 30 years ago, hepatitis A was widely spread in Mediterranean Europe, with a gradient of increasing endemicity from northern to southern countries. At this time, epidemiological conditions in southern Europe vary from country to country (and even from region to region within the same country), depending on the degree of social and healthcare system development. In fact, countries in this area can have a high, moderate, or low degree of endemicity for HAV infection. Turkey and the countries of the Balkan areas, for example, fall within the first group, and no strategies are envisaged to prevent HAV infection that carry any social and economic weight because of the high natural circulation (Franco and Vitiello, 2003). Turkey has only recently started to develop rapidly, and strong internal contrasts still exist among ethnic groups of different origin.

A cross-sectional study has recently been performed on the prevalence of HAV infection in a wide sample of refugee Kurds who arrived in southern Italy (Puglia region) as a consequence of ethnic conflict. The results of this study indicate that HAV infection seems to be clearly hyperendemic in Kurds from Turkey, as over

90% of the entire population tested was positive for anti-HAV and about 60% of seropositives were children up to 10 years old (Chironna et al., 2003a). The prevalence rate found in Kurdish refugee children from Turkey, however, is higher than that recently reported in indigenous Turkish children (Sidal et al., 2001), thus reflecting possible differences in socioeconomic, sanitary, and hygienic conditions among ethnic groups of the same country.

A similar pattern of HAV infection was previously observed in other immigrant populations coming into southern Italy, such as ethnic Albanians from Kosovo who arrived in Puglia (a southeastern region of Italy with a population of approximately 4 million) as a result of the 1999 war in the Balkans (Chironna et al., 2001). Also, data on the Albanian population have been obtained from seroepidemiological studies carried out among refugees who have arrived in southern Italy (Germinario et al., 1993; Chironna et al., 2000). The results of these studies indicate a very high circulation of HAV, with prevalence rates similar to those of hyperendemic areas. A seroepidemiological survey performed in Croatia showed a total anti-HAV prevalence of 68.5% in children from 1 to 15 years of age; an outbreak of hepatitis A in a refugee camp was stopped by vaccinating anti-HAV-negative children (Kaic et al., 2001).

Greece appears to be a transition area between countries with different levels of social and sanitary development; consequently, it has a moderate to high degree of HAV endemicity (Franco and Vitiello, 2003). The epidemiology of HAV infection has changed significantly in the last few decades in Spain and Italy due to the considerable improvement in both socioeconomic and health conditions. Spain was considered to be an area with a moderate degree of endemicity for HAV infection, but today this classification may no longer apply if one takes into account the results of current prevalence studies (Dal Re et al., 2000). In addition, the incidence of hepatitis A in Spain has dramatically decreased in recent years, with attack rates of 56 cases per 100,000 inhabitants in 1989 and 2 cases per 100,000 inhabitants in 2000 (Sanchez et al., 2002).

A similar pattern occurs in Italy, where in recent decades improvements in health and sanitation conditions have caused a progressive fall in the HAV infection rate among children under 14 years of age and an increase in susceptible teenagers and adults (Stroffolini et al., 2001), as well as a declining incidence rate from 10 cases per 100,000 inhabitants in 1985 to 3 cases per 100,000 inhabitants in 2001. Nevertheless, Puglia shows a completely different pattern from the rest of the country and is still a region of intermediate endemicity (Lopalco et al., 2000, 2004). Up to 60% of Italian cases of hepatitis A are reported from this region, where the incidence rate is high even in inter-epidemic periods (up to 30 cases per 100,000 inhabitants), and periodical epidemics have been described (Figure 4.3). In particular, between 1996 and 1997 in this region, over 11,000 cases of hepatitis A were reported, accounting for an annual incidence rate of over 130 per 100,000 inhabitants (Malfait et al., 1996; Lopalco et al., 1997). An economic study of the hepatitis A outbreak that occurred in 1996 in Puglia yielded useful information regarding costs to patients, the public health services, and society as a whole (Lucioni et al., 1998). The study concluded that the mean cost of infection for each patient was $662, equivalent to 6.6% of their mean annual income. Costs to the Italian National Health Service totaled $15.67 million, and costs to society were estimated at $24.45 million.

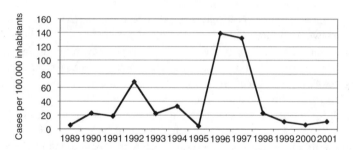

FIGURE 4.3 Incidence of hepatitis A in Puglia, Italy.

MODES OF TRANSMISSION

Hepatitis A infection is primarily transmitted by the fecal–oral route, either through direct contact with an infected person or through contaminated water and food. The role of the person-to-person transmission is exemplified by the high transmission rates among young children in developing countries, in areas where crowding is common and sanitation is poor, in households (Staes et al., 2000), and in childcare settings (Desenclos and MacLafferty, 1993). In the United States, fecal–oral transmission via person-to-person contact within a household is the predominant way in which the disease spreads; the incidence of secondary attack of clinically apparent infection among household members may approach 20 to 50% (Koff, 1998). Currently, in the United States, outbreaks across a community are thought to be the main source of HAV infection, as they affect schoolchildren, adolescents, and young adults. Outbreaks of hepatitis A occur periodically throughout the world, and fecally contaminated water and food are the main vehicles.

In North America, water contaminated by sewage has been associated with hepatitis A outbreaks (Bloch et al., 1990; De Serres et al., 1999); however, the long incubation period of HAV infection may obscure the relationship between illness and consumption of contaminated water, and the absence of an easily accessible test to detect HAV in water may make this source of transmission difficult to recognize (De Serres et al., 1999).

One of the earliest documented outbreaks of hepatitis A associated with consumption of contaminated food was the demonstration of a rising titer of specific antibody in members of a family who contracted acute hepatitis after eating mussels (Dienstag et al., 1976). Widespread foodborne outbreaks of hepatitis A have been recognized increasingly in recent years and are associated with uncooked or fresh food contaminated before distribution, including lettuce (Rosenblum et al., 1990), frozen raspberries (Reid and Robinson, 1987; Ramsey and Upton 1989), frozen strawberries (Niu et al., 1992; Anon., 1997; Hutin et al., 1999), and salad food items (Lowry et al., 1989; Pebody et al., 1998; Dentiger et al., 2001). The global movement of food items that cannot be heated for viral inactivation may be a major cause of outbreaks in developed countries in the future (Cuthbert, 2001).

In addition, HAV infection is the most serious viral infection linked to shellfish consumption (Lees, 2000; Potasman et al., 2002). The first documented outbreak of "infectious hepatitis" occurred in Sweden in 1955, when 629 cases were associated with raw oyster consumption (Roos, 1956). Since the early 1970s, the global consumption of shellfish has increased considerably and, with it, the reports of HAV outbreaks world-wide (Potasman et al., 2002). The largest known modern epidemic of hepatitis A, which occurred in 1988, was also due to consumption of contaminated seafood. In Shanghai, China, 292,301 cases of acute hepatitis were attributed to eating raw clams harvested from a sewage-polluted area (Halliday et al., 1991). Smaller outbreaks associated with shellfish consumption have been reported from the United States (Desenclos et al., 1991; Rippey, 1994), Australia (Conaty et al., 2000), Japan (Fujiyama et al., 1985), Spain (Sànchez et al., 2002), France (Costa-Mattioli et al., 2001), and Italy (Mele et al., 1989; Stroffolini et al., 1990; Leoni et al., 1998).

In Italy, shellfish consumption was the most frequently reported source of HAV infection over a 10-year surveillance (Mele et al., 1997). Recent estimates suggest that shellfish may be responsible for 70% of all hepatitis A cases in Italy (D'Argenio and Salamina, 1998). During the outbreak observed in Puglia in 1996, the largest epidemic of hepatitis A (5620 cases) in Italy since this disease became notifiable in 1989, a matched case-control study (Malfait et al., 1996) showed a strong association between illness and consumption of raw shellfish (odds ratio, 31.8; 95% confidence interval, 12.1 to 118). In addition, the storage of shellfish in seawater at the place of sale was also associated with an increased risk of illness (odds ratio, 41.4; 95% confidence interval, 11.79 to 145.1).

In Puglia, water for storage is usually seawater taken close to the urban coast, where sewage contamination is likely. This local custom has been blamed for the cases of cholera that occurred in this region in 1994, during the same period when a major epidemic was reported in Albania, on the opposite coast of Adriatic sea (Greco et al., 1995). Shellfish are largely consumed in this region, and they are commonly eaten raw or slightly cooked. Seafood marketed in Puglia is obtained from a variety of international providers, with a major proportion coming from countries within the European Union (EU) and from other Mediterranean countries. The significant detection of HAV in mussels imported in Puglia, complying with all European Union shellfish standards (Anon., 1991), has been recently demonstrated by experimental evidence (Chironna et al., 2002). This observation confirms the fact that hepatitis A cases have been associated with consumption of shellfish controlled through legal standards (Mele et al., 1989), and enteric viruses are often detected in shellfish with bacterial counts meeting the current criteria for public consumption (Bosch et al., 1994; Romalde et al., 2002).

Persons infected with HAV who handle food products that are not subsequently cooked can be a source of contamination, even if this handling occurs before retail distribution. Recent studies with molecular techniques (Youtsuyanagi et al., 1996) showed that infected foodhandlers may shed virus for longer periods of time than previously thought and therefore may remain infectious even after full recovery. Various outbreaks of hepatitis A have been associated with foods contaminated by infected foodhandlers (Koster et al., 1990; Weltman et al., 1996; Massoudi et al., 1999; Chironna et al., 2004).

Remarkably, large epidemics are still possible in developed countries. Witness the 1992 foodborne outbreak of hepatitis A in Denver, Colorado, where up to 5000 persons were exposed to HAV after consuming foods that were prepared by 9 ill employees (Dalton et al., 1996). It was calculated that the foodborne outbreak in Denver incurred costs of $689,314 for disease control. Occasional outbreaks of hepatitis A have been linked to sources shared by large number of people, such as contaminated drinking water or bathing areas (Koff, 1998). Travel to developing countries from low-prevalence areas is a well-defined risk; hepatitis A is the most frequently diagnosed form of hepatitis imported into developed countries from developing ones (Steffen et al., 1994). The infection with HAV is mainly transmitted via the enteric route, but parenteral transmission is also possible. Hepatitis A outbreaks among homosexual men have been reported (Henning et al., 1995), and another group at risk for HAV infection by parenteral transmission is the injected- drug-using population (Grinde et al., 1997). Finally, transmission of HAV via bloodborne biological products is unusual but has been reported in patients with cancer (Rosenberg et al., 1987) or hemophilia (Mannucci, 1992).

FOODBORNE HEPATITIS A

Many microbial pathogens can contaminate human food and water supplies and cause illness after they or their toxins are consumed. Foodborne pathogens include a variety of enteric bacteria, viral pathogens, and parasites. Viruses that are known to be transmissible through foods and are of some concerns to human health are shed in the feces of infected humans and transmitted via the fecal–oral route. The source of contamination for foods is through contact with human and animal fecal pollution. This contamination may occur directly, through poor personal hygiene practices of infected foodhandlers, or indirectly, through contact with fecally contaminated water or other cross-contamination routes. The enteric viruses are environmentally stable (Jaykus et al., 1994) and do not replicate in food or environmental samples but can be transmitted easily as they have notably low infectious doses (Haas et al., 1983); therefore, food serves as a vehicle for transmission of viruses, and the common practices for food storage and processing are not adequate to eliminate the risk of transmission.

Hepatitis A infection is the most serious viral infection transmitted by contaminated food, as it causes a debilitating disease and, occasionally death. The role of HAV as a cause of foodborne disease has been widely recognized, and it is likely to appear among the most frequent causes of viral foodborne disease (Koopmans et al., 2002). Many foodstuffs have been involved in HAV-associated outbreaks, but it is now clear that almost any food item can be the vehicle of the virus if contaminated. As previously mentioned, however, the fairly protracted incubation period of hepatitis A virus makes association with a particular food vehicle in individual or sporadic cases very difficult. Normally, the food is not available for testing, and consumption histories are inconclusive.

In the United States, about 5% of all 25,000 to 83,000 HAV cases annually seem to be related to foodborne transmission (Mead et al., 1999; Koopmans et al., 2002).

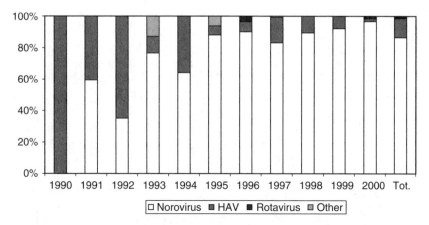

FIGURE 4.4 Distribution (%) of total cases in the United States (1990–2000) of viral-associated foodborne disease outbreaks as reported to the CDC through the Foodborne Disease Outbreak Surveillance System (listed by etiologic agent).

Also, in European countries, sporadic and epidemic cases of hepatitis A have been linked to contamination of food (Koopmans et al., 2002). A Foodborne Disease Outbreak Surveillance System has been activated at the Centers for Disease Control (CDC) in the United States. Based on data of the CDC, from 1990 to 2000 about 23,500 cases of viral-associated outbreaks were reported, and about 12% were caused by HAV (Figure 4.4), although a decrease in hepatitis A cases can be observed throughout those years (CDC, 2003). In more than 50% of cases, the vehicle of transmission is unknown. Among known vehicles, the most frequently implicated are contaminated fruits (primarily strawberries), vegetables (lettuce, carrots, etc.), and salads. Fruits and vegetables may act as vehicles of infection if they are fertilized with sewage sludge or are irrigated with sewage-contaminated water. Also, bread and bread-based products (e.g., sandwiches) are frequently involved in epidemic foci, whereas shellfish or seafood consumption is related only to a small number of cases.

The largest outbreak of HAV associated with contaminated fruit (Table 4.4) was reported in Michigan and Maine in 1997 (Hutin et al., 1999) and involved 242 primary cases, mainly children. The HAV was linked to consumption of frozen strawberries from one processor that were grown in Mexico and widely distributed to school-lunch programs. The study was not able to identify the point at which fecal contamination of the strawberries occurred (irrigation, harvesting, sorting or shipping, processing), as the fruits implicated in the outbreak had been processed approximately a year earlier. Also, apparently sporadic cases in other states could be traced and linked to the same source by viral genetic analysis, which revealed crucial information for the outbreak investigation.

Lettuce was the food implicated in a HAV epidemic in Kentucky in 1988 when 202 persons become ill after having consumed a green salad in three restaurants in Jefferson County. The source of the infection was probably fresh produce from one distributor that had been contaminated before distribution to the restaurants.

TABLE 4.4
Recent Foodborne Outbreaks of Hepatitis A

Year	State or Region/Country	No. of Cases	Food Vehicle	Methods	Refs.
1988	Shanghai/China	300,000	Raw clams	Case-control study	Halliday et al. (1991)
1988	Multistate/United States	61	Raw oysters	Case-control study + molecular techniques	Desenclos et al. (1991)
1988	Kentucky/United States	202	Lettuce	Case-control study	Rosenblum et al. (1990)
1991–1992	Loire–Atlantique–Morbihan/France	800	Shellfish	Molecular techniques	Apaire-Marchais et al. (1995)
1996–1997	Puglia/Italy	11,000	Raw shellfish	Case-control study	Malfait et al. (1996), Lopalco et al. (1997)
1997	Multistate/United States	242	Strawberries	Case-control study + molecular techniques	Hutin et al. (1999)
1997	New South Wales/Australia	467	Oysters	Case-control study + molecular techniques	Conaty et al. (2000)
1998	Ohio/United States	43	Onions	Case-control study + molecular techniques	Dentiger et al. (2001)
1999	North Bretagne/France	32	Raw shellfish	Case-control study + molecular techniques	Costa-Mattioli et al. (2001)
1999	Valencia/Spain	184	Imported coquina clams	Case-control study + molecular techniques	Sanchez et al. (2002)

An onions-associated hepatitis A outbreak involved patrons of one restaurant who ate menu items containing green onions (Dentiger et al., 2001). As in the case of the strawberries, the point at which contamination of the onions occurred was not identified. The implicated onions could have come from Mexico or California. The gene sequence of the outbreak strain was consistent with HAV acquired in Mexico, where hepatitis A is endemic, although no linkage was established with certainty between the onions and the cases by tracing HAV in the food.

The main food type associated with recent hepatitis A outbreaks, however, is molluscan shellfish, such as oysters, cockles, and mussels, which are usually found in shallow coastal or estuarine waters, commonly near sewage outlets (Lees, 2000; Potasman et al., 2002). The largest hepatitis A outbreak ever reported, as mentioned previously, occurred in Shanghai, China, in 1988, where almost 300,000 cases were linked to the consumption of clams harvested from a site impacted by human sewage pollution (Halliday et al., 1991). In this outbreak, the estimated attack rates in those who had and had not consumed clams were about 12% and 0.5%, respectively, with a very high overall hepatitis attack rate during the epidemic of 4083 per 100,000 populations. In the course of the epidemic, 47 people died.

In Southern Italy, particularly in the Puglia region, the very large outbreak of hepatitis A that began in 1996 involved about 11,000 people over 2 consecutive years (Malfait et al., 1996; Lopalco et al., 1997). Analysis of the risk factors showed a strong association with raw seafood consumption (odds ratio, 31.8; 95% confidence interval, 11.79 to 118). The sustained circulation of seafood contaminated locally and the accumulation of susceptible subjects in the population probably caused the occurrence of this large epidemic. The observed seasonal pattern for HAV in Puglia with a peak in February was explained by local habits of consuming raw seafood on special occasions, such as Christmas and New Year's Eve. In addition, case-control studies showed that the risk of illness increased when the mussels had been stored in water before purchase (odds ratio, 41.4; 95% confidence interval, 11.79 to 145.1). As noted earlier, water for such storage was usually seawater obtained close to the urban coast, where sewage contamination was likely.

An oysters-associated outbreak of hepatitis A was reported in Australia (Conaty et al., 2000). More than 450 cases were reported, and a matched case-control study and environmental investigation revealed that oysters grown in the Wallis Lake area (subsequently withdrawn from sale) represented the source of infection.

In addition to the large epidemic in Southern Italy from 1996 to 1997, other outbreaks of hepatitis A in the European region include those reported in France from 1991 to 1992 (Apaire-Marchais et al., 1995) and in 1999 (Costa-Mattioli et al., 2001) and in Valencia, Spain, in 1999 (Sànchez et al., 2002). The French epidemic from 1991 to 1992 involved around 800 cases and was associated with shellfish consumption, although definitive evidence was not available. The epidemic in North Bretagne, France, that occurred in 1999 involved 32 cases and was investigated through case-control studies and molecular analysis. The outbreak that occurred in Spain in 1999 involved 184 confirmed cases who had consumed imported coquina clams. An epidemiological study showed that the only positive association was found with the consumption of coquina clams imported from Peru (Sanchez et al., 2002). Genetic analysis of the 5′ non-coding region (5′NCR) demonstrated the occurrence of identical sequences in shellfish and patient serum samples, confirming the shell-fish-borne origin of the outbreak. All sequences of HAV strains belonged to genotype IB, although the overall homology was 98%. Generally, among patients involved in common-source outbreaks, complete identity among all isolates has been found (Hutin et al., 1999; Robertson et al., 2000); however, in this case, further molecular epidemiological analysis of fragments of the VP1/2A and 5′ end of the genome from shellfish and sera isolates revealed the presence of six variants (Bosch et al., 2001), thus confirming previous findings on the heterogeneity of HAV strains associated with the consumption of contaminated shellfish (Costa-Mattioli et al., 2001; Sànchez et al., 2002).

On the basis of these studies, it is likely that HAV strains characterized during shellfish-associated outbreaks are heterogeneous due to peculiar features of shellfish. In fact, bivalve shellfish are filter feeders and tend to accumulate whatever pollutants are in the water, which can result in viral contamination from a multitude of possible sources affecting many HAV-infected shedding individuals. Further studies are needed to clarify this issue.

The recent reports of HAV epidemics associated with shellfish consumption pose an important question with regard to public health. Most countries have shown a significant increase in shellfish catches during recent years (Potasman et al., 2002); nevertheless, current regulations regarding the commercialization of shellfish are unable to guarantee the protection of consumers. In fact, sanitary controls for bivalve shellfish rely on microbiological criteria to define the suitability of these products. In Europe, the commercialization of bivalve shellfish is regulated by the EU Council Directive 91/492/EEC, which establishes that shellfish that meet a microbiological standard of less than 230 *Escherichia coli*, or 300 fecal coliforms, in 100 g of shellfish flesh and in the absence of *Salmonella* spp. can be placed on the market for human consumption. In the United States, sanitary controls pertain to the waters in which shellfish are grown (Lees, 2000); however, no specific microbiological criteria concerning the presence of enteric viruses have been established.

It is well known that compliance with the routine microbiological standards of shellfish and harvesting water does not exclude the presence of enteric viruses. Several studies have demonstrated that no correlation exists between fecal indicators and the presence of enteric viruses (Gerba, 1979; Le Guyader et al., 1993; Chironna et al., 2002), and viruses can persist in shellfish grown in seawater with normal microbiological standards.

Depuration is the common method used to obtain marketable shellfish; never-theless, this method is inadequate for complete virus elimination, even if performed with advanced systems (De Medici et al., 2001). A recent study on the depuration dynamics of viruses in shellfish was conducted to evaluate the duration of the depuration treatment required to produce shellfish without viral genome detectable by polymerase chain reaction (PCR) (Muniain-Mujika et al., 2002). All shellfish samples become negative for human viruses by PCR only after 5 days of depuration treatment. The authors concluded that, realistically, the characteristics of the market do not permit shellfish to be kept in depuration tanks for long periods of time; therefore, the problem of sanitary control of shellfish commercialized for human consumption remains an important issue.

Also, foodhandlers are responsible of many epidemic foci of hepatitis A. Contamination of food by infected foodhandlers is probably the most common cause of viral foodborne illness. Food items such as salads and desserts that receive considerable handling during preparation and are not given any further heat treatment before consumption are often implicated in foodborne viral outbreaks. Examples of such outbreaks include the previously mentioned 1992 outbreak in Denver, Colorado, in which 43 secondary cases were reported and more than 5000 subjects were exposed to HAV due to the consumption of a variety of gourmets food prepared by infected foodhandlers (Dalton et al., 1996). In 1994, in Kentucky, a catering company foodhandler with hepatitis A was recognized as the source of infection of an outbreak of HAV involving 91 patrons attending events serving foods prepared from the catering company, and eating uncooked foods was strongly associated with the illness (Massoudi et al., 1999). To date, though, the association of foodhandlers with known hepatitis A outbreaks has been investigated only with classical epidemiological studies (case-control studies).

In 2002, an epidemic cluster of hepatitis A associated with a foodhandler occurred in Bari, Southern Italy, and involved 26 cases (Chironna et al., 2004). The outbreak was investigated by a case-control study that indicated that the source of HAV infection was an HAV-infected foodhandler employed in a delicatessen who had been handling foods until being hospitalized (odds ratio, 5.36; 95% confidence interval, 1.58 to 19.25). The outbreak was also investigated with the use of molecular analysis, which confirmed the previous findings. All of the cases had consumed foodstuffs prepared in the delicatessen. Also, the sequences of all cases were identical to one another and to the sequence of the HAV strain isolated from the foodhandler which belonged to genotype IB.

These studies further confirm the role of foodhandlers in the spread of foodborne diseases and underscore the need for appropriate training in safe foodhandling practices. Well-standardized surveillance networks together with virological studies could help to better document outbreaks of hepatitis A and could provider useful information to stop the spread of disease and to plan adequate preventive strategies.

DETECTION OF HAV IN FOOD

Epidemiological studies have shown that the major routes of contamination of foods with human enteric viruses include: (1) shellfish harvested from fecally contaminated estuaries, (2) fruits or vegetables irrigated or washed with fecally contaminated water, and (3) foods that become contaminated during preparation through contact with fecally contaminated surfaces or hands of infected foodhandlers (Jaykus, 2000). As a result, many efforts have been made to establish methodologies for detecting enteric viruses in food.

The detection of viral pathogens by conventional virological techniques (e.g., viral isolation in cell cultures) is quite difficult in samples of complex composition such as foodstuffs. In particular, detection of hepatitis A in food actually is not possible in a routine laboratory because of the requirement for a living host for growth. In addition, crude food extracts are highly cytotoxic and therefore not suitable for direct inoculation onto cells. Furthermore, the level of virus particles in a contaminated food is usually very low, and detection with molecular techniques (which are discussed in this section) still presents many difficulties. Such techniques cannot be applied for inspection of food for the presence of enteric viruses on a large scale. For many reasons, the detection of HAV in foods is difficult and is rarely attempted. Due to the low levels of contamination and the large sample sizes of implicated foods that must be tested, it is necessary to separate the viruses from the food matrix and concentrate them prior to application of detection methods such as cell culture infectivity assay or immunological and molecular techniques.

Recently, molecular techniques have become available that have greatly contributed to our understanding of the epidemiology of HAV and allowed the detection of viruses in both environmental and food samples (Le Guyader et al., 2000; Pina et al., 2001). Nevertheless, although acid amplification methods such as reverse transcription–polymerase chain reaction (RT–PCR) have shown great promise for detection of HAV in clinical samples, the lack of consensus on an ideal method for detecting HAV in food testifies to the difficulty of the task.

A review of the literature regarding the detection of HAV in foods (Lees, 2000; Sair et al., 2002) reveals two major areas for which methodological developments are needed. The first of these is the development of rapid, simple, and efficient methods to extract and concentrate HAV from food matrices. The second research need includes enhancement of RT-PCR amplification methods to increase speed, sensitivity, and specificity in the analysis of foods. This would include efforts to improve RNA extraction methods to eliminate possible inhibitors co-extracted from the complex food matrices (Hafliger et al., 1997; Dix and Jaykus, 1998; Shieh et al., 1999; Leggitt and Jaykus, 2000; Dubois et al., 2002).

A variety of methods have been reported regarding shellfish processing for the detection of viral RNA (Le Guyader et al., 1994; Atmar et al., 1995; Lopez-Sabater et al., 1997; Croci et al., 1999), and several studies have demonstrated the successful application of PCR to detect virus in shellfish artificially contaminated in the laboratory. In addition, recent studies have also reported the application of these methods to the detection of enteric viruses in naturally polluted bivalve mollusks (Le Guyader et al., 2000; Chironna et al., 2002; Sànchez et al., 2002).

Most of the current methods for detecting HAV have concentrated on refining virus extraction and or nucleic acid extraction and purification techniques to overcome the problem of inhibiting substances present in crude shellfish extracts (Figure 4.5). A common approach has been to base methods for virus extraction on those previously developed for detection of HAV in cell culture (Lees et al., 1994; Jaykus et al., 1996).

Following virus extraction, a variety of subsequent nucleic acid extraction and purification protocols have been employed (Kingsley and Richards, 2001; Shieh et al., 1999, Le Guyader et al., 2000; Chironna et al., 2002). Because PCR reaction volumes are small, these protocols generally must incorporate concentration steps. In addition, RT–PCR or a nested or hemi-nested RT–PCR has been used to amplify HAV RNA. It has been pointed out, however, that the use of RT–PCR does not differentiate between infectious and non-infectious viruses, as amplified nucleic acid could originate either from viable virus or damaged non-infectious virus and require additional confirmation (Lees, 2000). A recent study investigated the presence of

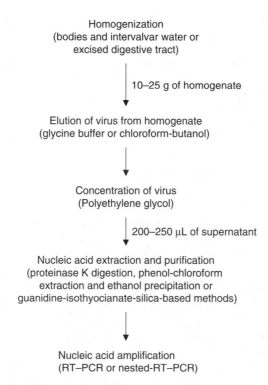

Homogenization
(bodies and intervalvar water or
excised digestive tract)

10–25 g of homogenate

Elution of virus from homogenate
(glycine buffer or chloroform-butanol)

Concentration of virus
(Polyethylene glycol)

200–250 µL of supernatant

Nucleic acid extraction and purification
(proteinase K digestion, phenol-chloroform
extraction and ethanol precipitation or
guanidine-isothyocianate-silica-based methods)

Nucleic acid amplification
(RT–PCR or nested-RT–PCR)

FIGURE 4.5 Scheme of steps needed to detect HAV in shellfish.

live virus in mussels, subjecting all samples that tested positive by PCR screening to a cell culture assay and using RT–PCR to detect the presence of HAV in culture supernatant (Chironna et al., 2002). This integrated method was applied because even virus not capable of producing the cytopathic effect can be detected in very low concentrations. In this study, about one third of mussels positive for the presence of HAV RNA were shown to be contaminated by live virus (Chironna et al., 2002). Also, previous reports have shown a correlation between the detection of viral RNA by PCR and the detection of infectious particle (Kopecka et al., 1993; Graff et al., 1993).

Some molecular methods for virus detection have been applied to other foods, such as fruits, vegetables, and hamburger (Leggitt and Jaykus, 2000; Dubois et al., 2002; Sair et al., 2002), but their application in the field requires further confirmation and standardization procedures. In addition, it remains unclear what the predictive value of a negative test is. This information is required before screening of such specimens can be done to monitor contamination.

The development of a robust, specific, and sensitive method to recover HAV from food remains a primary goal for researchers. Such a method would permit identification of contaminated food and improve our understanding of the modes of food contamination, thereby contributing useful information to improve public health policy and safety.

MEASURES TO CONTROL FOODBORNE HEPATITIS A

The strategy to control hepatitis A varies considerably in different areas and among various population groups. Suitable knowledge of the size and epidemiologic characteristics of the disease should be the first step toward developing an appropriate strategy. It is necessary to improve the rate of notification of all cases. Extensive seroepidemiologic surveys would accurately estimate the size of the problem and identify the specific epidemiologic characteristics and high-risk groups. Furthermore, the relative importance of the disease, pressure of other more important problems, existing health services organization, cost of the vaccine, economic conditions prevailing in the country, and positive political climate are important factors in planning a national or local strategy (Papaevangelou, 1997). Among the measures to control hepatitis A, improving sanitation and hygienic standards is the primary and permanent goal. The disease incidence should be monitored not only by passive but also by established active surveillance systems. This would enable the rapid detection and control of local community outbreaks. Attention should be given to determining the source of infection, the existing high-risk groups, and contacts made by patients. In addition, the high effectiveness and long-lasting immunity of the HAV vaccine (Table 4.5) represents the most promising measure for controlling the disease (Van Damme et al., 1994). Moreover, the hepatitis A vaccine is effective in the prevention of secondary infection of HAV and should be recommended for household contacts of primary cases of hepatitis A (Sagliocca et al., 1999).

Since safe, immunogenic, and effective vaccines became available, many guidelines and recommendation have been published about hepatitis A prevention in intermediate and low endemic countries. Priority and relevant use of these measures should be based on the established known main epidemiologic patterns. In the poorest of developing countries, where a lack of hygiene facilitates the transmission of HAV, hepatitis A is hyperendemic. In these countries, mass immunization of very young children, together with improvements in water supplies and sanitary standards, is the key to future control of HAV infection (Koff, 1998). Major obstacles include the cost of the vaccine, the absence in many areas of an appropriate healthcare infrastructure for vaccine delivery, and competing healthcare problems that may seem more urgent. In such countries, hepatitis A is not considered a very important healthcare problem. The mass immunization strategy could be reassessed when the vaccine becomes less expensive and the burden of the diseases increases with shifting to older age as a result of the improvement of sanitation (Papaevangelou, 1997).

In areas with a pattern of moderate endemicity, priority should be given to further improving sanitation conditions. Although the infection spreads mainly by person-to-person contact, community-wide epidemics among those of school age or early adulthood are common because transmission by water and food still occurs. In certain populations, cyclical trends may exist. An outbreak may occur after a period of several years when a new cohort of susceptible subjects emerges, thus promoting the return of high rates of viral infection and clinical disease.

Vaccination of high-risk population groups should be encouraged. The extent of vaccination would depend on the specific prevailing epidemiologic features and on the availability of seroepidemiologic data. The availability of appropriate funds and

TABLE 4.5

Comparison of the Effects of Active and Passive Immunization Against Hepatitis A

Characteristics	Human Immunoglobulin (Ig)	Hepatitis A Virus (HAV) Vaccine
Onset of protection?	Immediate	Immediate
Will also protect when given shortly after HAV exposure?	Yes	Yes
Long-term protection?	No	Yes
May stop epidemic outbreaks?	No	Yes

health services required to rapidly vaccinate and maintain an ongoing vaccination program should be considered. Vaccination of children 2 to 9 or 12 years old has been recommended, and these measures should be considered sufficient to drastically reduce the burden of the disease (Papaevangelou, 1997).

A vaccination program against hepatitis A was initiated in Puglia, Italy, in 1997, as part of a comprehensive program that also included health education and measures against environmental pollution (Germinario et al., 2000). According to the protocol, all children are vaccinated at 15 to 18 months of age, and all 12 years olds are also vaccinated with a combined hepatitis A and B vaccine during the mandatory hepatitis B vaccination phase. In addition, a pilot program of hepatitis A and B vaccination of preadolescents (12 years of age) in the schools of Catalonia, Spain, commenced during the 1998–1999 school year (Lopalco, 2000). These vaccination programs have taken advantage of the infrastructure and logistics of the hepatitis B vaccination program in schools. The routine vaccination against HAV in preadolescents is a public health intervention that not only is justified by avoiding the burdens of the disease but may also be defended from the perspective of its efficiency (Domìnguez et al., 2003).

The most recent recommendations for prevention of hepatitis A from the Advisory Committee on Immunization Practices (ACIP) broaden the target groups for vaccination (Anon., 1999). In the United States, routine vaccination is now recommended for children in states, counties, and communities with rates of hepatitis A that are twice the 1987 to 1997 national average of 10 cases per 100,000 population (Table 4.6). In addition, states, counties, and communities with rates exceeding the national average should consider routine childhood vaccination. An economic analysis indicated that either universal vaccination or screening and vaccination of 2-year-old children should be considered cost effective in developed countries (Das, 1999).

A pattern of low endemicity of hepatitis A is found in countries with very high levels of hygiene and living standards. The morbidity rate is very low (5 to 15 per 100,000 inhabitants) and applies primarily to adolescents and young adults; however, HAV still circulates, and the possibility of extensive outbreaks still exists through mass consumption of contaminated food or a compromised water supply system.

TABLE 4.6

Burden of Hepatitis A in States with Average Reported Incidence of ≥20 Cases per 100,000 Population (1987–1997)

State	Rate (per 100,000)	Cumulative Average Number of Cases per Year[a]
Arizona	48	1852
Alaska	45	2137
Oregon	40	3297
New Mexico	40	3916
Utah	33	4519
Washington	30	6007
Oklahoma	24	6786
South Dakota	24	6953
Idaho	21	7172
Nevada	21	7449
California	20	13,706

[a] Approximately 37% of these cases were among persons younger than 20 years old.

Note: The reported disease incidence in the United States from 1987 to 1997 was 10.8 cases per 100,000 population. Reported hepatitis A cases from the 11 states shown here accounted for an average of 50% of reported cases each year, yet the total population of these states represents 22% of the U.S. population.

Source: Adapted from Anon., *Morbid. Mortal. Wkly. Rep.*, 48(RR-12), 1–37, 1999.

Community-wide outbreaks may also occur among certain high-risk groups in young adults 20 to 30 years old. Illicit drug users and active homosexuals play a major role in such outbreaks. The vaccination of these specific groups would be an important control of such types of community-wide outbreaks. In areas of very low endemicity (infection rate <5 per 100,000 inhabitants), pre-exposure vaccination should be seriously considered for the following high-risk groups: travelers to endemic areas, children of selected populations, healthcare workers in neonatal intensive-care units, institutionalized patients, individuals with clotting-factor disorders, occupationally exposed persons, workers in plants for treating sewage and wastewater, active homosexuals, illicit drug users, and persons with chronic liver disease (Table 4.7).

How to manage foodhandlers has been an intriguing question (Koff, 1998). Foodhandlers are not at higher risk than other persons for becoming infected with HAV; however, foodhandlers do have the potential to infect hundreds of people if they work while infected with HAV, do not use good handwashing techniques, and have contact with ready-to-eat food. If a foodhandler is experiencing symptoms of hepatitis A, the foodhandler should immediately be excluded from food handling, seek medical care, and not return to food handling until 2 weeks after the beginning

---

TABLE 4.7

Pre-Exposure Vaccination Against Hepatitis A in High-Risk Groups

Groups

Travelers to endemic areas
Children of selected populations
Healthcare workers in neonatal intensive-care units
Institutionalized patients
Individuals with clotting-factor disorders
Occupationally exposed persons
Workers in plants for treating sewage and wastewater
Active homosexuals
Illicit drug users
Persons with chronic liver disease

---

of the illness. In the past, when hepatitis A was recognized in a foodhandler, co-workers were generally given immunoglobulin. The concern has been raised, however, that foodhandlers who have received immunoglobulin as post-exposure prophylaxis may develop asymptomatic infection and shed HAV, thereby continuing to infect those who eat the food. Pre-exposure HAV vaccination of foodhandlers is reasonable (Koff, 1998) and has been advocated (Dalton et al., 1996) and implemented in some cities in the United States. The high turnover of employees and the fact that many part-time foodhandlers have no health insurance or access to medical care have limited implementation of vaccination programs for this group. Moreover, such policies have not been shown to be cost effective and generally are not recommended in the United States or other developed countries (Koopmans et al., 2002). Personal hygiene is most important in preventing foodborne viral infection and includes frequent handwashing and wearing gloves. This should apply for all points in the food chain where foodstuffs are handled.

The globalization of the food market has hampered implementation of control measures to ensure the safety of food; however, for prevention of foodborne transmission of HAV, it also essential that food items are not grown or washed in fecally contaminated water. Among the high-risk foodstuffs, bivalve shellfish are notorious as a source of foodborne viral infections, because filter-feeding shellfish can concentrate the HAV up to 100-fold from large volumes of water, thus allowing accumulation of virus from fecally contaminated water (Leoni et al., 1998; Malfait et al., 1996; Normann et al., 1995). Depuration is a practice that may reduce bacterial contamination but is far less effective in reducing viral contamination (De Medici et al., 2001). Quality control of food and water on the basis of detecting indicator organisms for fecal contamination has proven to be an unreliable predictor of viral contamination (Croci et al., 2000; Chironna et al., 2002). Although several other foods (desserts, fruits, vegetables, salads, sandwiches) have also been implicated as vehicles of HAV transmission, most studies of virus detection in food have focused on shellfish, for which several groups have developed slightly different methods to be used for molecular tracing of virus strains (Lees, 2000).

Recently, some methods were reported for virus detection in other food (Bidawid et al., 2000; Schwab et al., 2000), but their application in the field remains anecdotal. Because a food can become contaminated at any point during its production and delivery to the consumer, a hazard analysis and critical-control points program (HACCP) or other systematic quality-control program is necessary to prevent HAV contamination (Koopmans et al., 2002). Food safety, at least in the developed world, is increasingly predicated on the HACCP system, along with appropriate general precautions.

Today, food safety is a top priority of WHO, and the member states have adopted a strongly worded resolution that recognizes food safety as an essential public health function (WHO, 2000). Many interesting challenges can be identified in the area of food safety that have spurred a new wave of solutions; however, these solutions will not materialize without support from all parts of the food production and consumption chain (Schlundt, 2002).

REFERENCES

Alter, M.J., Gallagher, M., Morris, T.T., Moyer, L.A., Meeks, E.L., Krawezynski, K., Kim, J.P., and Margolis, H.S. (1997) Acute non-A-E hepatitis in the United States and the role of hepatitis G virus infection: Sentinel Counties Viral Hepatitis Study Team, *N. Engl. J. Med.*, 336: 741–746.

Anderson, D.A. and Ross, B.C. (1990) Morphogenesis of hepatitis A virus: isolation and characterization of subviral particles, *J. Virol.*, 64: 5284–5289.

Anon. (1991). Council Directive of the July 15, 1991 (91/492/EEC): health conditions for the production and the placing on the market of live bivalves molluscs, *Off. J. Eur. Comm.*, L268: 1–14

Anon. (1997) Hepatitis A associated with consumption of frozen strawberries: Michigan, March 1997, *Morbid. Mortal. Wkly. Rep.*, 46: 288–295.

Anon. (1999) Prevention of hepatitis A through active or passive immunization: recommendations of the Advisory Committee on Immunization Practices (ACIP), *Morbid. Mortal. Wkly. Rep.*, 48(RR-12): 1–37.

Apaire-Marchais, V., Robertson, B.H., Aubineau-Ferre, V., Le Roux, M.G., Leveque, F., Schwartzbrod, L., and Billaudel, S. (1995) Direct sequencing of hepatitis A virus strains isolated during an epidemic in France, *Appl. Environ. Microbiol.*, 61: 3977–3980.

Arauz-Ruiz, P., Sundqvist, L., Garcia, Z., Taylor, L., Visona, K., Norder, H., and Magnius L.O. (2001) Presumed common source outbreaks of hepatitis A in an endemic area confirmed by limited sequencing within the VP1 region, *J. Med. Virol.*, 65: 449–456.

Atmar, R.L., Neill, F.H.., Romalde, J.L., Le Guyader, F., Woodley, C.M., Metcalf, T.G., and Estes, M.K. (1995) Detection of Norwalk virus and hepatitis A virus in shellfish tissues with PCR, *Appl. Environ. Microbiol.*, 61(8): 3014–3018.

Barzaga, B.N. (2000) Hepatitis A shifting epidemiology in South-East Asia and China, *Vaccine*, 18: S61–S64.

Berge, J.J., Drennan, D.P., Jacobs, R.J., Jakins, A., Meyerhoff, A.S., Stubblefield, W., and Weinberg, M. (2000) The cost of hepatitis A infections in American adolescents and adults in 1997, *Hepatology*, 31: 469–473.

Bidawid, S., Farber, J.M., and Sattar, S.A. (2000) Rapid concentration and detection of hepatitis A virus from lettuce and strawberries, *J. Virolog. Meth.*, 88: 175–185.

Bloch, A.B., Stramer, S.L., Smith, J.D., Margolis, H.S., Fields, H.A., McKinley, T.W., Gerba, C.P., Maynard, J.E., and Sikes, R.K. (1990) Recovery of hepatitis A virus from a water supply responsible for a common source outbreak of hepatitis A, *Am. J. Public Health*, 80: 428–430.

Bosch, A., Abad, F.X., Gajardo, R., and Pintò R.M. (1994) Should shellfish be purified before public consumption?, *Lancet*, 344: 1024–1025.

Bosch, A., Sanchez, G., Le Guyader, F., Vanaclocha, H., Haugarreau, L., and Pinto, R.M. (2001) Human enteric viruses in coquina clams associated with a large hepatitis A outbreak. *Water Sci. Technol.*, 43: 61–65.

Bruisten, S.M., Steenbergen, J.E., Pijl, A.S., Niesters, H.G.M., van Doornum, G.J.J., and Coutinho, RA. (2001) Molecular epidemiology of hepatitis A virus in Amsterdam, the Netherlands, *J. Med. Virol.*, 63: 88–95.

Byun, K.S., Kim, J.H., Song, K.J., Baek, L.J., Song, J.W., Park, S.H., Kwon, O.S., Yeon, J.E., Kim, J.S., Bak, Y.T., and Lee, C.H. (2001) Molecular epidemiology of hepatitis A virus in Korea, *J. Gastroenterol. Hepatol.*, 16: 519–524.

CDC (2003) http://www.cdc.gov/foodborneoutbreaks/report_pub.htm (accessed April 25, 2003).

Chen, Y., Mao, J., Hong, Y., Yang, L., Ling, Z., and Yu, W. (2001) Genetic analysis of wild-type hepatitis A virus strains, *Chin. Med. J. (Engl.)*, 114: 422–423.

Chironna, M., Germinario, C., Lopalco, P.L., and Quarto, M. (2000) Prevalence of enterically transmitted hepatitis in refugees in southern Italy, *Antiviral Ther.*, 5 (Suppl. 1): F.10.

Chironna, M., Germinario, C., Lopalco, P.L., Carrozzini, F., and Quarto, M. (2001) Prevalence of hepatitis virus infections in Kosovar refugees, *Int. J. Infect. Dis.*, 5: 209–213.

Chironna, M., Germinario, C., De Medici, D., Fiore, A., Di Pasquale, S., Quarto, M., and Barbuti, S. (2002) Detection of hepatitis A virus in mussels from different sources marketed in the Puglia region (South Italy), *Int. J. Food Microbiol.*, 75: 11–18.

Chironna, M., Germinario, C., Lopalco, P.L., Carrozzini, F., Barbuti, S., and Quarto, M. (2003a) Prevalence rates of viral hepatitis infections in refugee Kurds from Iraq and Turkey, *Infection*, 31: 93–97.

Chironna, M., Grottola, A., Lanave, C., Villa, E., Barbuti, S., and Quarto M. (2003b) Genetic analysis of HAV strains recovered from patients with acute hepatitis from Southern Italy, *J. Med. Virol.*, 70: 343–349.

Chironna, M., Lopalco, P.L., Prato, R., Germinario, C., Barbuti, S., Quarto, M. (2004) Outbreak of infection with hepatitis A virus (HAV) associated with a foodhandler and confirmed by sequence analysis reveals a new HAV genotype IB variant, *J. Clin. Microbiol.*, in press.

Cianciara, J. (2000) Hepatitis A shifting epidemiology in Poland and Eastern Europe, *Vaccine*, 18: S68–S70.

Ciocca, M. (2000) Clinical course and consequences of hepatitis A infection, *Vaccine*, 18(18, Suppl. 1): S71–S74.

Cohen, J.I., Ticehurst, J.R., Purcell, R.H., Buckler-White, A., and Baroudy B.M. (1987) Complete nucleotide sequence of wild-type hepatitis A virus: comparison with different strains of hepatitis A virus and other picornaviruses *J. Virol.*, 61: 50–59.

Conaty, S., Bird, P., Bell, G., Kraa, E., Grohmann, G., and McAnulty, J.M. (2000) Hepatitis A in New South Wales, Australia, from consumption of oysters: the first reported outbreak, *Epidemiol. Infect.*, 124: 121–130.

Costa-Mattioli, M., Monpoeho, S., Schvoerer, C., Besse, B., Aleman, M.H., Billaudel, S., Cristina, J., and Ferré, V. (2001) Genetic analysis of hepatitis A virus outbreak in France confirms the co-circulation of subgenotypes Ia, Ib and reveals a new genetic lineage, *J. Med. Virol.*, 65: 233–240.

Costa-Mattioli, M., Cristina, J., Romero, H., Perez-Bercof, R., Casane, D., Colina, R., Garcia, L., Vega, I., Glikman, G., Romanowsky, V., Castello, A., Nicand, E., Gassin, M., Billaudel, S., and Ferre, V. (2002) Molecular evolution of hepatitis A virus: a new classification based on the complete VP1 protein, *J. Virol.*, 76: 9516–9525.

Croci, L., De Medici, G., Morace, G., Fiore, A., Scalfaro, C., Beneduce, F., and Toti. L. (1999) Detection of hepatitis A virus in shellfish by nested reverse transcription–PCR, *Int. J. Food Microbiol.*, 48: 67–71.

Croci, L., De Medici, D., Scalfaro, C., Fiore, A., Divizia, M., Donia, D., Casentino, A.M., Moretti, P., and Costantini, G. (2000) Determination of enteroviruses, hepatitis A virus, bacteriophages, and *Escherichia coli* in Adriatic Sea mussels, *J. Appl. Microbiol.*, 88: 293–298.

Cuthbert, J. (2001) Hepatitis A: old and new, *Clin. Microbiol. Rev.*, 14: 38–58.

D'Argenio, P. and Salamina, G. (1998) Shellfish consumption and awareness of risk of acquiring hepatitis A among Neapolitan families: Italy, 1997, *Eurosurveillance*, 3: 97–98.

Dal Re, R., Garcia-Corbeira, P., and Garcia-de-Lomas, J. (2000) A large percentage of the Spanish population under 30 years of age is not protected against hepatitis A, *J. Med. Virol.*, 60: 363–366.

Dalton, C.B., Haddix, A., Hoffman, R.E., and Mast, E.E. (1996) The cost of food-borne outbreak of hepatitis A in Denver, Colorado, *Arch. Intern. Med.*, 156: 1013–1016.

Das, A. (1999) An economic analysis of different strategies of immunization against hepatitis A virus in developed countries, *Hepatology*, 29(2): 548–552.

De Medici, D., Ciccozzi, M., Fiore, A., Di Pasquale, S., Parlato, A., Ricci-Bitti, P., and Croci, L. (2001) Closed-circuit system for the depuration of mussels experimentally contaminated with hepatitis A virus, *J. Food Protect.*, 64: 877–880.

de Paula, V.S., Baptista, M.L., Lampe, E., Niel, C., and Gaspar, A.M. (2002) Characterization of hepatitis A virus isolates from subgenotypes IA and IB in Rio de Janeiro, Brazil, *J. Med. Virol.*, 66: 22–27.

De Serres, G., Cromeans, T.L., Levesque, B., Brassard, N., Barthe, C., Dionne, M., Prudhomme, H., Paradis, D., Shapiro, C.N., Nainan, O.V., and Margolis, H.S. (1999) Molecular confirmation of hepatitis A virus from well water: epidemiology and public health implications, *J. Infect. Dis.*, 179: 37–43.

Dentiger, C.M., Bower, W.A., Nainan, O.V., Cotter, S.M., Myers, G., Dubusky, L.M., Fowler, S., Salehi, E.D., and Bell, B.P. (2001) An outbreak of hepatitis A associated with green onions, *J. Infect. Dis.*, 183: 1273–1276.

Desenclos, J.C. and MacLafferty, L. (1993) Community wide outbreak of hepatitis A linked to children in day care centres and with increased transmission in young adult men in Florida 1988–1989, *J. Epidemiol. Commun. Health*, 47: 269–273.

Desenclos, J.C., Klontz, K.C., Wilder, M.H., Nainan, O.V., Margolis, H.S., and Gunn R.A. (1991) A multistate outbreak of hepatitis A caused by the consumption of raw oysters, *Am. J. Public Health*, 81: 1268–1272.

Diaz, B.I., Sariol, C.A., Normann, A., Rodriguez, L., and Flehmig, B. (2001) Genetic relatedness of Cuban HAV wild-type isolates *J. Med. Virol.*, 64: 96–103.

Dienstag, J.L., Gust, I.D., Lucas, C.R., Wong, D.C., and Purcell, R.H. (1976) Mussel-associated viral hepatitis, type A: serological confirmation, *Lancet*, i: 561–564.

Dix, A.B. and Jaykus, L.A. (1998) Virion concentration method for the detection of human enteric viruses in extracts of hard-shelled clams *J. Food Protect.*, 61: 458–465.

Domìnguez, Á., Salleras, L., Carmona, G., and Batalla, J. (2003) Effectiveness of a mass hepatitis A vaccination program in preadolescents, *Vaccine*, 21: 698–701.

Dubois, E., Agier, C., Traore, O., Hennechart, C., Merle, G., Cruciere, C., and Laveran, H. (2002) Modified concentration method for the detection of enteric viruses on fruits and vegetables by reverse transcriptase–polymerase chain reaction or cell culture, *J. Food Protect.*, 65: 1962–1969.

Feinstone, S.M., Kapikian, A.Z., and Purcell, R.H. (1973) Hepatitis A: detection by immune electron microscopy of a viruslike antigen associated with acute illness, *Science*, 182: 1026–1028.

Franco, E. and Vitiello, G. (2003) Vaccination strategies against hepatitis A in southern Europe, *Vaccine*, 21: 696–697.

Fujiyama, S., Akahoshi, M., Sagara, K., Sato, T., and Tsurusaki, R. (1985) An epidemic of hepatitis A related to ingestion of raw oysters, *Gastroenterol. Jpn.*, 20: 6–13.

Gerba, C.P., Goyal, S.M., LaBelle, R.L., Cech, I., and Bodgan, G.F. (1979) Failure of indicator bacteria to reflect the occurrence of enteroviruses in marine waters, *Am. J. Public Health*, 69: 1116–1119.

Germinario, C., Quarto, M., Barbuti, S., Greco, D., Squarcione, S., and Lo Caputo, S. (1993) Public Health emergency in Albania, *Eur. J. Public Health*, 3: 66.

Germinario, C., Lopalco, P.L., Chironna, M., and Da Villa, G. (2000) From hepatitis B to hepatitis A prevention: the Puglia (Italy) experience, *Vaccine*, 18: S83–S85.

Graff, J., Ticehurst, J., and Flehmig, B. (1993) Detection of hepatitis A virus in sewage sludge by antigen capture polymerase chain reaction, *Appl. Environ. Microbiol.*, 59: 3165–3170.

Greco, D., Luzzi, I., Sallabanda, A., Dibra, A., Kaccarricy, E., and Shapo, L. (1995) Cholera in the Mediterranean: outbreak in Albania, *Eurosurveillance*, 0: 1–2.

Grinde, B., Stene-Johansen, K., Sharma, B., Hoel, T., Jensenius, M., and Skaug, K. (1997) Characterisation of an epidemic of hepatitis A virus involving intravenous drug abusers: infection by needle sharing?, *J. Med. Virol.*, 53: 69–75.

Haas, C.N. (1983) Estimation of risk due to low doses of microorganisms: a comparison of alternative methodologies, *Am. J. Epidemiol.*, 118: 573–582.

Hafliger, D., Gilgen, M., Luthy, J., and Hubner, P. (1997) Seminested RT-PCR systems for small round structured viruses and detection of enteric viruses in seafood, *Int. J. Food Microbiol.*, 37: 27–36.

Halliday, M.L., Kang, L.-Y., Zhou, T.K., Hu, M.-D., Pan, Q.-C., Fu, T.-Y., Huang, Y.-S., and Hu, S.-L. (1991) An epidemic of hepatitis A attributable to the ingestion of raw clams in Shanghai, China, *J. Infect. Dis.*, 164: 852–859.

Henning, K.J., Bell, E., Braun, J., and Barker, N.D. (1995) A community-wide outbreak of hepatitis A: risk factors for infection among homosexual and bisexual men, *Am. J. Med.*, 99: 132–136.

Hutin, Y.J., Pool, V., Cramer, E.H., Nainan, O.V., Weth, J., Williams, I.T., Goldstein, S.T., Gensheimer, K.F., Bell, B.P., Shapiro, C.N., Alter, M.J., and Margolis, H.S. (1999) A multistate, foodborne outbreak of hepatitis A: National Hepatitis A Investigation Team, *N. Engl. J. Med.*, 340: 595–602.

Jaykus, L.A., (2000) Enteric viruses as emerging agents of foodborne disease, *Irish J. Agric. Food Res.*, 39: 245–255.

Jaykus, L.A., Hemard, M.T., and Sobsey MD. (1994) Human enteric pathogenic viruses, in *Environmental Indicators and Shellfish Safety*, Hackney, C.R. and Peirson, M.D., Eds., Chapman & Hall, New York.

Jaykus, L.A., De Leon, R., and Sobsey, M.D. (1996) A virion concentration method for detection of human enteric viruses in oysters by PCR and oligoprobe hybridization, *Appl. Environ. Microbiol.*, 62: 2074–2080.

Kaic, B., Borcic, B., Ljubicic, M., Brkic, I., and Mihaljevic, I. (2001) Hepatitis A control in a refugee camp by active immunization, *Vaccine*, 19(27): 3615–3619.

Kingsley, D.H. and Richards, G.P. (2001) Rapid and efficient extraction method for reverse transcription–PCR detection of hepatitis A and Norwalk-like viruses in shellfish, *Appl. Environ. Microbiol.*, 67: 4152–4157.

Koff, R.S. (1998) Hepatitis A, *Lancet*, 351: 1643–1649.

Koopmans, M., von Bonsdorff, C.H., Vinjé, J., de Medici, D., and Monroe, S. (2002) Food-borne viruses, *FEMS Microbiol. Rev.*, 26: 187–205.

Kopecka, H., Dubrou, S., Prevot, J., Marechal, J., and Lopez-Pila, J.M. (1993) Detection of naturally occurring enteroviruses in waters by reverse transcription, polymerase chain reaction, and hybridization, *Appl. Environ. Microbiol.*, 59: 1213–1219.

Koster, D., Hofmann, F., and Berthold, H. (1990) Hepatitis A immunity in food-handling occupations, *Eur. J. Clin. Microbiol. Infect. Dis.*, 9: 304–305.

Le Guyader, F., Apaire-Marchais, V., Brillet, J., and Billaudel, S. (1993) Use of genomic probes to detect hepatitis A virus and enterovirus RNAs in wild shellfish and relationship of viral contamination to bacterial contamination *Appl. Environ. Microbiol.*, 59: 3963–3968.

Le Guyader, F., Dubois, E., Menard, D., and Pommepuy, M. (1994) Detection of hepatitis A virus, rotavirus, and enterovirus in naturally contaminated shellfish and sediment by reverse transcription–seminested PCR, *Appl. Environ. Microbiol.*, 60: 3665–3671.

Le Guyader, F., Haugarreau, L., Miossec, L., Dubois, E., and Pommepuy M. (2000) Three-year study to assess human enteric viruses in shellfish, *Appl. Environ. Microbiol.*, 66: 3241–3248.

Lees, D. (2000) Viruses and bivalve shellfish, *Int. J. Food Microbiol.*, 59: 81–116.

Lees, D.N., Henshilwood, K., and Dore, W.J. (1994) Development of a method for detection of enteroviruses in shellfish by PCR with poliovirus as a model, *Appl. Environ. Microbiol.*, 60: 2999–3005.

Leggitt, P.R. and Jaykus, L.A. (2000) Detection methods for human enteric viruses in representative foods, *J. Food Protect.*, 63: 1738–1744.

Lemon, S.M. (1997) An overview of the molecular virology and pathogenesis of type A viral hepatitis, in *Viral Hepatitis and Liver Disease*, Rizzetto, M., Purcell, R.H., Gerin, J.L., and Verme, G., Eds., Minerva Medica, Turin, pp. 559–561.

Lemon, S.M. and Robertson, B.H. (1993) Current perspective in the virology and molecular biology of hepatitis A virus, *Semin. Virol.*, 4: 285–295.

Leoni, E., Bevini, C., Degli Esposti, S., and Graziano, A. (1998) An outbreak of intrafamiliar hepatitis A associated with clam consumption: epidemic transmission to a school community, *Eur. J. Epidemiol.*, 14: 187–192.

Lopalco, P.L., Malfait, P., Salmaso, S., Germinario, C., Quarto, M., and Barbuti, S. (1997) A persisting outbreak of hepatitis A in Puglia, Italy, 1996: epidemiological follow up, *Eurosurveillance*, 2(4): 31–32.

Lopalco, P.L., Salleras, L., Barbuti, S., Germinario, C., Bruguera M., Buti, M., and Dominguez, A. (2000) Hepatitis A and B in children and adolescents: what can we learn from Puglia (Italy) and Catalonia (Spain)?, *Vaccine*, 19: 470–474.

Lopalco, P.L., Malfait, P., Menniti-Ippolito, F., Prato, R., Germinario, C., Chironna, M., Quarto, M., and Salmaso, S. (2004) Determinants of acquiring hepatitis A virus in a large Italian region in endemic and epidemic periods, *J. Viral. Hepat.*, in press.

Lopez-Sabater, E.I., Deng, M.Y., and Cliver, D.O. (1997) Magnetic immunoseparation PCR assay (MIPA) for detection of hepatitis A virus (HAV) in American oyster (*Crassostrea virginica*), *Lett. Appl. Microbiol.*, 24: 101–104.

Lowry, P.W., Levine, R., Stroup, D.F., Gunn, R.A., Wilder, M.H., and Konigsberg, C., Jr. (1989) Hepatitis A outbreak on a floating restaurant in Florida, 1986, *Am. J. Epidemiol.*, 129: 155–164.

Lucioni, C., Cipriani, V., Mazzi, S., and Pannunzio, M. (1998) Cost of an outbreak of hepatitis A in Puglia, Italy, *Pharmacoeconomics*, 13(2): 257–266.

Malfait, P., Lopalco, P.L., Salmaso, S., Germinario, C., Salamina, G., Quarto, M., and Barbuti, S. (1996) An outbreak of hepatitis A in Puglia, Italy, 1996, *Eurosurveillance*, 1(5): 33–35.

Mannucci, P.M. (1992) Outbreak of hepatitis A among Italian patients with haemophilia, *Lancet*, 339: 819.

Massoudi, M.S., Bell, B.P., Paredes, V., Insko, J., Evans, K., and Shapiro, C.N. (1999) An outbreak of hepatitis A associated with an infected foodhandler, *Public Health Reports*, 114: 157–164.

Mbayed, V.A., Sookoian, S., Alfonso, V., and Campos, R.H. (2002) Genetic characterization of hepatitis A virus isolates from Buenos Aires, Argentina, *J. Med. Virol.*, 68: 168–174.

Mead, P.S., Slutsker, L., Dietz, V., Mc Caig, L.F., Bresee, J.S., Shapiro, C., Griffin, P.M., and Tauxe, R.V. (1999) Food-related illness and death in the United States, *Emerging Infect. Dis.*, 5: 607–625.

Mele, A., Rastelli, M.G., Gill, O.N., di Bisceglie, D., Rosmini, F., Pardelli, G., Valtriani, C., and Patriarchi, P. (1989) Recurrent epidemic hepatitis A associated with consumption of raw shellfish, probably controlled through public health measures, *Am. J. Epidemiol.*, 130: 540–546.

Mele, A., Stroffolini, T., Palumbo, F., Gallo, G., Ragni, P., Balocchini, E., Tosti, M.E., Corona, R., Marzolini, A., and Moiraghi, A. (1997) Incidence of and risk factors for hepatitis A in Italy: public health indications from a 10-year surveillance, SEIEVA Collaborating Group, *J. Hepatol.*, 26: 743–747.

Melnick, J.L. (1982) Classification of hepatitis A virus as enterovirus type 72 and of hepatitis B virus as hepadnavirus type 1, *Intervirology*, 18: 105–106.

Minor, P.D. (1991) Picornaviridae, in *Classification of Nomenclature of Viruses: Fifth Report of the International Committee on Taxonomy of Viruses*, *Archives of Virology*, Suppl. 2, Francki, R.I.B., Fauquet, C.M., Knudson, D.L., and Brown, F., Eds., Springer-Verlag, Wien, pp. 320–326.

Morace, G., Aulicino, F.A., Angelozzi, C., Costanzo, L., Donadio, F., and Rapicetta, M. (2002) Microbial quality of wastewater: detection of hepatitis A virus by reverse transcriptase–polymerase chain reaction, *J. Appl. Microbiol.*, 92: 828–836.

Muniain-Mujika, I., Girones, R., Tofino-Quesada, G., Calvo, M., and Lucena, F. (2002) Depuration dynamics of viruses in shellfish, *Int. J. Food Microbiol.*, 77: 125–133.

Nainan, O.V., Margolis, H.S., Robertson, B.H., Balayan, M., and Brinton, M.A. (1991) Sequence analysis of a new hepatitis A virus naturally infecting cynomolgus macaques (*Macaca fascicularis*), *J. Gen. Virol.*, 72: 1685–1689.

Najarian, R., Caput, D., Gee, W., Potter, S.J., Renard, A., Merryweather, J., Van Nest, G., and Dina, D. (1985) Primary structure and gene organization of human hepatitis A virus, *Proc. Natl. Acad. Sci. U.S.A.*, 82: 2627–2631.

Niu, M.T., Polish, L.B., Robertson, B.H., Khanna, B.K., Woodruff, B.A., Shapiro, C.N., Miller, M.A., Smith, J.D., Gedrose, J.K., Alter, M.J., Margolis H.S., and the National Hepatitis A Investigation Team (1992) Multistate outbreak of hepatitis A associated with frozen strawberries, *J. Infect. Dis.*, 166: 518–524.

Nordenfelt, E. (1992) Hepatitis A in Swedish travellers, *Vaccine*, 10 (Suppl. 1): S73–S74.

Nordenfelt, E. (1997) Current epidemiological trends of viral hepatitis in northern Europe, in *Viral Hepatitis and Liver Disease*, Rizzetto, M., Purcell, R.H., Gerin, J.L., and Verme, G., Eds., Minerva Medica, Turin, pp. 545–550.

Normann, A., Pfisterer-Hunt, M., Schade, S., Graff, J., Chaves, R.L., Crovari, P., Icardi, G., and Flehmig, B. (1995) Molecular epidemiology of an outbreak of hepatitis A in Italy, *J. Med. Virol.*, 47: 467–471.

Papaevangelou, G. (1997) Current recommendations for control of hepatitis A, in *Viral Hepatitis and Liver Disease*, Rizzetto, M., Purcell, R.H., Gerin, J.L., and Verme, G., Eds., Minerva Medica, Turin, pp. 720–723.

Pebody, R.G., Leino, T., Ruutu, P., Kinnunen, L., Davidkin I., Nohynek, H., and Leinikki P. (1998) Foodborne outbreaks of hepatitis A in a low endemic country: an emerging problem?, *Epidemiol. Infect.*, 120: 55–59.

Pina, S., Buti, M., Jardì, R., Clemente-Casares, P., Jofre, J., and Girones, R. (2001) Genetic analysis of hepatitis A virus strains recovered from the environment and from patients with acute hepatitis, *J. Gen. Virol.*, 82: 2955–2963.

Potasman, I., Paz, A., and Odeh, M. (2002) Infectious outbreaks associated with bivalve shellfish consumption: a worldwide perspective, *Clin. Infect. Dis.*, 35: 921–928.

Ramsay, C.N. and Upton, P.A. (1989) Hepatitis A and frozen raspberries, *Lancet*, 1: 43–44.

Redlinger, T.E., O'Rourke, K., and Van Derslice, J. (1997) Hepatitis A among schoolchildren in a U.S.–Mexico border community, *Am. J. Public Health*, 87: 1715–1717.

Reid, T.M. and Robinson, H.G. (1987) Frozen raspberries and hepatitis A, *Epidemiol. Infect.*, 98: 109–112.

Rippey, S.R. (1994) Infectious diseases associated with molluscan shellfish consumption, *Clin. Microbiol. Rev.*, 7: 419–425.

Robertson, B.H. and Nainan, O.V. (1997) Genetic and antigenic variants of hepatitis A virus, in *Viral Hepatitis and Liver Disease*, Rizzetto, M., Purcell, R.H., Gerin, J.L., and Verme, G., Eds., Minerva Medica, Turin, pp. 14–18.

Robertson, B.H., Jansen, R.W., Khanna, B., Totsuka, A., Nainan, O.V., Siegl, G., Widell, A., Margolis, H., Isomura, S., Ito, K., Ishizu, T., Moritsugu, Y., and Lemon, S.M. (1992) Genetic relatedness of hepatitis A virus strains recovered from different geographical regions, *J. Gen. Virol.*, 73: 1365–1377.

Robertson, B.H., Averhoff, F., Cromeans, T.L., Han, X., Khoprasert, B., Nainan, O.V., Rosenberg, J., Paikoff, L., DeBess, E., Shapiro, C.N., and Margolis, H.S. (2000) Genetic relatedness of hepatitis A virus isolates during a community-wide outbreak, *J. Med. Virol.*, 62: 144–150.

Romalde, J.L., Area, E., Sànchez, G., Ribao, C., Torrado, I., Abad, F.X., Pinto, R.M., Barja, J.L., and Bosch, A. (2002) Prevalence of enterovirus and hepatitis A virus in bivalve molluscs from Galicia (NW Spain): inadequacy of the EU standards of microbiological quality, *Int. J. Food Microbiol.*, 74: 119–130.

Romalde, J.L., Torrado, I., Ribao, C., and Barja, J.L. (2001) Global market: shellfish imports as a source of reemerging food-borne hepatitis A virus infections in Spain, *Int. Microbiology*, 4: 223–226.

Roos, R. (1956) Hepatitis epidemic conveyed by oyster, *Sven Lakartidningen*, 53: 989–1003.

Rosenberg, S.A., Lotze, M.T., Muul, L.M., Chang, A.E., Avis, F.P., Leitman, S., Linehan, W.M., Robertson, C.N., Lee, R.E., Rubin, J.T. et al. (1987) A progress report on the treatment of 157 patients with advanced cancer using lymphokine-activated killer cells and interleukin-2 or high-dose interleukin-2 alone, *N. Engl. J. Med.*, 316: 889–897.

Rosenblum, L.S., Mirkin, I.R., Allen, D.T., Safford, S., and Hadler, S.C. (1990) A multifocal outbreak of hepatitis A traced to commercially distributed lettuce, *Am. J. Public Health*, 80: 1075–1079.

Sagliocca, L., Amoroso, P., Stroffolini, T., Adamo, B., Tosti, M.E., Lettieri, G., Esposito, C., Buonocore, S., Pierri, P., and Mele, A. (1999) Efficacy of hepatitis A vaccine in prevention of secondary hepatitis A infection: a randomised trial, *Lancet*, 353: 1136–1139.

Sair, A.I., D'Souza, D.H., Moe, C.L., and Jaykus, L.A. (2002), Improved detection of human enteric viruses in foods by RT-PCR, *J. Virolog. Meth.*, 100: 57–69.

Sànchez, G., Pintò, R.M., Vanaclocha, H., and Bosch, A. (2002) Molecular characterization of hepatitis A virus isolates from a transcontinental shellfish-borne outbreak, *J. Clin. Microbiol.*, 40: 4148–4155.

Schlundt, J. (2002) New directions in foodborne disease prevention, *Int. J. Food Microbiol.*, 78: 3–17.

Schultheiss, T., Kusov, Y.Y., and Gauss-Muller, V. (1994) Proteinase 3C of hepatitis A virus (HAV) cleaves the HAV polyprotein P2–P3 et al. sites including VP1/2A and 2A/2B, *Virology*, 198: 275–281.

Schwab, K.J., Neill, F.H., Fankhauser, R.L., Daniels, N.A., Monroe, S.S., Bergmire-Sweat, D.A., Estes, M.K., and Atmar, R.L. (2000) Development of methods to detect "Norwalk-like viruses" (NLVs) and hepatitis A virus in delicatessen foods: application to a foodborne NLV outbreak, *Appl. Environ. Microbiol.*, 66: 213–218.

Shieh, Y.C., Calci, K.R., and Baric, R.S. (1999) A method to detect low levels of enteric viruses in contaminated oysters, *Appl. Environ. Microbiol.*, 65: 4709–4714.

Sidal, M., Unuvar, E., Oguz, F., Cihan, C., Onel, D., and Badur, S. (2001) Age-specific seroepidemiology of hepatitis A, B, and E infections among children in Istanbul, Turkey, *Eur. J. Epidemiol.*, 17: 141–144.

Staes, C. J., Schlenker, T.L., Risk, I., Cannon, K.G., Harris, H., Pavia, A.T., Shapiro, C.N., and Bell, B.P. (2000) Sources of infection among person with acute hepatitis A and no identified risk factors during a sustained community-wide outbreak, *Pediatrics*, 106(4): E54.

Steffen, R., Kane, M.A., Shapiro, C.N., Billo, N., Schoellhorn, K.J., and van Damme, P. (1994) Epidemiology and prevention of hepatitis A in travelers, *JAMA*, 272: 885–889.

Stene-Johansen, K., Jenum, P.A., Hoel, T., Blystad, H., Sunde, H., and Skaug, K. (2002) An outbreak of hepatitis A among homosexuals linked to a family outbreak, *Epidemiol. Infect.*, 129: 113–117.

Stroffolini, T., Bigini, W., Lorenzoni, L., Palazzesi, G.P., Divizia, M., and Frongillo, R. (1990) An outbreak of hepatitis A in young adults in central Italy, *Eur. J. Epidemiol.*, 6: 156–159.

Stroffolini, T., Mele, A., and Sagliocca, L. (2001) Vaccination policy against hepatitis A in Italy, *Vaccine*, 19: 2404–2406.

Tanaka, J. (2000) Hepatitis A shifting epidemiology in Latin America, *Vaccine*, 18: S57–S60.

Taylor, M.B. (1997) Molecular epidemiology of South African strains of hepatitis A virus: 1982–1996, *J. Med. Virol.*, 51: 273–279.

Tufenkeji, H. (2000) Hepatitis A shifting epidemiology in the Middle East and Africa, *Vaccine*, 18: S65–S67.

Van Damme, P. and Bell, B. (2001) Hepatitis A: how to match prevention strategies to changing epidemiology, *Vaccine*, 19: 999–1002.

Van Damme, P., Mathei, C., Thoelen, S., Meheus, A., Safary, A., and Andre, F.E. (1994) Single dose inactivated hepatitis A vaccine: rationale and clinical assessment of the safety and immunogenicity, *J. Med. Virol.*, 44: 435–441.

Vento, S., Garofano, T., Renzini, C., Cainelli, F., Casali, F., Ghironzi, G., Ferraro, T., and Concia, E. (1998) Fulminant hepatitis associated with hepatitis A virus superinfection in patients with chronic hepatitis C, *N. Engl. J. Med.*, 338: 286–290.

Weitz, M., Baroudy, B.M., Maloy, W.L., Ticehurst, J.R., and Purcell, R.H. (1986) Detection of a genome-linked protein (VPg) of hepatitis A virus and its comparison with other picornaviral VPgs, *J. Virol.*, 60: 124–130.

Weltman, A.C., Bennett, N.M., Ackman, D.A., Misage, J.H., Campana, J.J., Fine, L.S., Doniger, A.S., Balzano, G.J., and Birkhead, G.S. (1996) An outbreak of hepatitis A associated with a bakery, New York, 1994: the 1968 "West Branch, Michigan" outbreak repeated, *Epidemiol. Infect.*, 117: 333–341.

WHO. (2000). Resolution WHA53.15 on Food Safety, Fifty-Third World Health Assembly, World Health Organization, Geneva, Switzerland.

Wu, J., Zou, S., and Giulivi, A. (2001) Current hepatitis A in Canada, *Can. J. Infect. Dis.*, 12: 341–344.

Yotsuyanagi, H., Koike, K., Yasuda, K., Moriya, K., Shintani, Y., Fujie, H., Kurokawa, K., and Iino, S. (1996) Prolonged fecal excretion of hepatitis A virus in adult patients with hepatitis A as determined by polymerase chain reaction, *Hepatology*, 24: 10–13.

5 β-Nitropropionic Acid in the Diet: Toxicity Aspects

*Madhusudan G. Soni, Ioana G. Carabin,
James C. Griffiths, and George A. Burdock*

CONTENTS

Abstract   Various fungi of the genus *Arthrinium*, as well as *Aspergillus* and *Penicillium*, are known to produce β-nitropropionic acid (NPA), and the presence of NPA has been detected in at least four families of higher plants. Although consumption of foods containing NPA is widespread, human poisoning by NPA is rare and limited to situations involving egregious mishandling of food products. As a fungal metabolite, NPA has poisoned both people and grazing animals. In northern China, fungi growing on sugarcane stored over the winter were responsible for at least 885 cases of poisoning and 88 deaths between 1972 and 1989. Orally ingested NPA is rapidly absorbed from the gastrointestinal tract into the circulation and is metabolized to nitrite, although in certain conditions NPA may bind succinate dehydrogenase upon oxidation. The primary mechanism of toxicity of NPA is as an irreversible inhibitor of a mitochondrial membrane enzyme, succinate dehydrogenase, which catalyzes the oxidation of succinate to fumarate. This inhibition in experimental animals is manifested as a pathological change in striatal areas of the brain that resembles the course of Huntington's disease in humans. In recent years, this resemblance has been extensively exploited to understand the mechanisms of neurodegeneration. Ingestion of sub-threshold doses of NPA does not result in irreversible damage nor does the NPA accumulate in the body. The oral LD_{50} dose of NPA for mice and rats is between 77 and 100 mg/kg. In chronic experimental studies, NPA has not exhibited carcinogenicity or chronic toxicity. Based on the results of chronic rat studies, the no-observed-adverse-effect level (NOAEL) for NPA has been determined to be 2.5 mg/kg/day. Results of genotoxicity studies are equivocal, but positive assays can be traced back to the use of a single impure sample of NPA. On the basis of a NOAEL of 2.5 mg/kg/day from the chronic rodent bioassay and applying a safety factor of 100, an acceptable daily intake (ADI) of 25 µg/kg/day, or 1.5 mg/day for a 60-kg individual, is appropriate.

Key Words   *excitotoxicity, Huntington's disease, mitochondrial toxin, neurodegeneration, β-nitropropionic acid, safety*

HISTORICAL PERSPECTIVE

Mycotoxins, produced by several genera of molds, are natural contaminants of cereals and other commodities throughout the world, particularly in tropical countries. One of the mycotoxins, β-nitropropionic acid (CAS No. 504-88-1; also referred to as 3-nitropropionic acid, NPA, or hiptagenic acid) is also found in at least four families of higher plants and in insects. NPA may be unique among toxins because of its common, widespread occurrence in nature. Further, although the method of biosynthesis may vary between life forms (i.e., via aspartate or malonate), the evolutionary purpose of this substance in all species appears to be as a defense against predators.

Livestock poisoning via consumption of forage plants containing high amounts of NPA (e.g., as much as 26,000 ppm) can produce significant toxic effects, up to and including death. Much of the research on NPA has been driven because of the economic losses sustained from loss of pasture as the result of NPA-containing plants, many of which had been mistakenly introduced as a source of forage. Humans have a history of exposure to NPA because of its natural presence in certain food preparations and as a contaminant in foods. Human exposure to NPA has also occurred for centuries from (processed) karaka tree nuts in New Zealand, where the nuts were eaten as a dietary staple by Maori tribesmen, and from the fungi *Aspergillus* and *Penicillium* used in the production of Oriental dietary staples including *miso* (fermented soybean paste) and *katsuobushi* (fermented dry bonito). Accidental poisonings of NPA have been reported resulting from consumption of unprocessed karaka tree nuts and moldy sugarcane.

β-Nitropropionic acid has been extensively studied for its mechanism of action, and it has been shown to act as a reversible inhibitor of fumarase and aspartase and as an irreversible, non-competitive inhibitor of succinate dehydrogenase, an electron acceptor and a part of mitochondrial Complex II. The specific site of toxicity in mammals is a high-energy consumptive portion of the brain, which undergoes irreversible change upon receiving a threshold dose. No irreversible effects of sub-threshold doses of NPA exposure have been found, and no accumulation of NPA in the body has been reported. This review highlights the toxicological aspects of NPA found in the diet and critically evaluates the information available on the safety of NPA in animals and humans, including nonclinical studies and published case reports.

DESCRIPTION

β-Nitropropionic acid is a white crystalline solid with a melting point of 63 to 65°C. It has the empirical formula $C_3H_5NO_4$ (Figure 5.1) and has been assigned CAS Registry Number 504-88-1. The name given for NPA by CAS in the 9th Collective Index of Chemical Names is *propionic acid, 3-nitro-*, but several legitimate synonyms are commonly used (Table 5.1). NPA has been isolated from *Streptomyces* found in soil and occurs as a metabolite of a number of fungal species of *Aspergillus* and *Penicillium* (fungi make only NPA, not the esters as do higher plants) (Gustine, 1979). These fungal genera are commonly present in several Oriental fermented foodstuffs in which NPA has been identified. NPA has also been isolated from plants and nuts. General descriptive parameters of NPA along with physical and chemical properties are summarized in Table 5.1.

$$O_2N-CH_2-CH_2-COOH$$

FIGURE 5.1 Chemical structure of β-nitropropionic acid (NPA); note the attachment of the nitro function on the β-carbon.

TABLE 5.1

General Descriptive Characteristics of β-Nitropropionic Acid

Parameter	Description
Primary name	3-Nitropropionic acid
Chemical formula	$C_3H_5NO_4$
Synonyms	β-Nitropropionic acid; BNP; bovinocidin; hiptagenic acid; NCI-C03076; 3-nitropropionic acid; propionic acid, 3-nitro; propanoic acid, 3-nitro
Physical description	Crystals; gold crystalline solid
Molecular weight	119.08
Melting point	63 to 65°C
Solubility	Water; ethanol; chloroform

OCCURRENCE Of β-NITROPROPIONIC ACID

Glucose esters of NPA found in the *Coronilla*, *Astragalus*, and *Indigofera* genera of the Leguminosae family of plants, as well as other families (Table 5.2), are the primary source of the toxic nitroaliphatic compounds producing animal toxicity. The glucoside of β-nitropropionic alcohol (NPOH), a miserotoxin, was first isolated from *Astragalus miser* var. *oblongifolius* by Stermitz et al. (1969). Subsequently, it has been detected in a number of other species. In these plant species, the amount of NPA (as NPA, NPOH, or as NO_2, depending on the method of analysis) ranges from <1 ppm to 26,000 ppm. Williams and Gomez-Sosa (1986) have identified 32 species of *Astragalus* specific to Argentina with 2000 to 13,000 ppm NPA (as NO_2) in the leaves. Recently, Ebrahimzadeh et al. (1999) detected nitro compounds in concentrations of 2 to 25 mg NO_2 per g (2000 to 25,000 ppm NO_2) of plants in 37 of 440 (8.4%) of species of *Astragalus* tested from Iran. As early as 1822, the presence of NPA-bearing forage plants from all countries has been documented (Williams, 1981). Most of the livestock losses have been attributed to consumption of crownvetch (*Coronilla varia*, Fabaceae), milkvetch (*Astragalus* spp.), and creeping indigo (*Indigofera endeca-phylla*). Some of these plants had been introduced as sources of forage prior to the knowledge that they were capable of producing the toxin (Williams and Davis, 1982).

The ester variants of NPA (glucose esters) in *Coronilla varia* are the six mono-esters, two diesters (cibarian and coronarian), and three triesters (coronillin, karakin, and corollin). Concentrations of the esters, when measured in freeze-dried plant material, reached a maximum of 20 mg NO_2 per g in the flowers and 12 mg NO_2 per g in the leaves, with lower levels found in the stems and roots. One of the diesters (cibarian) and one triester (karakin) comprised approximately two thirds of the total esters in the leaves and were present in nearly equal amounts (Gustine, 1979). NPA is also found as an ester in the glycoside hiptagen in the bark of the Javanese *Hiptage mandablanta* tree (Alston et al., 1985).

β-Nitropropionic acid (as NPOH) is an exocrine chemical defense of the chry-somelid beetle (*Chrysomela tremulae*). The beetle secretes two δ-3-isoxazolin-5-one glucosides, one of which hydrolyzes to yield NPOH upon ingestion by the predator.

TABLE 5.2
Higher Plants Reported To Contain β-Nitropropionic Acid

Family	Genus and Species	
Malpighiaceae	*Hiptage mandablanta*	
	Hiptage benghalensis (L.) Kurz	
	Heteropteris angustifolia Gris.	
Corynocarpaceae	*Corynocarpus similes*	
	Corynocarpus laevagatus J.R. and G. Forst.	
Violaceae	*Viola odorata*	
Leguminosae	*Astragalus candadensis* L.	*Astragalus robbinsii* (Oakes) Gray
	Astragalus cibarius Sheld.	*Indigofera spicata* Forsk.
	Astragalus collinus Dougl.	*Indigofera suffruticosa*
	Astragalus emoryanus Rydb.	*Indigofera endecaphylla*
	Astragalus falcatus	*Coronilla varia* L.
	Astragalus flexuosis (Hook.) Don	*Lotus corniculatus*
	Astragalus hamosus	*Lotus pedunculatus*
	Astragalus miser	

Source: Adapted from Gustine, D.L., *Crop Science*, 19, 197–203, 1979.

The toxins are stored in extracellular vesicles and secreted onto the dorsum of the gold-metallic-colored beetle (Pasteels et al., 1989). The nitrogen source for the glycosides and the NPA in beetles was found to be L-aspartic acid (Randoux et al., 1991). The beetles convert the aspartate to β-aminopropanoic acid or *N*-hydroxyaspartic acid, then either of these to *N*-hydroxy-β-aminopropanoic acid, and from there to β-nitropropanoic acid or isoxazolidin-5-one and to δ-3-isoxazolin-5-one (Pasteels et al., 1989).

Other natural sources of NPA include an unidentified fungus from zinnia (*Zinnia elegans*) leaves (Kamikawa et al., 1980), the fungus *Melanconis thelebola* from red alder trees (*Alnus rubra* Bong.) and tomato plants (Evidente et al., 1992), and the fungus *Septoria cirsii*, introduced to control Canada thistle (Hershenhorn et al., 1993). NPA is also found in the karaka tree, the distribution of which is confined to New Zealand and the Chatham Islands. At one time, karaka nuts were used as a staple vegetable by the indigenous Maori tribes, but in recent years the tree is primarily used for decorative purposes. Karaka nuts were prepared by baking the fruit in earthen ovens for several hours, washing them for a day or two to remove the toxin and to loosen and remove the skin and flesh, and then drying the karaka kernels in the sun (Bell, 1974). The concentration of the toxin ranges from 0.025% in green berries and 0.08% in ripe berries to 0.03% in fresh nuts (Bell, 1974). An early report, in 1871, described the toxicity in children following consumption of the unprocessed nuts. In 1886, karaka nut toxicity in cattle was reported, and in 1918 it was reported for pigs. A report of honeybee mortality as the result of attraction to the flowers of the karaka tree (Bell, 1974) indicates that the toxin may not be confined to the nuts alone. Carter (1951) described the toxin extracted from nuts as a glucoside, 1,4,6-tris-(β-nitropropionyl) D-glycopyranose ($C_{15}H_{21}O_{15}N_3$), which could be hydrolyzed to yield three molecules of NPA.

Another source of NPA exposure for humans is by economically valuable fungi, such as *Aspergillus* sp. and *Penicillium* sp., which are used in starter cultures (called *tane-koji*) for the fermentation of soy bean paste for *miso*, dried bonito fish flesh for *katsuobushi*, and other products (Kinosita et al., 1968; Orth, 1977). Although not all *miso* contains NPA, the average daily *miso* consumption is reported to be 32.7 g by rural Japanese and 26.1 g by city dwellers (Kinosita et al., 1968). For another possible NPA-containing product, *katsuobushi*, no quantitative data on consumption are available, although consumption in rural areas is "fairly large" (Kinosita et al., 1968). Processing plants manufacturing the *katsuobushi* also produce a widely eaten appetizer called *shuto* or *shiokara*, which is made from the washed and fermented intestines of the bonito. The fermentation organism used is the same for *katsuobushi*, but consumption data for *shuto* are not available. Other products produced by the same starter cultures may include soy sauce (*shoyu*) and *sake* or rice wine (Kinosita et al., 1968).

In a series of studies, Kinosita et al. (1968) investigated the presence of mycotoxins in fermented foods. These investigators isolated *Aspergillus oryzae* from starter cultures from a commercial production facility in Los Angeles, California, and from starter cultures and food samples obtained from commercial food production facilities in Japan, from rural areas where small shops maintain fungal cultures, and from households where cultures of wild strains are kept and passed down from one generation to another. Starter cultures were also obtained from Honolulu, Hawaii, and fermented soybean paste was obtained from South Korea. A total of 37 strains of fungi were isolated from 24 samples of foodstuffs, and the amount of NPA in each was determined (Table 5.3). Kinosita et al. (1968) reported "trace" amounts of NPA in several of these samples. Assuming that "trace" is equal to one tenth of the lowest reported amount (0.1 mg/kg), the cultures found to have trace amounts contained 0.01 mg NPA per liter. This being the case, and if those cultures producing zero are excluded, then the average potential NPA production in these fermented foods is approximately 0.17 mg/mL. Based on these assumptions and a daily reported consumption of 29.4 g of *miso*, the daily intake of NPA from *miso* alone could be as much as 5.0 mg/day. Disappearance data indicate that Japanese consume approximately 9.8 L soy sauce (*shoyu*) per person per year (Uchida, 1989) and 500 mL per person per year in the United States (Burdock et al., 2001). On the basis of a Japanese consumption rate of 2.7 mL/day (assuming that only one tenth of the soy sauce is actually consumed, and the remainder is left on plates and utensils), the daily intake of NPA from soy sauce would be approximately 0.46 mg/day. Thus, NPA consumption from *miso* and soy sauce would be approximately 5.5 mg/day.

Cheese is also a good medium for the growth of fungi. Iwasaki and Kosikowski (1973) identified NPA in 5 of 18 cheeses they examined: Fontina, Geitmelshe Kaas, Le Sanglier, Pave De Moyan, and Fontinelli (Table 5.4). Orth (1977) also studied the growth of 16 different strains of *Aspergillus oryzae* and found that seven strains produced from 1.9 to 43.6 mg NPA per liter of culture. Using *Aspergillus oryzae* ATCC 12892 and *Aspergillus oryzae* Higati, Iwasaki and Kosikowski (1973) and Penel (1977) examined the potential for these molds to produce NPA on commonly

TABLE 5.3
Reported Occurrence of β-Nitropropionic Acid in *Katsuobushi*, *Miso*, and *Shoyu*

Natural Source	Source Organism	NPA (mg/mL medium) Medium 1[a]	Medium 2[a]
Katsuobushi	*Penicillium cyclopium*	Trace	0
Miso and *shoyu*	*Aspergillus* sp.	Trace	0
Miso and *shoyu*	*A. glaucus* group	Trace	0
Miso and *shoyu*	*Aspergillus* sp.	0.3	0
Miso and *shoyu*	*A. versicolor* group	0.2	0
Miso and *shoyu*	*P. chrysogenum*	Trace	0
Miso and *shoyu*	*A. oryzae*	Trace	0
Miso and *shoyu*	*A. soyae*	0.2	0
Miso and *shoyu*	*A. soyae*	Trace	0
Miso and *shoyu*	*A. oryzae*	Trace	0
Miso and *shoyu*	*A. soyae*	0.1	Trace
Miso and *shoyu*	*A. soyae*	0.4	0
Miso and *shoyu*	*A. candidus* group	1.1	Trace
Miso and *shoyu*	*A. flavus* group	0	Trace

[a] Medium 1, glucose-ammonium nitrate; medium 2, supplemented Czapeck Dox medium.

Source: Adapted from Kinosita, R. et al., *Cancer Res.* 28, 2296–2311, 1968.

eaten foods (Table 5.5). These studies indicate that contaminated foods also provide a source of NPA exposure. Liu et al. (1989, 1992) reported that these species produced as much as 1600 to 1700 ppm NPA in culture. In another study, Wei et al. (1994) demonstrated production of NPA by the strains identified by Liu and his associates and by other ATCC fungal strains (Table 5.6). Wei et al. (1994) also demonstrated

TABLE 5.4
Levels of β-Nitropropionic Acid Detected in Stock Cultures

Mold	NPA (mg/L culture)
Aspergillus oryzae ATCC 12892	1279
A. oryzae Higati	111
A. oryzae ATCC 7252	40
A. flavus (oryzae) ATCC 11500	17
A. oryzae ATCC 11494	1

Source: Adapted from Iwasaki, T. and Kosikowski, F.V., *J. Food Sci.*, 38, 1162–1165, 1973.

TABLE 5.5
β-Nitropropionic Acid Production
by *Aspergillus oryzae* ATCC 12892
in Commonly Consumed Foods

Substrate	NPA (mg/kg)
Cheese	248
Cheese[a]	111
Banana	20
Peanut	15
Cheddar cheese	12
White potato	5
Yellow sweet potato	1

[a] Produced by *A. oryzae* Higati.

Source: Adapted from Iwasaki, T. and Kosikowski, F.V., *J. Food Sci.*, 38, 1162–1165, 1973; Penel, A.J., β-Nitropropionic Acid in Foods with Reference to *Aspergillus oryzae* (ATCC 12892), UMI Dissertation Services, Ann Arbor, MI, 1977.

NPA production by *Arthrinium sacchari* in several media under different conditions of growth. Porter and Bright (1987) reported that *Penicillium atrovenetum* produced 2000 mg NPA per liter of culture. Majak and Pass (1989) confirmed NPA production by *P. atrovenetum*. *Arthrinium* species, including *A. sacchari*, *A. saccharicola*, and *A. phaeospermum*, have been shown to be the organisms responsible for mass poisonings in China through production of NPA in improperly stored sugarcane.

These studies suggest that consumption of NPA by humans is likely through consumption of both commercially and domestically prepared foodstuffs using fungi and through unintentional exposure from fungi-contaminated foods. The National Cancer Institute (NCI), in its rationale for suggesting a carcinogenicity study on NPA, also raised the question of long-term consumption of NPA from food preparations and as a contaminant in foods (NCI, 1978).

BIOSYNTHESIS

In 1920, Gorter first isolated NPA as hiptagenic acid, which was later correctly identified by Carter and McChesney (1949). Glucose esters of NPA have been characterized from several plant species, including creeping indigo (*Indigofera endecaphylla*), *Viola odorata*, various *Astragalus* species, crownvetch, and *Lotus pedunculatus*. It is also produced by a number of fungi, including *Aspergillus flavus*, *A. wentii*, *A. oryzae*, *Penicillium atrovenetum*, *Arthrinium sacchari*, *A. saccharicola*, and *A. phaeospermum* (Hamilton et al., 2000). Biosynthesis studies of NPA were originally conducted with the ascomycete fungus *Penicillium atrovenetum* (Majak

TABLE 5.6
Species of *Arthrinium* Reported To Produce
β-Nitropropionic Acid

Fungi	ATCC Strains	Maximum NPA Concentrations (μg/mL)
Arthrinium sacchari	76289	716
	76290	295
	76981	1716
Arthrinium phaeospermum	24357	1620
	76291	1593
Arthrinium sereaenis	24358	1527
Arthrinium aureum	56042	1211
Arthrinium terminalis	76309	692

Source: Adapted from Wei, D.-L. et al., *Curr. Microbiol.*, 28, 1–5, 1994.

and Pass, 1989). Shaw (1967) studied incorporation of radiolabeled amino acids into NPA by growing cultures of *P. atrovenetum*. Both the amino group and the carbon skeleton of aspartic acid were found to be involved in the synthesis of NPA.

Shaw and McCloskey (1967) reported that in cultures of *P. atrovenetum* grown on ^{15}N- and ^{18}O-labeled substrates, ammonium ion was used for the synthesis of the nitro group in preference to nitrate. The amino group of aspartic acid was utilized in preference (approximately 2:1) to the ammonium ion for the synthesis of the nitro group. Also, [3-^{14}C]- and [4-^{14}C]-aspartic acids were incorporated equally well into NPA; L-[4-^{14}C]-aspartic acid, but not the corresponding D-isomer, was incorporated into the nitro compound. These studies supported the earlier conclusions that both the amino group and the carbon skeleton of aspartic acid are involved in the synthesis of NPA. Baxter et al. (1992) hypothesized that the *P. atrovenetrum* biosynthetic pathway involved conversion of L-aspartate to nitrosuccinate via oxidation of the amino group, followed by decarboxylation of the nitrosuccinate to NPA.

These and other investigators also reported that the biosynthesis of NPA appears to occur by very different routes in fungi compared to higher plants (Baxter et al., 1992; Candish et al., 1969). In higher plants (*Indigofera spicata*), malonate and malonylhydroxamate were likely precursors of NPA. In earlier studies, Gustine (1979) suggested that malonate may play a role in nitroaliphatics of *I. spicata* and demonstrated that ^{15}N-labeled nitropropanol was incorporated into cibarian ester in *Astragalus cibarius*. Shaw and DeAngelo (1969) concluded that NPA synthesis is probably not directly associated with the metabolism of inorganic nitrogen compounds and that an organic pathway for the formation of the nitro group is more likely.

The influence of growth temperature on the concentration of NPA in various plant parts of crownvetch forage (*Coronilla varia*) was studied by Faix et al. (1978). With increasing growth temperature, NPA formation increased, and the most consistent increase occurred in the stem tips and leaflets. These investigators concluded that higher growth temperatures can increase NPA production in crownvetch forage and that the overall yield can be a function of the leafiness of the forage. In *Penicillium atrovenetum*, abrupt and reproducibly large quantities (2 g/L) of NPA secretion were noted on day 5 after inoculation into medium (Porter and Bright, 1987). Becker (1967) reported degradation of NPA by mold, and the rate of oxidation of NPA to nitrate by cultures of *Aspergillus flavus* was linear. For each micromole of NPA assimilated by the mold, 1 μmol of nitrate was detected. NPA was readily oxidized at pH 3.8 but not at pH 6.8. In the presence of glucose, nitrate was not detected until after all of the glucose had been utilized. Becker (1967) attributed the effect of glucose to the inhibition of NPA uptake and also to its role as an electron donor for a nitrate reductase. Gruner et al. (1972) reported that an enzyme system found in *P. atrovenetum* extracts catalyzes the degradation of NPA to nitrite, nitrate, and unidentified carbon compounds. These investigators suggested that more than one enzyme is involved in the degradation of NPA and that this system may be responsible for the production of nitrite and nitrate by growing cultures of *P. atrovenetum*.

CHEMICAL ANALYSIS

β-Nitropropionic acid in plants, animals, and microorganisms can be determined by one of three analytical techniques: thin-layer chromatography (TLC), gas–liquid chromatography (GLC), or high-performance liquid chromatography (HPLC).

THIN-LAYER CHROMATOGRAPHY

As extensive removal of interfering substances is generally not necessary in this procedure, many of the interferences from the sample matrix are well separated from and do not mask the NPA spot. Moskowitz and Cayle (1974) identified NPA in crude biological extracts by TLC. The sample is extracted with ether at pH 2.0 to 2.5 and evaporated to dryness. The residue is dissolved in 1.0 mL acetone and spotted on silica gel plates for either one- or two-dimensional TLC. This approach can detect a quantity as small as 30 μg in a large excess of contaminating materials. Several different solvent systems can be employed in these determinations. Paterson (1986) used TLC on silica gel with a toluene–ethyl-acetate–90% formic acid eluting solvent. The author determined and compared the retention factors of 107 secondary metabolites (including NPA) of 304 *Penicillium* strains. Benn et al. (1989) employed silica gel TLC using a solvent system of chloroform–acetone containing 1% water to quantitate NPA. In this method, the compound is visualized with diazotized *p*-nitroaniline spray. In another method, Evidente et al. (1992) employed TLC on silica gel with an *n*-butanol–acetic-acid–water eluting solvent, and the NPA spot was developed with iodine and/or by spraying with 0.5% ninhydrin in acetone, followed by heating at 110°C for 10 minutes.

GAS CHROMATOGRAPHY

In these methods, removal or clean-up of the sample matrix and other interferences is critical, as the signal from trace amounts of the compound of interest may be covered up or rendered difficult to detect. Gilbert et al. (1977) developed a sensitive GLC method for quantitation of NPA based on extraction, isolation, and derivatization of the compound to its pentafluorobenzyl derivative and detection by an electron affinity detector. The method was applied to mold filtrates and cheeses with limits of detection of approximately 1 and 3 ppm, respectively.

HIGH-PERFORMANCE LIQUID CHROMATOGRAPHY

This method has the potential for determining a wide variety of substances, as it does not require the volatility needed for GLC and is usually far more sensitive than TLC. Muir and Majak (1984) separated and determined NPA in plasma by reverse-phase HPLC on 15- and 30-cm octadecylsilane on silica columns protected by guard columns. Plasma samples were obtained by low-speed centrifugation of heparinized whole blood treated with cold 0.6-*N* perchloric acid and chilled. The supernatant of the centrifuged sample was used for analysis. Elution was performed isocratically with 0.15% orthophosphoric acid (adjusted to pH 2.0) at 1 mL/min. NPA was quantified using an external standard and a variable wavelength detector set at 210 nm. Frisvad and Thrane (1987) developed a method for the analysis of mycotoxins and other fungal metabolites based on HPLC with an alkylphenone retention index and photodiode-array detection combined with TLC in two different eluents. The investigators reported retention characteristics of NPA and 181 other mycotoxins and related compounds.

MECHANISM OF ACTION

The primary mechanism of the toxic action of NPA is as a "suicide" substrate of succinate dehydrogenase, a mitochondrial membrane enzyme that catalyzes the oxidation of succinate to fumarate. NPA toxicity is manifested as a pathological change in the striatal areas of the brain. It also induces reversible inhibition of fumarase and aspartase (an enzyme not present in humans). Other enzymes inhibited by NPA include isocitrate lyase and possibly rat brain acetylcholinesterase (Ludolph et al., 1991). Systemic administration of NPA to rodents results in clinical symptoms similar to those observed in Huntington's disease (HD) (Brouillet et al., 1993a; Ludolph et al., 1991). NPA preferentially affects the basal ganglia (Vecsei et al., 1998). NPA induces selective lesions in the striatum by a process that appears to involve secondary oxidative stress followed by a loss of adenosine triphosphate (ATP). Its toxicity also appears to be age dependent.

INHIBITION OF SUCCINATE DEHYDROGENASE

At physiological pH, the isoelectronic form of NPA can be converted to the highly reactive dianion, which irreversibly inhibits succinate dehydrogenase (Hamilton et al., 2000). This inhibition has been proposed as the biochemical basis of NPA toxicity. Alston et al. (1977) reported that NPA is an isoelectronic analog of succinate. Based on the results of a series of *in vitro* studies, these investigators demonstrated that 3-nitropropionate carbanion is a highly specific, time-dependent, and irreversible inhibitor of succinate dehydrogenase. By analogy, with regard to the reaction of nitroethane with D-amino acid oxidase, the results of these investigations are consistent with the hypothesis that the carbanionic inhibitor forms a covalent N-5 adduct with the active site, flavin. Hence, toxicity of NPA is due to the irreversible blockage of the Krebs cycle by 3-nitropropionate carbanion.

Subsequent experiments by Coles et al. (1979) confirmed the proposed mechanism of action of NPA. In these experiments, purified, soluble preparations of succinate dehydrogenase (SDH) from beef heart and a stoichiometric amount of 3-nitropropionate carbanion were used. It was found that the inhibition of SDH developed slowly and that nearly complete inactivation occurred. 3-Nitroacrylate, the expected product of dehydrogenation by the enzyme, inactivates the SDH rapidly and irreversibly. Several lines of evidence have suggested that the oxidation product, 3-nitroacrylic acid, reacted with an essential sulfhydryl (–SH) group at the substrate site. Pretreatment of SDH with NPA prevented the binding of ^{14}C-labeled oxaloacetate at the substrate site and, conversely, prior binding of oxaloacetate to the enzyme prevented the irreversible inactivation by a twofold excess of NPA. Inactivation of the enzyme by NPA also prevented the alkylation of one –SH group by N-ethyl[14C]-maleimide. The –SH group in question is located in the 70,000-Da subunit and is known from prior studies to be the combining site of succinate and of oxaloacetate. Coles et al. (1979) have suggested that the inactivation step involves a nucleophilic attack by this essential –SH group on the double bond of 3-nitroacrylate.

Erecinska and Nelson (1994) described their observations on the mechanism of NPA toxicity and its relationship to the neurodegenerative disease. A fall in creatine phosphate/creatine ratio is a very early and sensitive indicator of a mismatch between the energy supply and demand. Although the majority of striatal neurons have a low level of electrophysiological activity, the striatum receives a rich blood supply and exhibits a rather high metabolic rate; therefore, it is sensitive to mitochondrial toxins, such as NPA. Additionally, as the rate of energy use in younger animals appears to be lower compared to adults, degenerative changes may affect adults more. Stimulation of lactate synthesis is another early indicator of the mitochondrial dysfunction. Second, a fall in energy generation results in a decrease in guanosine triphosphate (GTP)/guanosine diphosphate (GDP) that substantially curtails protein production due to effects at the level of initiation; hence, even a small block in ATP generation might lead to the inability of a cell to maintain a normal contingent of protein and explain rapid neuronal death. Third, glutaminase initiates the metabolism of amino acids and the generation and release of the potent excitotoxin glutamate; even at the early stages of inhibition of the respiratory chain, the release of glutamate might exert an excitotoxic action. This also provides an explanation for the apparent effectiveness of blocking the glutamate receptor in the treatment of the consequences of inhibition of mitochondrial function. In addition to glutamate, the level of *gamma*-aminobutyric acid (GABA) also increases and should be detectable as an early indication of mitochondrial dysfunction (Erecinska and Nelson, 1994).

Spencer et al. (1993) also reported decreased energy levels in mouse cortical explants treated with NPA and the development of comparable patterns of neuronal pathology. These changes were attenuated by prior treatment with glutamate antagonists (MK-801, kynurinic acid) (Kim et al., 1999). These observations suggest that NPA blocks ATP production and thus renders nerve cells susceptible to the excitotoxic effects of the glutamate neurotransmitter. In a recent study, Dautry et al. (2000) investigated the depletion of N-acetylaspartate as a marker of neuronal dysfunction in rats and primates treated with NPA. The results of this study suggest that early N-acetylaspartate depletion reflects a reversible state of neuronal dysfunction preceding cell degeneration, and *in vivo* quantification of N-acetylaspartate may be a valuable tool for assessing early neuronal dysfunction (Dautry et al., 2000).

The precise mechanism of NPA-induced neuronal degeneration is not well understood. Administration of NPA to mice and rats produces brain injury consistent with an excitotoxic mechanism observed in ischemia/hypoxia (Gould and Gustine, 1982; Hamilton and Gould, 1987b). As glutamate receptor antagonists show protection from NPA-induced toxicity without changes in extracellular glutamate (Ludolph et al., 1992), it has been proposed that NPA-induced neurodegeneration is a consequence of secondary excitotoxic mechanisms, or indirect activation of glutamate receptors (Riepe et al., 1992; Zeevalk et al., 1995).

Recent studies have suggested the involvement of reactive oxygen species and oxidative stress in NPA-induced neurotoxicity (Beal et al., 1995; Binienda and Kim, 1997; Fu et al., 1995). Lesions produced by the systemic administration of NPA increased the production of hydroxyl-free radicals in the striatum, and NPA neurotoxicity was attenuated in copper/zinc superoxide dismutase transgenic mice (Beal et al., 1995). Binienda et al. (1998) reported that the administration of NPA resulted in the depletion of glutathione levels and the induction of antioxidant enzyme activities, suggesting conditions favorable for oxidative stress. Alexi et al. (1998) reported that NPA-induced metabolic compromise causes neurodegeneration that involves three interacting processes: energy impairment, excitotoxicity, and oxidative stress. This triplet of cooperative pathways of neurodegeneration helps to explain the regional selectivity of NPA for neurotoxicity to basal ganglia.

Administration of NPA has also been found to result in apoptosis in the rat striatum (Sato et al., 1997). This striatal apoptosis might be related to excitotoxicity; however, *in vitro* studies do not support this hypothesis (Pang and Geddes, 1997). Kim et al. (1999) suggested that the apoptotic neuronal death initially involved in striatal damage caused mild failure and created more energy failure with subsequent NPA treatment, eventually leading to neuronal necrosis. In *in vitro* experiments, cells might be lacking organized glutamatergic input. Kim et al. (1999) demonstrated that removal of the corticostriatal glutamate pathway reduced superoxide production and apoptosis induction in the denervated striatum of decorticated mice after NPA treatment. Additionally, the N-methyl-D-aspartate (NMDA) receptor antagonist, MK-801, prevented apoptosis in the striatum after NPA treatment for 5 days, whereas a non-NMDA receptor antagonist was ineffective. These investigators also evaluated the initial type of neuronal death by NPA treatment from 1 to 5 days. In early striatal damage, apoptotic neuronal death initially occurred after NPA treatment. These results show that excitotoxicity related to oxidative stress initially induces apoptotic neuronal death in mouse striatum after treatment with NPA.

ABSORPTION, DISTRIBUTION, METABOLISM, AND EXCRETION

As the presence of nitroaliphatic compounds in forage has the potential for considerable economic impact, several studies on the absorption of these compounds have appeared in the literature. In the rumen of cattle dosed with timber milkvetch (*Astragalus miser* var. *serotinus*), miserotoxin was rapidly hydrolyzed to 3-nitropropanol (NPOH) (Majak et al., 1984). The miserotoxin showed a rapid rate of disappearance from the rumen, with an average half-life of 1.24 hours. Increased plasma levels of NPA and inorganic nitrite suggest rapid absorption of NPOH from the rumen; however, conversion of NPOH to NPA was not observed to any significant extent in the rumen. It has been suggested that the difference in toxicity between NPA and NPOH is related to the rate of its absorption from the gastrointestinal tract (James et al., 1980). Miserotoxin is hydrolyzed to glucose and NPOH in ruminants, whereas in monogastric animals it is hydrolyzed to glucose and NPA under the acidic conditions of the stomach (Mosher et al., 1971). In non-ruminants, NPA esters can be rapidly hydrolyzed by mammalian tissue esterases to release NPA, while NPOH is oxidized by hepatic alcohol dehydrogenase to NPA (Hamilton et al., 2000).

Infusion of 3-nitropropanol (NPOH) into the rumen (30 mg/kg), abomasum (10 mg/kg), or small intestine (10 mg/kg) of sheep resulted in rapid absorption and conversion of NPOH into NPA (Pass et al., 1984). The major site of absorption for the miserotoxin aglycone was the reticulo-rumen; however, the abomasum and small intestine can also absorb NPOH. Injection of NPA into different regions of the alimentary tract also showed the reticulo-rumen to be the primary site of absorption. Compared to the abomasum, absorption of NPA or NPOH from the small intestine was much more rapid. Plasma levels of NPA and inorganic nitrite were higher after dosing with NPOH than with NPA, indicating a more rapid rate of uptake of the aglycone (Pass et al., 1984). Upon absorption from the alimentary tract, NPOH is rapidly converted to NPA by an irreversible reaction. Studies in sheep, cattle, and rats demonstrate that oxidation probably occurs in the liver (Majak and Pass, 1989). Supplementation of cattle diet with protein resulted in enhanced degradation of NPA by ruminal microorganisms. The protein supplement increased nitropropanol degradation by approximately 40% and promoted *in vitro* cellulose digestion (Majak, 1992).

Several investigators have attempted to unravel the mechanism of metabolism of NPOH in *in vitro* studies. Alston et al. (1981) hypothesized that NPOH is oxidized to 3-nitropropanal (NPAL) by equine alcohol dehydrogenase (ALDH), which decomposes to nitrite and acrolein, the proximate toxin, which irreversibly binds succinate dehydrogenase (SDH). McDiarmid et al. (1986) tested this hypothesis by employing equine ALDH and found the products of NPOH to be NPA (12%) and nitrite (50%). An intermediate generated in this series was thought to be 3-nitropropanal. By employing HPLC techniques, Benn et al. (1989) further examined the oxidation of NPOH by equine ALDH. The intermediate product, NPAL, was synthesized and was also trapped in the reaction mixture as the semicarbazone. At neutral pH, NPAL spontaneously decomposed to nitrite and acrolein; however, in the presence of ALDH, NPAL was partially oxidized to NPA. Prior administration of ethanol or 4-methylpyrazole to inhibit ALDH suppressed the conversion of NPOH to NPA and protected rats from intoxication (Pass et al., 1985); however, if the ALDH inhibitors were given after the nitroalcohol, toxicity still developed. Administration of an aldehyde dehydrogenase inhibitor, diethyldithiocarbamic acid, had little effect on the conversion of NPOH to NPA and did not alter the toxicity of NPOH. These studies suggest that NPOH and NPA are equally toxic to rats, and NPOH toxicity is due to its rapid conversion to NPA (Pass et al., 1985).

Majak and Cheng (1981) investigated the mechanism for conversion of NPOH to NPA and subsequent detoxification by ruminal bacteria. Although NPA has been reported to be present in seven genera representing four different families of higher plants, NPOH is detected only in a group of *Astragalus* species of the family Leguminosae. Bound forms of NPA and NPOH are usually isolated, with NPA occurring as the mono-, di-, or triester of glucose and NPOH as the β-glucoside miserotoxin. Of the 33 strains of rumen bacteria tested, five degraded both NPOH and NPA under anaerobic conditions, and another five strains degraded only NPA (Majak and Cheng, 1981). Pure cultures of rumen bacteria and mixed rumen microorganisms metabolize NPA faster than NPOH. The presence of nitrite was detected during incubation of both NPOH and NPA with resting cells, but not with growing cultures of active strains of rumen bacteria. Nitrite was metabolized much faster compared to the nitrotoxins by both pure cultures of rumen bacteria and mixed rumen microorganisms. These studies suggest that the nitro group of either NPA or NPOH is metabolized to inorganic nitrite, which is reduced to ammonia by rumen microorganisms, thereby resulting in its detoxification (Majak and Cheng, 1981).

In another study, Anderson et al. (1993) explored the concept that the rates of detoxification reactions are critical to the acquisition of tolerance to nitroaliphatic-containing plants. These investigators examined the detoxified end products of NPA and NPOH by ruminal organisms. The rates of disappearance of NPA and NPOH varied somewhat among samples of ruminal fluid but were approximately 0.4 and 0.1 μmol/mL of ruminal fluid per hour, respectively. Rates with threefold-concentrated cells from rumen fluid were correspondingly higher. Ruminal microbes from both cattle and sheep reduced the nitro groups *in situ*, NPA was converted to β-alanine (which, in turn, was converted to other products) and NPOH was converted to 3-amino-1-propanol (87% conversion). Addition of sulfide and ferrous ions to suspensions of ruminal microbes increased the rate of NPOH reduction approximately threefold, but the rates of NPA reduction were not proportionately increased.

TOXICOLOGICAL STUDIES

The toxicity of nitroaliphatic compounds has been extensively studied; however, several inconsistencies can be noted in the results obtained. These inconsistencies stem from an uncertainty of the qualitative and quantitative nature of the nitroaliphatic substance administered and the ability of ruminants to detoxify the NPA. In studies with nitroaliphatic-containing plants, the plants were often dried or frozen and stored for various periods of time or extracted in various solvents before use. Additionally, it is often difficult to determine from the study description exactly which nitroaliphatic substances the animals received — as the glucoside (miserotoxin), as NPA or NPOH, or as some combination of these three. Finally, indications are that more than one toxin may be present in some higher plants. Yet another source of inconsistency arises from the use of NPA produced from a synthetic process involving β-propiolactone (a mutagen and carcinogen), which may have been present as a contaminant in some experimental studies.

Williams and James (1976) reported that the amount of nitroaliphatic substances in plants diminished with time and storage. Further, the amount of nitroaliphatic substances varies with the growing conditions of the plants and the portion of the plant used (Aylward et al., 1987; Cooke, 1955; Gold and Brodman, 1991). The difficulty stemming from these observations is twofold: First, studies were often expressed only in terms of the quantity of plant administered to the animal as opposed to the amount of NO_2 present in the sample, and, second, the quantitative analysis (of NO_2, NPA, etc.) was not conducted on the substance immediately prior to administration. Additionally, as noted in the NCI report on the bioassay study, NPA itself was determined not to be stable in feed (NCI, 1978). The form of the toxin is important because animals vary in their ability to hydrolyze the toxin from the glucoside, thus making it available for absorption and toxicity. Hutton et al. (1958) demonstrated that when seeds of *Indigofera endecaphylla* were fed to mice, liver toxicity was produced, but the seeds did not give a positive reaction for NPA and that NPA-free extracts of leaves still produced the hepatotoxicity. Ludolph et al. (1991) noted that not all species of *Astragalus* contain NPA or NPOH and that others may be selenium accumulating and some may produce 8α,β-indolizidine-1α,2α,8α triol, the likely toxic constituent in locoweed poisoning. As noted previously, NPA produced from a synthetic process involves β-propiolactone, which may be present as a contaminant (Hansen, 1984). This lactone would not be present from naturally derived NPA, as biosynthesis takes place via a different route. NPA used in the NCI study was manufactured via the β-propiolactone process and had an impurity level of approximately 5% (NCI, 1978). All of these observations suggest that much of the data from feeding plant stuffs to animals, as well as much of the data involving the administration of synthetic NPA, should be considered only qualitatively.

ACUTE TOXICITY STUDIES

A fairly consistent LD_{50} value in rats given NPA or NPOH either intraperitoneally or orally in the range of 60 to 80 mg/kg was reported in the literature (Table 5.7). A dose of 100 mg/kg was reported to be quickly fatal (Bell, 1974). The subcutaneous LD_{50} is approximately half the amount for other routes (30 mg/kg). Toxicity in mice was fairly consistent for an oral or subcutaneous dose with a range of approximately 165 to 250 mg/kg, although refined sugarcane toxin had a slightly lower LD_{50} (68 to 100 mg/kg). The approximate lethal dose of 1600 mg/kg reported by Shafer and Bowles (1985) is at least a factor of 20 greater than those reported by other authors, although no explanation could be determined from the original publication.

Age-dependent toxicity of NPA was studied by Bossi et al. (1993). At a dose of 30 mg/kg, NPA produced 50% mortality in rats 11 to 14 weeks of age, but no deaths were noted in rats 3 to 6 weeks or 7 to 10 weeks of age. Contrary to these observations in rats, Tan et al. (1990) could not find any significant difference in the

TABLE 5.7
Acute (Single-Dose) Studies with β-Nitropropionic Acid (NPA) or β-Nitropropionic Alcohol (NPOH)

Species	Route/Dose	Substance	Findings	Refs.
Rat	Oral	NPA	No deaths at 125 mg/kg; 100% mortality at 200, 250, and 500 mg/kg; histological changes in liver, lungs, kidneys	Penel (1977)
Rat	Oral	NPOH	$LD_{50} = 77$ mg/kg	Bell, (1974)
Rat	Oral	NPA	60 mg/kg, animals subdued; 100 mg/kg, quickly fatal	Majak et al. (1983)
Rat	Intraperitoneal	NPOH	$LD_{50} = 61$ mg/kg (95% CL = 51–70)	Bell (1974)
Rat	Intraperitoneal	NPA	$LD_{50} = 67$ mg/kg (95% CL = 63–72)	Pass et al. (1985)
Rat	Subcutaneous	NPA	$LD_{50} = 22$ mg/kg	Pass et al. (1985)
Rat	Subcutaneous (30 mg/kg)	NPA	Group 1, ages 3–6 weeks, 0 deaths; group 2, ages 7–10 weeks, 0 deaths; group 3, ages 11–14 weeks, 50% deaths; group 4, ages 16–20 weeks, 64% deaths	Bossi et al. (1993)
Rat	Subcutaneous	NPA	Brain lesions, 10 mg/kg for 1 to 4 days or 30 mg/kg single dose	Gould et al. (1985)
Rat	Subcutaneous	NPA	Brain lesions, 30 mg/kg	Hamilton (1986)
Mouse	Oral	NPA	$LD_{50} = 221$ mg/kg (range, 166–295 mg/kg)	Hamilton and Gould (1987a,b)
Mouse	Oral	Refined sugarcane toxin	$LD_{50} = 100$ mg/kg in males; $LD_{50} = 68.1$ mg/kg in females	Tan et al. (1990)
Mouse	Oral	NPA	LD_{50} for young mice = 221 mg/kg (95% CL = 166–295); LD_{50} for old mice = 205 mg/kg (95% CL = 169–249); No significant difference between the two age groups	Tan et al. (1989)
Mouse	Oral	NPA	Approximate lethal dose = 1600 mg/kg	Schafer and Bowles (1985)
Mouse	Subcutaneous	NPOH	$LD_{50} = 190$ mg/kg	Gould et al. (1985)
Mouse	Injection	NPA	Lethal dose = 300 mg/kg	Drummond et al. (1975)
Pigeon	Gavage	NPA	Lethal dose = 60–70 mg/kg (range, 38–80 mg/kg)	Bell (1974)

LD_{50} between "young" and "old" mice with a single dose. Beal et al. (1993b) produced age-dependent striatal lesions that were significantly greater in 4- and 12-month old animals than in 1-month old animals with malonate, a reversible inhibitor of succinate dehydrogenase.

In a recent study, Hickey and Morton (2000) reported that young mice transgenic for the Huntington's disease mutation (R6/2 mice) are resistant to chronic NPA-induced striatal toxicity, compared to their wild-type littermates. Further, fewer R6/2 than wild-type mice developed striatal lesions; however, adult R6/2 mice (12 weeks of age) were found to have increased vulnerability to NPA. These results indicate that in young R6/2 mouse brain, compensatory mechanisms exist that protect them against the toxic effect of the transgene and coincidentally protect against exogenous toxin. The existence of similar compensatory mechanisms may explain why, in humans, HD is a late-onset disorder, despite early expression of the genetic mutation.

Contrary to the results of several investigators, Penel (1977) reported no deaths within 5 days of a single oral dose of NPA at 125 mg/kg. At doses 200 mg/kg and higher, 100% lethality was noted. Interestingly, when the surviving animals were again dosed at 125 mg/kg, following 5 days' abstinence from NPA, all died within 75 minutes of administration. Histopathologic findings from the study were also at odds with other investigators, who reported histological changes in the liver, lungs, and kidneys but no changes in the brain. Penel (1977) also reported that the pathological findings were consistent with nitrite poisoning. Gould et al. (1985) and Hamilton et al. (1984) also noted the formation of methemoglobin in rats and mice, but the levels were below the threshold for lethality. Further, James et al. (1980) demonstrated that methemoglobinemia occurred in cattle fed *Astragalus*, and, although this formation may contribute to the respiratory distress of the animal, death still occurs even if the formation of methemoglobin is prevented by administration of methylene blue.

Acute effects of NPA on activities of endogenous antioxidants in the rat brain were studied by Binienda et al. (1998). Rats were administered 30 mg/kg NPA subcutaneously and killed at 30, 60, 90, and 120 minutes after injection. At 90 and 120 minutes after administration, catalase activity was increased in the hippocampus. At 120 minutes, cytosolic copper/zinc superoxide dismutase (SOD) and mitochondrial manganese–SOD levels were increased in the frontal cortex. The activity of glutathione peroxidase and levels of reduced glutathione were decreased in the hippocampus at 120 minutes. Depletion of glutathione and induction of antioxidant enzyme activities after NPA exposure suggest conditions favorable to oxidative stress. In an earlier study, Binienda and Kim (1997) reported that acute administration of NPA increases free fatty acid in the frontal cortex and hippocampus of rats, thus providing a substrate for free-radical formation. In another study, Nony et al. (1999) reported that subcutaneous administration of a single dose of NPA (30 mg/kg) to adult male Sprague-Dawley (SD) rats resulted in progressive hypothermia, with a loss of 3°C or more in core body temperature by 3 hours after dosing.

Fu et al. (1995) noted an increase in free-radical signals in rat livers at 15, 30, and 45 minutes after oral administration of 80 mg/kg NPA. In treated rats, the activities of liver SOD and glutathione peroxidase, as well as the content of malondialdehyde, were significantly increased. Klivenyi et al. (1999) studied the susceptibility of mice deficient in cellular glutathione. Systemic administration of NPA resulted in a significantly greater striatal damage and increases in 3-nitro-tyrosine concentration in glutathione peroxidase knock-out mice as compared to wild-type control mice. These investigators concluded that glutathione peroxidase plays an important role in detoxifying the increases in oxygen radicals after NPA administration.

Several animal studies show variable susceptibility to NPA toxicity, yet the reasons remain elusive (Alexi et al. 2000; Fukuda et al. 1998; Guyot et al., 1997). An age-related variation to NPA toxicity in experimental animals has been demonstrated; however, variability still is observed within each age group as well as between age groups (Beal et al., 1993a; Brouillet et al. 1993b). Alexi et al. (2000) reported that a single intraperitoneal injection of NPA (30 mg/kg) caused mortality in 21.7% of rats within 16 hours of injection. After 7 days, the brain activity of SDH, the biochemical target of NPA, was severely decreased in all animals receiving NPA; however, the majority of the animals did not develop neurological damage as assessed by histochemical staining. These investigators claimed that a rapid (1-day) decline in brain SDH activity induces neurological damage in the striatum, whereas a gradual (7-day) decline does not. This distinction occurred despite the fact that absolute levels of SDH decline were almost identical. The rapid decline in susceptible rats was associated with a striatal pocket of fully depleted SDH activity with neurological lesions, which were associated with both the pocket and the peripheral region surrounding the pocket. The fast decline in SDH activity in vulnerable rats was followed by cell death, whereas the slower decline in resilient rats was not.

In a cattle and sheep study, James et al. (1980) examined the effects of nitro-aliphatic-bearing plants and NPA or NPOH at both single and multiple intervals. Various species of *Astragalus* (*A. pterocarpus*, *A. canadensis*, *A. falcatus*, or *A. emoryanus*) were gathered from the field, dried, ground, and stored frozen. The plant material was mixed with water and administered by stomach tube. Administration of a single dose of dried *A. pterocarpus* to a cow (200 mg of NO_2 per kg body weight) resulted in no effect, but subsequent administration of two doses of NPA (10 mg/kg) over a 6-day period resulted in a rapid respiratory rate, central nervous system depression, and incoordination. When the same animal was dosed four times over 17 days with another species of *Astragalus* (3 mg NO_2 per kg body weight), the animal exhibited general body weakness and incoordination and was killed on the day of the last dose. In another cow, administration of a single dose of *A. canadensis* (275 mg of NO_2 per kg body weight) resulted in frothing at the mouth and generalized weakness. A third cow, dosed once with *A. falcatus* (350 mg of NO_2 per kg body weight) exhibited weakness and died (James et al., 1980).

Results from the study by James et al. (1980) indicate that the no-observed-effect level (NOEL) is 200 mg NO_2 per kg; however, several variables are involved in the intoxication of ruminants. Susceptibility of ruminants to NPA toxicity depends on factors such as the ability of the ruminant to absorb the intact miserotoxin followed by subsequent hydrolysis of the NPOH and reduction to NPA, as well as ruminal hydrolysis of the NPOH from the glycoside followed by absorption and reduction of the hydrolyzed NPOH to nitrite. Additional experiments by James et al. (1980), wherein cattle were orally dosed once with NPA (15 mg NO_2 per kg body weight) or NPOH (15 mg NO$_2$ per kg body weight) support these factors as being responsible for the variable susceptibility of ruminants. In this case, both animals experienced incoordination, nervousness, weakness, and stiffness and eventually died. Two sheep treated in a similar manner with NPA (20 and 30 mg NO$_2$ per kg body weight) also died (James et al., 1980).

Vasodilatory and antihypertensive effects of NPA in dogs were studied by Hong et al. (1990). Mongrel dogs were orally administered 1.0, 3.1, or 10 mg/kg of NPA, and changes in blood pressure and heart rate were monitored at 0, 1, 2, 4, 6, and 8 hours following dosing. A dose-dependent decrease in maximal systolic and diastolic arterial blood pressures was noted at approximately 2 hours following drug administration. Recovery from the antihypertensive effect of NPA was slow; however, within 8 hours of ingestion, symptoms completely disappeared. A slight, but long-lasting decrease in heart rate was observed after the administration of 1.0 and 3.1 mg/kg of NPA; however, at the highest dose (10 mg/kg), NPA provoked a modest and brief tachycardia (described by the authors as reflex tachycardia, common with nitrite-type antihypertensives) (Hong et al., 1990). In another study, Castillo et al. (1993) reported a mild but consistent decrease in both systolic and diastolic arterial blood pressure after oral NPA administration to renal hypertensive dogs.

Cooke (1955) force fed ether-extracted juice from creeping indigo (*Indigofera endecaphylla* Jacq.) to 1-day-old (0.5 mL) and 4-day-old (1 mL) chicks. The 1-day-old chicks died within 1 minute; the 4-day-old chicks died in 3 to 4 hours. Synthetic NPA (1 mL of a 0.2% solution) was force fed to several 2-week-old chicks, and chicks receiving synthetic NPA died within 0.5 hour. Yin et al. (1992) irradiated suckers of crownvetch, producing new varieties with lower NPA contents. The mortality rate of chicks given diets containing 10% dry meal of the new varieties was lower by 20 to 40% compared to the original crownvetch varieties.

SUBACUTE TOXICITY STUDIES

Rat Studies

Intraperitoneal administration of 10, 20, or 25 mg NPA/kg twice daily for up to 4 days resulted in decreased growth in rats at 20 and 25 mg/kg; food and water intake decreased at all dose levels. Neurological signs of hind limb paresis progressing to paralysis were evident within 2 days in the most severely affected rats. The severity of the symptoms was related to the dose of NPA. Ten of the 12 animals administered NPA at 25 mg/kg died and two recovered. Two of six rats at 10 mg/kg developed slight hind leg incoordination, but did not die. Intraperitoneal administration of thiamin hydrochloride (10 mg/kg daily for 4 days) to NPA-treated rats did not alleviate toxicity (Pass et al., 1988).

In a series of investigations, Hamilton (1986) characterized the stages of NPA toxicity. Sprague-Dawley rats were injected subcutaneously with either a single dose of 30 mg/kg NPA in saline or 10 mg/kg/day over 1 to 4 days. The majority of the rats at the high dose immediately became recumbent, while others at the high, as well as the low (10 mg/kg), dose exhibited increased spontaneous motor activity and/or uncoordinated gait. Progression of NPA toxicity was roughly divisible into three stages, characterized by somnolence in stage I, uncoordinated gait with stereotypical paddling and rolling movements in stage II, and ventral or lateral recumbency in stage III. The length of time to a specific stage was inversely proportional to the dose. Pathologic lesions in the brains were bilateral and symmetrical, affecting the caudate–putamen, the hippocampus (including the dentate gyrus), and the thalamus. At both dose regimens, the lesions were common. The severity was proportional to the length of time spent in what the author described as the most advanced stage of symptoms (stage III, recumbency), but not with the dose. Of the 40 rats that became recumbent, all had injuries of the caudate–putamen, and 63% had injury at all three sites. Brain damage in these rats was similar but not identical to rats with hypoxic brain damage from other causes (ischemia and hypoglycemia) (Hamilton and Gould, 1987a). The rats with typical brain lesions were not hypotensive or hypoxemic, indicating that neither of these conditions was necessary for the development of the morphologic lesions (Hamilton et al., 1984).

In the above-described study, no evidence of selective effects on neuronal subpopulations in the caudate–putamen or thalamus was noted, but in the hippocampus the neurons in the granule cell layer were relatively resistant to injury in comparison with the neurons in the pyramidal cell layer (Hamilton, 1986). No gradients of susceptibility were observed in the pyramidal cell layer. Neuronal alterations ranged from chromatin clumping with increased cytoplasmic lucency to severe cellular shrinkage or swelling with marked mitochondrial swelling. White matter changes included axonal swelling and axonal splitting of myelin lamellae. Vascular alterations included perivascular deposits of proteinaceous material (presumably from the leakage of serum proteins), variable electron lucency of endothelial cell cytoplasm, an apparent increase in pinocytotic vesicles, rare platelet thrombosis of capillaries, and rare intravascular blebs of luminal plasma membrane (Hamilton, 1986; Hamilton and Gould, 1987a). A uniform reduction in SDH was noted by histochemical staining of frozen sections of the brain. In another study, Nishino et al. (1997) reported that NPA-induced striatal damage was associated with astrocyte cell death and dysfunction of the blood–brain barrier. Nishino et al. (2000) proposed that the striatum-specific lesion caused by NPA is due to the cumulative insults characteristic of the striatum, including glutamatergic excitotoxicity, dopaminergic toxicity, vulnerability of the lateral striatal artery, and high activity in the glutamate transporter.

In a NCI (1978) range-finding study, the effects of NPA in rat diet were studied at 0, 100, 150, 250, 500, and 900 ppm. Five males and 5 females in each group were dosed for 6 weeks and then observed for 2 weeks. In male rats, the mean body weight gain at 100 ppm (0.5 mg/kg/day), 150 ppm (7.5 mg/kg/day), and 250 ppm (12.5 mg/kg/day) was 77, 59, and 59% of controls, respectively. At higher levels of NPA, 500 (25 mg/kg/day) and 900 ppm (45 mg/kg/day), all of the males died. In female rats, the mean body weight gain was 97% of controls at 100 ppm, 87% at 150 ppm, 71% at 250 ppm, and 62% at 500 ppm. At levels of 250, 500, and 900 ppm, 2, 4, and 5 females died, respectively. Histological examination revealed testicular atrophy with spermatogenic arrest in male rats and malacia in the midbrain in both sexes given doses of 150 ppm and above. Based on these results, doses for the chronic study were set at 25 and 50 ppm for males and 50 and 100 ppm for females (NCI, 1978).

Manipulating the number of NPA administrations to rats can result in either increased nocturnal spontaneous locomotor activity (hyperactivity) or nocturnal akinesia (hypoactivity). Two intraperitoneal injections (one injection every 4 days) of NPA (10 mg/kg) resulted in hyperactivity, while four or more injections of NPA produced hypoactivity (Borlongan et al., 1997).

Gender differences in the vulnerability to NPA of the lateral striatal artery in rats were studied by Nishino et al. (1998). Subcutaneous administration of NPA (20 mg/kg once a day for 2 days) resulted in striatal selective lesions associated with motor symptoms in half of the male rats, while female rats were resilient. The motor and histological disturbances were highly sex dependent. Castration had little effect, but ovariectomy enhanced vulnerability. Replacement therapy with testosterone increased, while estradiol or tomoxifen suppressed, the vulnerability in ovariectomized females.

In a recent study, Ouary et al. (2000) investigated the strain differences to NPA in rats. Three different strains of rats (Sprague-Dawley, Lewis, and Fisher 344) were treated initially with 7 mg/kg/day NPA; the dose was increased by 15% every day until all of the animals died. The animal deaths were recorded every day before NPA injection. All rats from all strains died within 7 days, except one of the SD strain. Doses resulting in first deaths in the Fisher, SD, and Lewis rats suggest that these rats exhibited high, intermediate, and low vulnerability to NPA, respectively. The survival curve indicated a more heterogeneous response to NPA toxicity in SD rats than observed in either Fisher and Lewis rats. The differences between SD and Lewis rats were further confirmed in a subcutaneous NPA study using osmotic minipumps, where doses up to 36 to 45 mg/kg/day for 5 days were necessary to induce striatal lesions in Lewis rats as compared to 12 to 14 mg/kg/day for 5 days in SD rats. The results of these investigations suggest that susceptibility to NPA may depend on genetic factors (Ouary et al., 2000).

In another study, Guyot et al. (1997) studied motor abnormality in rats treated with NPA. Subacute administration of 15 mg/kg/day NPA by the intraperitoneal route resulted in dramatic motor symptoms associated with extensive neuronal loss and gliosis in the lateral striatum, as well as severe hippocampal degeneration in 50% of the rats. However, subcutaneous treatment of rats with 10 mg/kg/day NPA for 1 month led to more subtle, excitotoxic-like lesions that were selective for the dorsolateral striatum and more closely resembled Huntington's disease in humans. Subcutaneously treated rats showed spontaneous motor symptoms, including mild dystonia, bradykinesia, and gait abnormalities. The degree of striatal neuronal loss was significantly correlated with the severity of spontaneous motor abnormalities, as is the case in Huntington's disease.

Mouse Studies

In a toxicity and repellency study in house and deer mice, Schafer and Bowles (1985) screened 933 chemicals for the approximate lethal dose (ALD) and the dose promoting food reduction in mice. For the ALD determinations, the animals were dosed and observed for 3 days. The authors reported an ALD for NPA in deer mice to be (a previously unreported high of) 1600 mg/kg. The dose of NPA, which approximated the LD_{50} when mixed with seeds and fed to animals on a subacute basis, was 613 mg/kg. The authors appeared to have exceeded doses given under similar conditions by a factor of at least 20. The article does not indicate the basis of this difference.

Adult mice (25 to 30 g) fed dried timber milkvetch (*Astragalus* spp.) exhibited symptoms within 36 hours, with death following approximately 24 hours thereafter. Consumption of 7 g milkvetch per 100 g body weight over a period of 2 to 12 days was sufficient to kill the mice. Initially, a loss of equilibrium was noted and then the mice rolled over frequently and were generally unsteady on their feet. The mice assumed a characteristic arching of the back with a drop in body temperature and a slowing of the heart rate. Massive hemorrhage on the mucosal lining of the stomach was noted (Mosher et al., 1971). Similar findings were noted in rats with symptoms of poisoning evident at 36 hours and deaths occurring approximately 24 hours later; other symptoms, including the occurrence of gastric hemorrhages, were similar to those noted in the mouse experiments. A significant increase in serum glutamic oxaloacetate transferase (SGOT) and serum isocitrate dehydrogenase (ICD) was also reported. In order to determine the toxic principal, mice were treated with deproteinized blood and intestinal contents of rats fed timber milkvetch, water extract of milkvetch, or NPA. Mice treated with the protein-free filtrate of intestinal contents died in 2 hours, while mice treated with protein-free filtrate of blood of milkvetch-fed rats died within 4 hours. Mice treated with milkvetch water extracts (orally, daily for 5 days) died in 5 days. Intraperitoneal injection of 2 mg neutralized NPA killed mice in 3 hours (Mosher et al., 1971).

Contrary to the observation that NPA-induced mortality in rats is correlated with age (Bossi et al., 1993), Tan et al. (1990) found the opposite effect in mice undergoing chronic administration. The chronic, repeated gavage administration (30 days) LD_{50} was significantly higher in old (LD_{50} = 138 mg/kg) compared with young (LD_{50} = 49 mg/kg) mice. Beal et al. (1993a) studied the relationship between age and striatal lesions by employing subcutaneously implanted osmatic pumps for subacute systemic administration of NPA. The NPA was administered at a dose of 20 mg/kg for 5 days. Subacute systemic administration of NPA produced age-dependent bilateral striatal lesions. Chronic administration of NPA over 1 month produced selective striatal lesions that replicated many of the characteristic histologic and neurochemical features of Huntington's disease (Beal et al., 1993a).

Brouillet et al. (1993b) studied the effects of age on striatal lesions produced by local administration of NPA to rats. A marked increase in striatal lactate concentrations that significantly correlated with increasing age was noted, as measured by *in vivo* chemical shift magnetic resonance imaging. Histological and neurochemical studies revealed a striking age dependence of the lesions, with 4-and 12-month-old animals being much more susceptible compared to 1-month-old animals. Administration of low doses of NPA for 1 month resulted in striatal lesions showing growth-related changes in dendrites of striatal spiny neurons. In a recent study, Page et al. (2000) found that, while producing striatal lesions that bear a similarity to those seen in Huntington's disease, the consequences of NPA for striatopallidal and striatonigral efferent projections do not reflect the reported neurodegenerative changes seen in a HD brain.

In a range-finding study, NPA was added to mouse feed in concentrations ranging from 150 to 800 ppm (NCI, 1978). Five males and five females were fed for 6 weeks and then observed for 2 weeks. Males receiving 150 or 600 ppm (21 to 85 mg/kg) had no effect on body weight gain. At the highest dose, an early weight depression was observed, but these animals recovered to control levels. In females, mean body weights were not affected at any dose tested. One male each in the 600- and 800-ppm group died. Hydronephrosis was noted in nine mice; however, the incidence was not dose related. Based on the results of this study, the low and high doses for males and females for the chronic studies were determined as 75 and 150 ppm (10 and 21 mg/kg), respectively.

Rabbit Studies

In a series of studies, Hutton et al. (1958) studied the active toxic principle of *Indigofera endecaphylla*. Gavage administration of synthetic NPA to 2 rabbits for 22 and 34 days at dose levels approximating 53 and 84 mg/kg/day, respectively, resulted in a decrease in body weight. Both rabbits were described as "lively" at the end of the experiment and when examined postmortem were without any remarkable histopathological changes. In an additional experiment, 2 rabbits were fed dried *I. endecaphylla* at a dose of 7.73 or 7.40 mg NPA/kg/day. Both rabbits died, and liver pathology indicated fine nodular cirrhosis. Continuing this series of experiments, groups of 2 to 3 rabbits were fed a combination of standard meal and dried plant material from different strains of *I. endecaphylla* for 5 to 32 days. One of the animals, surviving only 5 days, showed acute liver degeneration and necrosis. The remaining animals survived from 14 to 32 days, and all exhibited diffuse nodular cirrhosis. All the animals showed a decrease in body weight during the period of treatment. In a follow-up study, rabbits fed seeds of *I. endecaphylla* exhibited similar hepatic damage, but the seeds were negative for NPA. As the animals fed NPA had greater survival and different pathology from those fed plant parts with comparable or lesser amounts of NPA, the operative toxin in *I. endecaphylla* in this animal model was not NPA (Hutton et al., 1958).

Studies in Other Mammals

Feeding of weanling voles with a diet containing crownvetch (0.47% of the diet being NPA) resulted in both decreased food intake and weight gains compared to the controls fed alfalfa. The early clinical indications of intoxication were decreased activity and a hunched-up appearance. Symptoms of toxicity appeared within 2 days of initiation, and all of the animals died. In a follow-up study, feeding voles with diets containing crownvetch (0.008 to 0.15% NPA) resulted in mortality at the highest dose. The exact doses of NPA could not be determined, as the method for estimation of the nitroaliphatic compounds was not specific for NPA (Shenk et al., 1976). In another experiment, feeding a diet containing crownvetch to pigs resulted in a decrease in body weight and serious signs of incoordination and staggering from day 8 to day 15. The condition was first noticeable in the rear quarters and at later stages seemed to affect the entire body. Blood analysis revealed an increased packed cell volume and decreased glucose levels compared to controls which may have been a result of decreased food and water intake. Plasma urea nitrogen was normal. The pigs were returned to alfalfa diets on Day 11 and, after several days of normal diet, the symptoms of toxicity disappeared.

In a series of field and experimental studies, James et al. (1980) gathered various species of *Astragalus* (*A. pterocarpus*, *A. canadensis*, *A. falcatus*, and *A. emoryanus*) from the field, then dried, ground, and stored (frozen) the plant material. The plant material was mixed with water and administered to cattle by gavage at a dose level of 2 to 200 mg NO_2 per kg body weight daily for several days to 98 days (irregular administration). Several animals exhibited the characteristic signs of NPA toxicity, but the time of onset and the severity of symptoms varied. Some animals did not show any symptoms of toxicity. The variations in symptoms are likely due to differences in the susceptibility of ruminants to NPA toxicity, which can depend on several factors, including the ability of the ruminant to (1) absorb the intact toxin, followed by hydrolysis of the NPOH and reduction to NPA; (2) hydrolze the NPOH to glycoside, followed by absorption and reduction; and (3) reduce the hydrolyzed NPOH to nitrite.

James et al. (1980) also reported pathological differences between acutely and chronically intoxicated animals. In most cases, acute toxicity resulted in severe respiratory distress, pelvic limb weakness, prostration, and death with severe lung lesions, lobular alveolar emphysema, and collapsed and constricted bronchioles, often with interlobular edema. Some of the acutely intoxicated cattle also had widespread, small, focal hemorrhages in the central nervous system. Chronic or delayed intoxication of cattle presented mainly neurological signs such as knuckling and pelvic limb incoordination, as well as similar, but milder, lung lesions compared to animals with acute intoxication. Mild Wallerian degeneration of the spinal cord was noted in both acutely and chronically intoxicated cattle. An increase in methemoglobin was also noted in chronically treated animals, but the level returned to baseline within 24 hours of feeding. In acutely intoxicated cattle, the increase in methemoglobin was less pronounced.

Employing similar procedures, James et al. (1980) also examined sheep for nitroaliphatic intoxication using various species of *Astragalus*. The dose of *A. falcatus* administered ranged from 150 to 500 mg NO_2 per kg in as many as 4 doses over 10 days. The amount of *A. emoryanus* administered was 38 mg NO_2 per kg (7 doses in 9 days). The sheep exhibited depression, respiratory distress, weakness, and other symptoms characteristic of NPA toxicity. All the sheep died or were killed *in extremis*. The majority of sheep that were exposed showed similar acute symptomology with respiratory distress. The only pulmonary symptom observed on autopsy was edema. Some of the animals with physical incoordination showed mild Wallerian degeneration of the spinal cord and some also had kidney damage, such as subcapsular nephrosis. Sheep receiving oral doses ranging from 10 to 30 mg NO_2 per kg per day (NPA or NPOH) for 1 to 6 doses over as many as 28 days exhibited one or more signs characteristic of poisoning from the use of these compounds, and all died or were killed in extremis (James et al., 1980).

In another experiment, Williams and James (1976) collected Emory milkvetch when it was in the pod stage of growth and then dried, ground, and stored the plant material at 2°C. A ewe weighing 60 kg was fed 400 g of the milkvetch (38.9 mg NO_2 per kg body weight) for 7 days. On day 6 of the feeding, the ewe became weak and unsteady in the hindquarters. On day 7, the animal rapidly became weaker and more uncoordinated and was killed. Three hours after feeding on the first and third days, a blood sample tested for methemoglobin showed values of 4.6 and 4.3% of the total hemoglobin, respectively. Comparison of this animal with animals treated intravenously with NPA and NPOH (20 mg NO_2 per kg) revealed that the NPA-infused sheep became depressed and uncoordinated in the hindquarters 3 hours after treatment; 24 hours after the infusion, one sheep became weak and very uncoordinated and fell frequently, displaying symptoms consistent with NPA toxicity. One sheep was killed after one infusion, while the other was infused a second time and died later. Intravenous infusion of two sheep with NPOH resulted in weakness and incoordination in the hindquarters, 2 hours after treatment. Approximately 4 hours after treatment, both animals collapsed and died. Methemoglobin levels were relatively low (2 to 2.5%) in the NPA/NPOH-treated animal. The syndrome produced by NPOH was similar to that produced by NPA except that the time lapse between the onset of toxic signs and collapse and paralysis was more rapid and the knuckled fetlock stage was not evident with NPOH. The authors concluded that the toxicities produced in sheep with Emory milkvetch and NPA were identical.

Non-Mammalian Studies

β-Nitropropionic acid is also known to affect other species, as well. An approximately 60- to 70-mg/kg dose of NPA was lethal to pigeons (Bell, 1974). Shenk et al. (1976) reported that feeding a diet containing crownvetch (NPA, 0.05%) to chicks resulted in "mild" symptoms. Yin et al. (1992) reported a decreased mortality in chicks fed irradiated crownvetch compared to non-irradiated crownvetch. Administration of the leaf extract of *Astragalus hamosus* and *A. sesameus* to chicks produced signs of toxicity, and deaths occurred at high doses; however, the level of NO_2 was not provided in the article (Williams, 1980). In an *in vivo* study, Panigrahi (1993) tested the susceptibility of brine shrimp (*Artemia salina* L.) to NPA. Shrimp larvae were exposed to a paper disc inoculated with NPA. At a concentration of 90 µg NPA per disc, 35% of the brine shrimp died (Panigrahi, 1993). Feeding insects, *Sparganothis* fruitworms and *Sparganothis sulfureana*, a pinto bean diet containing low levels of NPA significantly increased the mortality of the larvae and reduced the pupal weight of both males and females over four generations (Byers et al., 1986).

SUBCHRONIC STUDIES

In an oral gavage study, Tan et al. (1989) administered 20, 40, and 80% of the LD_{50} (221 mg/kg) dose of NPA (approximately 44, 88, and 177 mg/kg, respectively) to mice daily for up to 99 days. The control group was similarly treated with water. During the first 10 days of the study, all of the mice treated with NPA lost weight, but surviving mice fed the lowest dose of NPA gained weight thereafter. Chronic symptoms observed were decreased open field behavior, tremulousness, and some hind limb weakness on grasping. Neuropathology as evaluated by light and electron microscopy showed variable adaxonal changes in lateral and ventral spinal cord myelinated axons, but no motor neuron degeneration. The chronic (30-day) oral dose LD_{50} was determined as 49 mg/kg. In another study, Wullner et al. (1994) investigated the systemic effects of NPA in doses ranging from 12 to 16 mg/kg/day for 30 days on striatal cytoarchitecture in rats. NPA at a dose of 16 mg/kg/day resulted in large lesions with a central necrotic core that was depleted of both neurons and glial cells. At lower doses of NPA (12 to 15 mg/kg/day), neither the area nor the binding density of the patches was affected.

Dopamine toxicity has been suggested as playing a role in NPA-induced brain damage. Johnson et al. (2000) investigated dopamine metabolism following long-term exposure to low doses of NPA in rats. Adult male SD rats were given 10 and 20 mg NPA per 40 mL in drinking water for 3 months. Dopamine and its metabolites were measured in the frontal cortex and caudate nucleus. Following 2 months of exposure, an increase in dopamine turnover was observed in the caudate nucleus of the high-dose group. The results of this study suggest an activation of the dopaminergic system after long-term, intermittent exposure to NPA. The production of radical oxygen species associated with dopamine metabolism may contribute to the NPA-induced neurotoxicity.

CHRONIC TOXICITY AND CARCINOGENICITY STUDIES

The National Cancer Institute (NCI, 1978) conducted a carcinogenicity study in rats and mice by administering NPA via gavage 5 days a week (104 weeks for mice and 110 weeks for rats). As NPA was determined to be unstable in feed, it was administered by gavage. The dose levels of NPA were determined from the results of the subchronic study. The low and high doses for rats were set at 25 and 50 ppm for males and 50 and 100 ppm for females. In the mice studies, for both males and females, the low and high doses were set at 75 and 150 ppm. Doses were converted from parts per million to milligrams per animal per day (mg/animal/day) and were used throughout the study. The study design is presented in Table 5.8.

In the rat study, NPA administration did not change the general appearance, body weights, and mortalities compared to controls. In both control and treated animals, a variety of neoplasms occurred. The neoplasms noted were spontaneous and common in rats (NCI, 1978). A slight, but not significant, increase in hepatic neoplastic nodules was noted in male rats and was within the normal range for the Fischer 344 strain (Haseman et al., 1990). Similarly, an increase (not statistically significant) in the incidence of pancreatic islet cell adenomas was noted in NPA-treated males. No such changes were noted in female rats or mice of either sex treated with NPA. Based on the results of these studies, NPA was determined to be non-carcinogenic in rats and mice.

In rats gavaged with NPA, focal myocardial fibrosis was observed. This may be a result of the stress of administration, as it was only seen in gavaged rats and not in control rats (not gavaged). In F344 rats, clinically silent degenerative myocardial changes of unknown etiology are common and may be produced by stress, diet, or the environment (MacKenzie and Alison, 1990). Further, the myocardial changes were not dose related.

TABLE 5.8
β-Nitropropionic Acid Bioassay Study Design

Animal Species	Sex	Dose[a] (mg/animal/day)	Duration of Study (weeks)
Rats (Fischer 344)	Males	Control[b]	
		0.425	110
		0.85	110
	Females	Control[b]	
		0.6	110
		1.2	110
Mice (B6C3F1)	Males	Control[b]	
		0.375	104
		0.75	104
	Females	Control[b]	
		0.375	104
		0.75	104

[a] Doses are equivalent to 25 and 50 ppm for male rats, 50 and 100 ppm for female rats, and 75 and 150 ppm for both sexes of mice.

[b] Control groups were not gavaged.

The administration of NPA to both male and female mice at 75 and 150 ppm resulted in decreased body weight gains compared to controls during the greater part of the study. No changes in mortalities were noted compared to controls. A variety of neoplasms were noted in both the control and NPA-treated groups. Chronic inflammatory, degenerative, and other non-neoplastic conditions were noted in all of the groups and were not related to NPA administration. In both sexes of mice, proliferative hepatocellular lesions occurred, but there was no indication that these changes were related to NPA administration. Based on the results of the rat and mouse studies, which did not show any effect attributed directly to the administration of NPA, the no-observed-adverse-effect level (NOAEL) for NPA in this chronic bioassay was determined as 50 ppm (2.5 mg/kg/day). The NOAEL was based on the male rat study, as this was the highest level used and was assumed to be safe in the most sensitive animal model.

In a chronic NPA study in baboons, Palfi et al. (1996) investigated the cognitive performances using the object retrieval detour task (ORDT) test. *Papio anubis* baboons were injected intramuscularly with NPA or saline (control) for 20 weeks. The dose regimen for the injection of NPA was designed to yield a linear increase in doses until obvious spontaneous abnormal movements could be observed (mean starting dose, 14 mg/kg/day; mean final dose, 33 mg/kg/day). After 3 to 6 weeks of treatment, a significant impairment in the ORDT was observed in the NPA-treated animals, occurring in the absence of spontaneous abnormal movements but in the presence of apomorphine-inducible dyskinesias. Continued administration of NPA resulted in the progression of spontaneous abnormal movements. Selective bilateral caudate–putamen lesions with a sparing of the cerebral cortex, notably the prefrontal cortex, were noted by histological observation. Chronic NPA administration in primates was found to replicate the basic pathophysiological triad of Huntington's disease, including spontaneous abnormal movements, progressive striatal degeneration, and a frontostriatal syndrome of cognitive impairment. In earlier studies, these investigators have shown that the chronic systemic injection of NPA to baboons can produce various dyskinetic movements and dystonic postures associated with selective striatal lesions (Brouillet et al., 1993a, 1995; Ferrante et al., 1993).

REPRODUCTIVE STUDIES

In a NCI range-finding study, NPA was given to five male and female rats through diet at concentrations ranging from 100 to 900 ppm (NCI, 1978). All of the animals were treated for 6 weeks, then observed for 2 weeks. In the male rats, histological examinations revealed testicular atrophy with spermatogenic arrest at 150 ppm, although no incidence data or statistical analyses were presented (NCI, 1978). This finding should not be regarded as definitive, because the finding occurred with nearly equal incidence in the controls and the treated groups in the chronic bioassay, where the animals were exposed to NPA for 110 weeks; NPA was found to be unstable in the diet so the changes may have been induced by a degradation product; no occurrence of testicular atrophy or spermatogenic arrest was noted in mice in the range-finding or chronic studies; the observed effect may be the result of arrested development in the range-finding animals; and these finding have not been corroborated by other investigators.

GENOTOXICITY STUDIES

The scientific literature concerning the mutagenicity of NPA is controversial. An impure commercial sample of NPA was reported as being mutagenic to *Salmonella typhimurium* strains TA1535 and TA100. Hansen (1984) reported that a sample from the impure lot of NPA was mutagenic in strain TA100 without metabolic activation, but this activity was diminished after recrystallization. Earlier, Dunkel and Simmon (1980) also reported that a sample of NPA used in the NCI study was found to be mutagenic in strain TA100 (1500 µg/plate) without metabolic activation. Hansen (1984) showed that a new, pure sample of NPA was non-mutagenic in strains TA98, TA100, and TA1538, with or without metabolic activation. These studies demonstrate that the reported mutagenicity of NPA may have been due to the presence of impurities. The impurities in the NPA samples may have included β-propiolactone, from which NPA is synthesized and which also produces base-pair mutagenicity. The mutagenic impurity is not expected to be present in the natural state, as natural synthesis of NPA occurs by a different route. Based on this information, it is possible to divide mutagenicity studies into two categories: those that used the NCI sample and those that did not.

A summary of the mutagenicity studies on NPA is presented in Table 5.9. Investigators who did not use the contaminated NCI NPA material have shown that NPA was not mutagenic in the experimental system utilized (Hansen, 1984; Myhr et al. 1988; Oshiro et al., 1991). Caspary et al. (1988b) found that NPA was

TABLE 5.9
Mutagenicity Assays with β-Nitropropionic Acid

Assay	Results	Sample Origin	Refs.
TA100	Positive	NCI	Dunkel and Simmon
TA1537	Positive	NCI	(1980)
TA100	Positive	NCI	Zeiger (1987)
TA1535	Positive	NCI	
TA98	Negative	NCI	
TA1537	Negative	NCI	
TA100	Positive	NCI	Hansen (1984)
TA98	Negative	NCI	
TA100	Negative	Commercial	Hansen (1984)
TA98	Negative	Commercial	
TA1538	Negative	Commercial	
CHO cell HGPRT assay	Negative	Commercial	Oshiro et al. (1991)
CHO cell HGPRT assay	Negative	Commercial	Myhr et al. (1988)
CHO micronucleus assay	Negative	Commercial	Oshiro et al. (1991)
Survival assay (Rauscher-leukemia-virus-infected rat embryo cells)	Positive	NCI	Traul et al. (1981)
Mouse lymphoma	Positive	NCI	Caspary et al. (1988a)
Human lymphoblast	Positive	NCI	
CHO SCE	Positive	NCI	
CHO chromosomal aberrations	Positive	NCI	
Mouse lymphoma	Positive	NCI (?)	Caspary et al. (1988b)[a]
Mouse lymphoma	Positive	NCI (?)	
Rat hepatocyte DNA repair	Positive	NCI	Williams et al. (1989)

[a] A summary of two studies performed at different laboratories.

mutagenic; however, it is possible that these investigators used the NPA sample from NCI, as other studies published by these investigators used the NCI sample. It has been shown that β-propiolactone acts as a positive mutagen in these test systems (RTECS, 1994). Based on these observations, it appears that purified NPA is not mutagenic.

Batiste-Alenton et al. (1995) investigated the genotoxicity of NPA in three *Drosophila* short-term somatic assays. The somatic mutation and/or recombination in *D. melanogaster* was studied by *zeste-white*, *white ivory*, and *wing spot* assays. In the *zeste-white* assay, the frequency of eye color mosaicism was studied in adult *Drosophila* males of the UZ strain after larval treatment with 0, 5, and 10 mM NPA. Similar assays were performed in the *white ivory* test using the (wi)4 strain of *Drosophila*. The induction of mosaicism was studied in *Drosophila* after larval treatment with NPA at 0-, 5-, 10-, and 20-mM concentrations in the *wing spot* assay. Although no dose response was observed, NPA did produce positive results in both the *zeste-white* and the *wing spot* tests. The authors classified NPA only as weakly genotoxic because of the lack of a dose response.

CYTOTOXICITY

The presence of a nitro group on an aliphatic chain has raised questions as to the ability for substances such as NPA to affect smooth muscle. In isolated guinea pig atria, NPA treatment resulted in a concentration-dependent decrease in contractile force and heart rate. The investigators speculated that the cardiodepressor activity of NPA may be explained by an interference with the availability of cytosolic free Ca^{2+} (Castillo et al., 1994). In other *in vitro* studies using rabbit aortic rings, it was found that NPA did not produce relaxation via endothelial receptors and was not mediated by muscarinic, β-adrenergic, or histaminergic (H_1) receptors (Castillo et al., 1993; Hong et al., 1990). Preincubation of the aortic rings with KCl resulted in less sensitivity to the relaxation mediated by NPA, suggesting that at least part of the mechanism of vasodilation is not related to an inhibition of calcium influx through the voltage-dependent Ca^{2+} channel. Similar to nitrovasodilators, NPA exerts a relaxant effect through guanylate cyclase stimulation and the subsequent increase in cyclic guanosine monophosphate (cGMP) levels into the vascular smooth muscle cells. Hong et al. (1990) suggested that the antihypertensive effect of NPA in renal hypertensive dogs may be attributed mainly to the vasodilating action of NPA.

In isolated, spontaneously beating atria, NPA (10^{-4} *M*) was found to decrease the heart rate by 62% (Lopez et al., 1998). NPA treatment did not decrease the amplitude or duration of the action potentials; however, exposure to 10^{-2} *M* NPA prolonged the duration of the intervals between the two action potentials from 530 to 1400 msec. NPA exposure inhibited the oxygen consumption by heart mitochondria when either malate/glutamate or succinate was used as the metabolism substrate. NPA exposure resulted in decreased atrial ATP levels by approximately 62% without affecting cytochrome C oxidase activity. These results show that NPA decreases the atrial rate by increasing the action potential phase 4, probably by inhibiting mitochondrial respiration, thereby decreasing cardiac ATP content, thus suggesting that NPA-induced bradycardia might be related to intracellular ATP depletion.

In an *in vitro* study using brain homogenate, NPA was found to inhibit synaptosomal respiration in a dose-dependent manner. The degree of inhibition was greater when respiration was stimulated by a concomitant increase in ATP usage. The addition of NPA resulted in a rapid decrease in the creatine phosphate/creatine ratio and an increase in the lactate/pyruvate ratio. Initially, a fall in the ATP/ADP and GTP/GDP ratios was less prominent but closely followed the creatine phosphate/creatine ratio. In the absence of glutamine, NPA caused a significant decrease in the internal concentrations of aspartate and a small reduction in glutamate levels, whereas GABA levels rose. The sum of these three amino acids inside synaptosomes decreased without any increase in their external levels. In the presence of glutamine in the medium, the decrease in intra-synaptosomal aspartate was accompanied by an increase in intra-synaptosomal glutamate and GABA. In the presence of NPA, the external concentration of glutamate was substantially increased. NPA had no effect on the basal release of either glutamate (and GABA) or biogenic amines; however, the addition of non-saturating concentrations of depolarizing agents, such as veratridine and KCl, increased the efflux.

In another *in vitro* study, Deshpande and Nishino (1998) investigated protection against the NPA-induced toxicity of astrocytes by basic fibroblast growth factor (bFGF) and thrombin. Addition of NPA at concentrations of 0.017 to 1.7 mM to astrocyte cultures produced a dose- and time-dependent astrocyte loss, as measured by a decrease in the number of glial fibrillary acidic protein (GFAP)-positive cells and an increase in the levels of lactate dehydrogenase (LDH). The NPA-induced decrease was noticed within 12 hours after the addition and was maximally affected at 24 hours. NPA-induced cell loss was attenuated by the presence of bFGF (10 ng/mL). At a concentration of 0.01 nM, thrombin protection against the toxicity of NPA was noted, while at higher concentrations thrombin (10 to 100 nM) produced greater cell loss. These results indicate that bFGF and low concentrations of thrombin attenuate NPA-induced acute astrocyte toxicity.

The NPA-induced toxicity in primary cultures of cerebellar granule cells and astrocytes was studied by Olsen et al. (1999). In both neurons and astrocytes, NPA inhibited SDH and the tricarboxylic acid cycle activity to the same extent. Although the extent of the inhibition of these biochemical markers was similar, NPA was 16 times more toxic to neurons compared to astrocytes. The LC$_{50}$ of NPA for neurons and astrocytes was determined to be 0.7 and 11 mM, respectively. The authors suggested that the relative resistance of astrocytes to NPA may be related to their low tricarboxylic acid cycle activity (5 to 10%) compared to the neuronal activity and also to the inability of NPA to cause astrocytic calcium overload. These studies demonstrate that NPA is predominantly an astrocyte-sparing neurotoxin.

In an organ bath of the brain tissues from Sprague-Dawley rats, Riepe et al. (1992) investigated the effects of NPA on energy metabolism and ATP-sensitive potassium channels. NPA at a concentration of 1 mM was found to produce a hyperpolarization for variable lengths of time before evoking an irreversible depolarization in the pyramidal cell layer of the hippocampal region CA1. The hyperpolarization was found to be a result of increased potassium conductance, which was attenuated by a selective antagonist of ATP-sensitive potassium channels (glibenclamide, 1 to 10 μM). In contrast, an agonist at this channel (diazoxide, 0.5 mM) induces a hyperpolarization in CA1 neurons of rat hippocampal slices. The transient hyperpolarization induced by prolonged (~1 hour) application of NPA is followed by a depolarization that is incompletely reversed by a brief application of glutamate antagonists, such as D-2-amino-5-phosphonopentanoic acid (APV); 6,7-dichloro-quinoxaline-2,3-dione (CNQX); 3-(±)-2-carboxypiperazin-4-yl)propyl-1-phosphonic acid (CPP); and 7-chloro-kynurenic acid (7CI-KYN). Application of glibenclamide within 5 minutes of NPA blocked or reduced hyperpolarization and accelerated depolarization. These results suggest that the metabolic inhibition by NPA initially activates ATP-sensitive potassium channels.

Siedel et al. (2000) investigated the possible involvement of intercellular adhesion molecule 1 (ICAM-1) in NPA-mediated neurodegeneration. Neuroblastoma cells were treated with different concentrations of NPA, and changes in gene expression were analyzed by mRNA differential display (DDRT–PCR). By employing 18 primer combinations, these investigators identified a set of 33 candidate cDNA derived from 29 excised DDRT bands for which the expression appeared to be changed in response to the NPA insult. The differential mRNA expression of ribosomal proteins (S6 and

L40), the protein kinase A catalytic *beta* subunit, and ICAM were verified using northern hybridization and RT–PCR techniques. The results of the differential display may be useful in elucidating the multiple processes causing neurodegeneration subsequent to NPA-induced lesions.

HUMAN OBSERVATIONS

Several reports of accidental NPA poisoning, also referred as "moldy sugarcane poisoning" or "deteriorated sugarcane poisoning," in China have appeared in the literature (Liu, 1993; Liu et al., 1989, 1992; Peraica et al., 1999). Initially, this poisoning was reported as an acute food poisoning of unknown etiology occurring in 13 provinces in China. The poisoning occurred seasonally, with most cases occurring from February to April, and was reported to primarily affect the central nervous system. From 1972 to 1988, 847 cases of poisoning were reported; 84 of the affected individuals died, and several were left "lifelong disabled" (Liu et al., 1989). By 1989, the total was up to 885 cases, with 88 deaths. The victims of these outbreaks were mostly children and young individuals (Liu et al., 1992). Following consumption of the moldy sugarcane, the incubation period (until signs of intoxication) was generally from 10 minutes to 8 hours; in most cases, the incubation period was between 2 and 3 hours (Liu et al., 1989) and less than 5 hours (Ming, 1995). Clinical signs of poisoning included a sudden onset of nausea, vomiting, abdominal pain, and diarrhea. The development of double vision, somnolence, nystagmus, convulsions, decerebrate rigidity, and coma was also reported in some patients. The patients who regained consciousness were mute and incontinent. In some patients, the development of a delayed dystonia 7 to 40 days later was noted. Clinical signs in these patients included grimacing, sustained athetosis of hands and fingers, torsion spasm, spasmodic torticollis, hemiballismus, and painful spasms of the extremities. Computed axial tomography (CAT) scan of these individuals revealed bilateral hypodensity of the putamen and, to a lesser extent, the globus pallidum. Occasional involvement of the caudate and claustrum was also noted. Similar to the spastic parapareses of lathyrism and cassavism, the clinical symptoms of toxic dystonia were permanent (Spencer et al., 1993). Changes in electroencephalographic recordings were noted, but body temperature, heart, liver, lung, cerebrospinal fluid, blood, urine, and feces were all normal (Liu et al., 1992).

The characteristic injuries observed in rats described previously (Hamilton and Gould, 1987b) were very similar to the lesions in bilateral lenticular nuclei shown in the CAT scans of patients with moldy sugarcane poisoning (Liu et al., 1992). Based on the abnormalities identified in the basal ganglia on cranial CAT scans, the development of delayed symptoms was predicted (Ming, 1995). Ludolph et al. (1991) reported that NPA caused gastrointestinal symptoms in adults, whereas signs of severe encephalopathy were not common. Curiously, the majority of the reported poisoning cases were children, a finding that contradicts the animal studies of Brouillet et al. (1993b) and others, who reported that older animals were more susceptible to NPA compared to the younger ones. The difference in age-related susceptibility in the Chinese poisoning was interpreted as being a result of a cultural factor rather than a biological one. Liu et al. (1992) and Spencer et al. (1993) reported that sugarcane is traditionally given to children as a seasonal and holiday confectionary and as a substitute for fresh fruit in the spring, at a time when fruit prices are high.

Liu et al. (1992) reported that the examination of the samples of sugarcane that caused the poisoning did not appear normal, as the bark had lost its normal luster, the color of the pulp had changed to light brown, and several samples smelled of moldy food and alcohol. In deteriorated sugarcane sampled from food markets in the areas of reported poisoning, strains of *Arthrinium* were found. In the deteriorated sugarcane samples, the presence of NPA as the toxin was identified (Liu et al., 1989). In these samples, levels of NPA ranged from 285 to 6660 ppm (Liu et al., 1992). The amount of sugarcane consumed by the patients was not determined. The maximum NPA concentration detected in cultures from the sugarcane was 4000 ppm (Liu et al., 1992).

NPA AND HUNTINGTON'S DISEASE

Huntington's disease (HD) is a genetic neurodegenerative disorder characterized clinically by both motor and cognitive impairments and striatal lesions. NPA provides an animal model of HD that closely resembles the human aspects of the disease, in terms of both pathology and symptomatology (Alexi et al., 1998). Blum et al. (2002a) determined the time course of neurochemical changes occurring following metabolic impairments produced by NPA in a rat model of HD. The similarities between the NPA animal model and HD in humans are summarized in Table 5.10; however, in a recent study, Sun et al. (2002) reported that the differential vulnerability of striatal projection neurons in NPA-treated rats does not match that typical of adult-onset HD. These investigators suggested that the NPA rat model does not fully mimic the adult-onset of HD pathogenesis. Although the mechanisms of metabolic dysfunction induced by NPA may not be the specific culprit in human HD, these models provide deeper insight into neurodegenerative disorders. Currently, no pharmacological treatments are available to prevent or arrest the HD process; however, these animal models also provide additional avenues for therapeutic intervention in neuronal damage resulting from metabolic compromise (Blum et al., 2002b).

SUMMARY AND CONCLUSIONS

Ubiquitous molds such as *Aspergillus*, *Penicillium*, and, to a lesser extent, *Arthrinium* are known to produce β-nitropropionic acid (NPA). The presence of NPA has also been reported in at least four families of higher plants. A long history exists of use and exposure to NPA as a result of the use of *Aspergillus* as an economic mold in the production of certain foods and the accidental contamination of foods. It is estimated that as much as 5.5 mg/day (79 µg/kg/day for a 70-kg person) of NPA is consumed by the Japanese population through *miso* and soy sauce alone. This consumption of NPA may be considerably higher if *sake* and other sources are taken into consideration. Despite the ubiquity of the presence of molds capable of the synthesis of NPA and the widespread consumption of foods containing NPA, human poisonings of NPA are confined to a specific set of circumstances. The major accidental poisonings with NPA occurred in China during late winter in 13 northern provinces as a consequence of ingesting sugarcane that had been stored for at least 2 months and

TABLE 5.10
Similarities Between β-Nitropropionic Acid Animal Model and Huntington's Disease

Neuropathology	Huntington's Disease	β-Nitropropionic Acid (NPA)
GABA	↓	↓
NADPHd/NOS/SST/NPY	↓=	↓=
ChAT	↓=	↓=[a]
Calbindin	↓	↓
Substance P	↓	↓
Fibers of passage	=	=
Dendritic alterations	Yes	Yes
Movement Dysfunction		
Chorea	Yes	Yes
Dystonia	Yes	Yes
Dyskinesia	Yes	Yes

[a] Results were not quantified.

Note: Results for Huntington's disease are from published postmortem results. Arrows indicate a decrease in phenotype marker, an equal sign indicates no change, and an arrow combined with an equal sign indicates that the change was relatively less severe than those of other markers. ChAT, choline acetyltransferase; GABA, γ-aminobutyric acid; NADPHd, nicotinamide adenine dinucleotide phosphate diaphorase; NOS, nitric acid synthase; NPY, neuropeptide Y; SST = somatostatin.

Source: Adapted from Alexi, T. et al., *NeuroReport* 9, R57–R64, 1998.

which was infested with *Arthrinium* spp. The poisoning cases are a result of the gross mishandling of sugarcane and the sale of discolored and off-odor product.

Absorption of NPA takes place in the gastrointestinal tract. Once absorbed, NPA enters the circulation and is metabolized to nitrite, although some may bind to succinate dehydrogenase upon oxidation. Most of the orally ingested NPA is likely to be metabolized in the liver. No published data on the excretion of NPA were found in the literature. The pathologic sequelae following NPA administration are reported to be consistent among all species. Once the threshold dose for the particular species is achieved and succinate dehydrogenase bound, the cell is energetically depleted and ischemia in certain organs ensues. In acute NPA toxicity, striatal muscle damage occurs and neuromuscular sequelae are manifested. NPA has been used in animal studies for the investigation of various neurodegenerative diseases in humans, such as HD.

The LD_{50} value of NPA for mice and rats has been found to be between 60 and 120 mg/kg. In rabbits and other mammals, the LD_{50} of NPA may be slightly higher. The 30-day LD_{50} of NPA in mice is approximately 50 mg/kg. In a chronic study in rats and mice, NPA did not exhibit carcinogenicity or chronic toxicity. The NOAEL in the chronic toxicity study in rats was determined to be 50 ppm (2.5 mg/kg/day) for males and 75 ppm for females (3.75 mg/kg/day). Mutagenicity test results of NPA are mixed; however, all of the positive tests can be traced to the use of a single impure sample of NPA. Mutagenicity assays with purified or recrystallized samples from the impure NPA were negative. Similarly, newly manufactured NPA was also negative. Chemically synthesized NPA may contain a mutagen, β-propiolactone, as a contaminant, which would not be present in samples from naturally derived NPA, as biosynthesis takes place via a different route.

On the basis of the extensive toxicity information available on NPA and on the basis of a chronic bioassay of NPA in rats and mice, an allowable daily intake (ADI) of NPA can be determined. Based on the NOAEL of 2.5 mg/kg/day from a chronic toxicity study in male rats, a tolerable intake of NPA in humans can be calculated. Using these experimental data and uncertainty factors of 10 for intraspecies differences and 10 for interspecies differences, a tolerable intake for ingestion of NPA by humans of 25 µg/kg per day or 1.5 mg/kg/day for a 60-kg individual is posited. This tolerable intake is lower than the current estimated daily intake of NPA from *miso* and soy sauce in the Japanese population which is approximately 5.5 mg/day. On the basis of the available information and toxicity data, an ADI of 25 µg/kg/day or 1.5 mg/kg/day of NPA is appropriate.

REFERENCES

Alexi, T., Hughes, P.E., Faull, R.L.M., and Williams, C.E. (1998) 3-Nitropropionic acid's lethal triplet: cooperative pathways of neurodegeneration, *NeuroReport*, 9: R57–R64.

Alexi, T., Faull, R.L.M., and Hughes, P.E. (2000) Variable susceptibility to neurotoxicity of systemic 3-nitropropionic acid, in *Mitochondrial Inhibitors and Neurodegenerative Disorders*, Sanberg, P.R., Nishino, H., and Borlongan, C.V., Eds., Contemporary Neuroscience Series, Humana Press, Totowa, NJ, pp. 129–140.

Alston, T.A. (1981) Suicide substrates for mitochondrial enzymes, *Pharmac. Ther.*, 12: 1–41.

Alston, T.A., Mela, L., and Bright, H.J. (1977) 3-Nitropropionate, the toxic substance of *Indigofera*, is a suicide inactivator of succinate dehydrogenase, *Proc. Natl. Acad. Sci. USA*, 74: 3767–3771.

Alston, T.A., Porter, D.J.T., and Bright, H.J. (1985) The bioorganic chemistry of the nitroalkyl group, *Biorg. Chem.*, 13: 375–403.

Anderson, R.C., Rasmussen, M.A., and Allison, M.J. (1993) Metabolism of the plant toxins nitropropionic acid and nitropropanol by ruminal microorganisms, *Appl. Environ. Microbiol.*, 59: 3056–3061.

Andrich, M. (1995) Personal conversation with Mary Andrich, Kikkoman Foods, Walworth, WI, Jan. 27, 1995.

Aylward, J.H., Cort, R.D., Haydock, K.P., Strickland, R.W., and Hegarty, M.P. (1987) *Indigofera* spp. with agronomic potential in the tropics: rat toxicity studies, *Austral. J. Agric. Res.* 38: 177–186.

Batiste-Alentorn, M., Xamena, N., Creus, A., and Marcos, R. (1995) Genotoxicity testing of five compounds in three *Drosophila* short-term somatic assays, *Mutation Res.*, 341: 161–167.

Baxter, R.L., Hanley, A.B., Chan, H.W.S., Greenwood, S.L., Abbot, E.M., McFarlane, K.J., and Milne, K. (1992) Fungal biosynthesis of 3-nitropropanoic acid, *J. Chem. Soc. Perkin Trans.*, 19: 2495–2502.

Beal, M.F., Brouillet, E., Jenkins, B., Henshaw, R., Rosen, B., and Hyman, B.T. (1993a) Age-dependent striatal excitotoxic lesions produced by the endogenous mitochondrial inhibitor malonate, *J. Neurochem.*, 61(3): 1147–1150.

Beal, M.F., Brouillet, E., Jenkins, B.G., Ferrante, R.J., Kowall, N.W., Miller, J.M., Storey, E., Srivastava, R., Rosen, B.R., and Hyman, B.T. (1993b) Neurochemical and histologic characterization of striatal excitotoxic lesions produced by the mitochondrial toxin 3-nitropropionic acid, *J. Neurosci.*, 13: 4181–4192.

Beal, M.F., Ferrante, R.J., Henshaw, W., Mathews, R.T., Chan, P.H., Kowal, N.W., Epstein, C.J., and Schultz, J.W. (1995) 3-Nitropropionic acid neurotoxicity is attenuated in copper/zinc superoxide dismutase transgenic mice, *J. Neurochem.*, 65: 919–922.

Becker, G.E. (1967) Effect of glucose on the oxidation of beta-nitropropionic acid by *Aspergillus flavus*, *J. Bacteriol.*, 94: 48–52.

Bell, M.E. (1974) Toxicology of karaka kernel, karakin, and beta-nitropropionic acid, *New Zeal. J. Sci.*, 17: 327–334.

Benn, M.H., McDiarmid, R.E., and Majak, W. (1989) *In vitro* biotransformation of 3-nitropropanol (miserotoxin aglycone) by horse liver alcohol dehydrogenase, *Toxicol. Lett.*, 47: 165–172.

Binienda, Z. and Kim, C.S. (1997) Increase in levels of total free fatty acids in rat brain regions following 3-nitropropionic acid administration, *Neurosci. Lett.* 230: 199–201.

Binienda, Z., Simmons, C., Hussain, S., Slikker, W., Jr., and Ali, S.F. (1998) Effect of acute exposure to 3-nitropropionic acid on activities of endogenous antioxidants in the rat brains, *Neurosci. Lett.*, 251: 173–176.

Blum, D., Galas, M.C., Gall, D., Cuvelier, L., and Schiffmann, S.N. (2002a) Striatal and cortical neurochemical changes induced by chronic metabolic compromise in the 3-nitropropionic model of Huntington's disease, *Neurobiol. Dis.*, 10: 410–426

Blum, D., Gall, D., Galas, M.C., d'Alcantara, P., Bantubungi, K., and Schiffmann, S.N. (2002b) The adenosine A1 receptor agonist adenosine amine congener exerts a neuroprotective effect against the development of striatal lesions and motor impairments in the 3-nitropropionic acid model of neurotoxicity, *J. Neurosci.*, 22: 9122–9133.

Borlongan, C.V., Koutouzis, T.K., Freeman, T.B., Hauser, R.A., Cahill, D.W., and Sanberg, P.R. (1997) Hyperactivity and hypoactivity in a rat model of Huntington's disease: the systemic 3-nitropropionic acid model, *Brain Res. Protocols*, 1: 253–257.

Bossi, S.R., Simpson, J.R., and Isacson, O. (1993) Age dependence on striatal neuronal death caused by mitochondrial dysfunction, *NeuroReport*, 4: 73–76.

Brouillet, E, Jenkins, B.G., Hyman, B.T., Ferrante, R.J., Kowall, N.W., Srivastava, R., Roy, D.S., Rosen, B.R., and Beal, M.F. (1993a) Age-dependent vulnerability of the striatum to the mitochondrial toxin 3-nitropropionic acid, *J. Neurochem.*, 60: 356–359.

Brouillet, E., Hantraye, P., Dolan, R., Leroy-Willig, A., Bottalanderr, M., Isacson, O., Maziere, M., Ferrante, R.J., and Beal, M.F. (1993b) Chronic administration of 3-nitropropionic acid induced selective striatal degeneration and abnormal choreiform movements in monkeys, *Soc. Neurosci. Abstr.*, 19: 409.

Brouillet, E., Hantraye, P., Ferrante, R.J., Dolan, R., Leroy-Willig, A., Kowall, N.W., and Beal, M.F. (1995) Chronic mitochondrial energy impairment produces selective striatal degeneration and abnormal choreiform movement in primates, *Proc. Natl. Acad. Sci. USA* 92: 7105–7109.

Burdock, G.A., Carabin, I.G., and Soni, M.G. (2001) Safety assessment of β-nitropropionic acid: a monograph in support of an acceptable daily intake in humans, *Food Chem.*, 75: 1–27.

Byers, R.A., David, L., Moyer, B.G., and Bierlein, D.L. (1986) 3-Nitropropionate in crown-vetch: a natural deterrent to insects?, in *Natural Resistance of Plants and Pests: Roles of Allelochemicals*, Green, M.B. and Hedin, P.A., Eds., ACS Symposium Series No. 296, American Chemical Society, Washington, D.C., pp. 95–105.

Candish, E., La Croix, J., and Unrau, A.M. (1969) Biosynthesis of 3-nitropropionic acid in creeping indigo (*Indigofera spicata*), *Biochemistry*, 8: 182.

Carter, C.L. (1951) The constitution of karakin, *J. Sci. Food Agric.*, 2: 54–55.

Carter, C. L. and McChesney, W. J. (1949) Hiptagenic acid identified as β-nitropropionic acid, *Nature*, 164: 575–576.

Caspary, W.J., Langenback, R., Penman, B.W., Crespi, C., Myhr, B.C., and Mitchell, A.D. (1988a) The mutagenic activity of selected compounds at the TK locus: rodent vs. human cells, *Mutat. Res.* 196: 61–81.

Caspary, W.J., Daston, D.S., Myher, B.C., Mitchell, A.D., Rubb, C.J., and Less, P.S. (1988b) Evaluation of the L5178Y mouse lymphoma cell mutagenesis assay: interlaboratory reproducibility and assessment, *Environ. Mol. Mutagen.*, 12: 195–225.

Castillo, C., Valencia, I., Reyes, G., and Hong, E. (1993) An analysis of the antihypertensive properties of 3-nitropropionic acid, a compound from plants in the genus *Astragalus*, *Arch. Inst. Cardiol. Mex.*, 63: 11–16.

Castillo, C., Reyes, G., Rosas-Lezama, M.A., Valencia, I., and Hong, E. (1994) Analysis of the cardiodepressor action of 3-nitropropionic acid, *Proc. West. Pharmacol. Soc.*, 37: 41–42.

CHEMID (2000) National Library of Medicine database, Bethesda, MD.

Coles, C.J., Edmondson, D.E., and Singer, T.P. (1979) Inactivation of succinate dehydrogenase by 3-nitropropionate, *J. Biol. Chem.*, 254: 5161–5167.

Cooke, A.R. (1955) The toxic constituent of *Indigofera endecaphylla*, *Arch. Biochem. Biophys.*, 55: 114–120.

Dautry, C., Vaufrey, F., Brouillet, E., Bizat, N., Henry, P., Conde, F., Bloch, G., and Hantraye, P. (2000) Early *N*-acetylaspartate depletion is a marker of neuronal dysfunction in rats and primates chronically treated with the mitochondrial toxin 3-nitropropionic acid, *J. Cereb. Blood Flow Metab.*, 20: 789–799.

Deshpande, S. B. and Nishino, H. (1998) *In vitro* protection of 3-nitropropionic acid-induced toxicity of astrocytes by basic fibroblast growth factor and thrombin, *Brain Res.*, 783: 28–36.

Drummond, R.J., Gustine, D.L., and Phillips, A.T. (1975) Alterations of gamma-amino butyric acid metabolism in brain by 3-nitropropionic acid, *Fed. Proc.*, 34: 283.

Dunkel, V.C. and Simmon, V.F. (1980) Mutagenic activity of chemicals previously tested for carcinogenicity in the National Cancer Institute Bioassay Program, in *Molecular and Cellular Aspects of Carcinogen Screening Tests*, Montesano, R., Bartsch, H., and Tomatis, L., Eds., International Agency for Research on Cancer, Lyon.

Ebrahimzadeh, H., Niknam, V., and Maassoumi, A.A. (1999) Nitro compounds in *Astragalus* species from Iran, *Biochem. System. Ecol.*, 27: 743–751.

Erecinska, M. and Nelson, D. (1994) Effects of 3-nitropropionic acid on synaptosomal energy and transmitter metabolism: relevance to neurodegenerative brain diseases, *J. Neurochem.*, 63: 1033–1041.

Evidente, A., Capretti, P., Giordano, F., and Surico, G. (1992) Identification and phytotoxicity of 3-nitropropanoic acid produced *in vitro* by *Melanconis thelebola*, *Experientia*, 48: 1169–1172.

Faix, J.J., Gustine, D.L., and Wright, M.J. (1978) Beta nitropropionic acid concentration of crownvetch plant parts as affected by growth–temperature–maturation variables, *Agron. J.*, 70: 689–691.

Ferrante, R.J., Hantraye, P., Brouillet, E., Kowall, N.W., and Beal, M.F. (1993) Striatal pathology of impaired mitochondrial metabolism in primates profiles Huntington's disease, *Soc. Neurosci. Abstr.*, 19: 408.

Frisvad, J. and Thrane, U. (1987) Standardized high performance liquid chromatography of 182 mycotoxins and other fungal metabolites based on alkylphenone retention indexes and UV–VIS spectra (diode array detection), *J. Chromatogr.*, 404: 195–214.

Fu, Y., He, F., Zhang, S., and Zhang, G. (1995) Lipid peroxidation in rats intoxicated with 3-nitropropionic acid, *Toxicon*, 33: 327–333.

Fukuda, A., Deshpande, S.B., Shimano, Y., and Nishino, H. (1998) Astrocytes are more vulnerable than neurons to cellular Ca^{2+} overload induced by a mitochondrial toxin, 3-nitropropionic acid, *Neuroscience*, 87: 497–507.

Gilbert, M., Penel, A., Koskowski, F.V., Henion, J.D., Maylin, G.A., and Lisk, D.J. (1977) Electron affinity gas chromatographic determination of beta-nitropropionic acid as its pentafluorobenzyl derivative in cheeses and mold filtrates. *J. Food Sci.*, 42: 1650–1653.

Gold, K. and Brodman, B.W. (1991) Studies on the distribution of a naturally occurring nitroaliphatic acid in crownvetch (*Coronilla varia*, Fabaceae), *Econ. Bot.*, 45: 334–338.

Gould, K. and Gustine, D.L. (1982) Basal ganglia degeneration, myelin alteration and enzyme inhibition induced in mice by the plant toxin 3-nitropropionic acid, *Neuropathol. Appl. Neurobiol.*, 8: 377–391.

Gould, D.H., Wilson, M.P., and Hamar, D.W. (1985) Brain enzyme and clinical alterations induced in rats and mice by nitroaliphatic toxicants, *Toxicol. Lett.*, 27: 83–89.

Gruner, B.J., DeAngelo, A.B., and Shaw, P.D. (1972) Isolation and some properties of an enzyme system which catalyzes the degradation of beta-nitropropionic acid, *Arch. Biochem. Biophys.*, 148: 107–114.

Gustine, D.L. (1979) Aliphatic nitro compounds in crownvetch: a review, *Crop Sci.*, 19: 197–203.

Guyot, M.C., Hantraye, P., Dolan R., Palfi, S., Maziere, M., and Brouillet, E. (1997) Quantifiable bradykinesia, gait abnormalities and Huntington's disease-like striatal lesions in rats chronically treated with 3-nitropropionic acid, *Neuroscience*, 79: 45–56.

Hamilton, B.F. (1986) Clinical signs and morphologic brain lesions in rats intoxicated with 3-nitropropionic acid, in *3-Nitropropionic Acid Neurotoxicity in Rats: A Type of Hypoxic (Energy-Deficient) Brain Damage*, UMI Dissertation Services, Ann Arbor, MI, pp. 26–59.

Hamilton, B.F. and Gould, D.H. (1987a) Correlation of morphologic brain lesions with physiologic alterations and blood–brain barrier impairment in 3-nitropropionic acid toxicity in rats, *Acta Neuropathol.*, 74: 67–74.

Hamilton, B.F. and Gould, D.H. (1987b) Nature and distribution of brain lesions in rats intoxicated with 3-nitropropionic acid: a type of hypoxic (energy deficient) brain damage, *Acta Neuropathol.*, 72: 286–297.

Hamilton, B.F., Gould, D.H., Wilson, M.P., and Hamar, D.H. (1984) Enzyme and structural alterations in brains of rats intoxicated with 3-nitropropionic acid, *Fed. Proc.*, 43: 558.

Hamilton, B.F., Gould, D.H., and Gustine, D.L. (2000) History of 3-nitropropionic acid: occurrence and role in human and animal disease, in *Mitochondrial Inhibitors and Neurodegenerative Disorders*, Sanberg, P.R., Nishino, H., and Borlongan, C.V., Eds., Humana Press, Totowa, NJ, pp. 21–33.

Hansen, T.J. (1984) Ames mutagenicity tests on purified 3-nitropropionic acid, *Food Chem. Toxicol.*, 22: 399–401.

Haseman, J.K., Arnold, J., and Eustis, S.L. (1990) Tumor incidences in Fischer 344 rats: NTP historical data, in *Pathology of the Fischer Rat: Reference and Atlas*, Boorman, G.A., Eustis, S.L., Elwell, M.R., Montgomery, C.A., Jr., and MacKenzie, W.F., Eds., Academic Press, New York, pp. 555–564.

Hershenhorn, J., Vurro, M., Zonno, M.C., Stierle, A., and Strobel, G. (1993) *Septoria cirsii*, a potential biocontrol agent of Canada thistle and its phytotoxin: beta-nitropropionic acid, *Plant Sci.*, 94: 227–234.

Hickey, M.A. and Morton, A.J. (2000) Mice transgenic for the Huntington's disease mutation are resistant to chronic 3-nitropropionic acid-induced striatal toxicity, *J. Neurochem.*, 75: 2163–2171.

Hong, E., Castillo, C., Rivero, I., and Somanathan, R. (1990) Vasodilator and antihypertensive actions of 3-nitropropionic acid, *Proc. West. Pharmacol. Soc.*, 33: 209–211.

Hutton, E.M., Windrum, G.M., and Kratzing, C.C. (1958) Studies on the toxicity of *Indigofera endecaphylla*. I. Toxicity for rabbits, *J. Nutr.*, 64: 321–337.

Iwasaki, T. and Kosikowski, F.V. (1973) Production of beta-nitropropionic acid in foods, *J. Food Sci.*, 38: 1162–1165.

James, L.F., Hartley, W.J., Williams, M.C., and Van Kampen, D.R. (1980) Field and experimental studies in cattle and sheep poisoned by nitro-bearing *Astragalus* or their toxins, *Am. J. Vet Res.*, 41: 377–382.

JECFA (1974) *Evaluation of Certain Food Additives*, 18th Report of the Joint FAO/WHO Expert Committee on Food Additives, Technical Report Series No. 557, Geneva, Switzerland, p. 20.

JECFA (1987) *Evaluation of Certain Food Additives and Contaminants*, 31st Report of the Joint FAO/WHO Expert Committee on Food Additives, Technical Report Series No. 759, Geneva, Switzerland, pp. 16–17.

Johnson, J.R., Robinson, B.L., Ali, S.F., and Binienda, Z. (2000) Dopamine toxicity following long term exposure to low doses of 3-nitropropionic acid (3-NPA) in rats, *Toxicol. Lett.*, 116: 113–118.

Kamikawa, T., Higuchi, F., Taniguchi, M., and Asaka, Y. (1980) Toxic metabolites of an unidentified filamentous fungus isolated from *Zinnia* leaves, *Agric. Biol. Chem.*, 44: 691–692.

Kim, G.W., Copin, J.C., Kawase, M., Chen, S.F., Sato, S., Gobbel, G.T., and Chan, H.P. (1999) Excitotoxicity is required for induction of oxidative stress and apoptosis in mouse striatum by mitochondrial toxin, 3-nitropropionic acid, *J. Cereb. Blood Flow Metab.*, 20: 119–129.

Kinosita, R., Ishiko, T., Sugiyama, S., Seto, T., Igarasi, S., and Goetz, I.E. (1968) Mycotoxins in fermented food, *Cancer Res.*, 28: 2296–2311.

Kitchin, K.T., Brown, J.L., and Kulkarni, A.P. (1993) Predicting rodent carcinogenicity of Ames test false positives by *in vivo* biochemical parameters, *Mutat. Res.*, 290: 155–164.

Klivenyi, P., Andreassen O.A., Ferrante, R.J., Dedeoglu, A., Mueller, G., Lancelot, E., Bogdanov, M., Andersen, J.K., Jaing, D., and Beal, M.F. (1999) Mice deficient in cellular glutathione peroxidase show increased vulnerability to malonate, 3-nitropropionic acid, and 1-methyl-4-phenyl-1:2:5:6-tetrahydropyridine, *J. Neurosci.*, 20: 1–7.

Liu, X.J. (1993) An observation on the regularity of mould invasion into sugarcane and its prevention, *Chung Hua Yu Fang I Hsueh Tsa Chih*, 27: 198–200.

Liu, X.J., Luo, X.Y., and Hu, W.J. (1989) *Anthrinium* spp. and the etiology of deteriorated sugarcane poisoning, in *Bioactive Molecules*, Vol. 10, Natori, S., Hashimoto, K., and Ueno, Y., Eds., Elsevier, Amsterdam, pp. 109–118.

Liu, X.J., Luo, X.Y., and Hu, W.J. (1992) Studies on the epidemiology and etiology of moldy sugarcane poisoning in China, *Biomed. Environ. Sci.*, 5: 161–177.

Lopez, P.S., Castillo, C.H., Pastellin, G.H., Hernandez, M.R., Suarez, M.J., Sanchez, M.L., and Escalante, B.A. (1998) Characterization of 3-nitropropionic acid-induced bradycardia in isolated atria, *Toxicol. Appl. Pharmacol.*, 148: 1–6.

Ludolph, A.C., He, F., Spencer, P.S., Hammerstad, J., and Sabri, M. (1991) 3-Nitropropionic acid: exogenous animal neurotoxin and possible human striatal toxin, *Can. J. Neurol. Sci.*, 18: 492–498.

Ludolph, A.C., Seelig, M., Ludolph, A., Novitt, P., Allen, C.N., Spencer, P., and Sabri, M.I. (1992) 3-Nitropropionic acid decreases cellular energy levels and causes neuronal degeneration in cortical explants, *Neurodegeneration*, 1: 155–161.

MacKenzie, W.F. and Alison, R.H. (1990) Heart, in *Pathology of the Fischer Rat*, Boorman, G.A., Eustis, S.L., Elwell, M.R., Montgomery, C.A., Jr., and MacKenzie, W.F., Eds., Academic Press, New York, pp. 461–472.

Majak, W. (1992) Further enhancement of 3-nitropropanol detoxification by ruminal bacteria in cattle, *Can. J. Animal Sci.*, 72: 863–870.

Majak, W. and Cheng, K.J. (1981) Identification of rumen bacteria that anaerobically degrade aliphatic nitrotoxins, *Can. J. Microbiol.*, 27: 646–650.

Majak, W. and Clark, L.J. (1980) Metabolism of aliphatic nitro compounds in bovine rumen fluid, *Can. J. Animal Sci.*, 60: 319–325.

Majak, W. and Pass, M.A. (1989) Aliphatic nitrocompounds, in *Toxicants of Plant Origin*, Vol. II, Cheeke, P.R., Ed., CRC Press, Boca Raton, FL, pp. 143–159.

Majak, W., Pass, M.A., and Madryga, F.J. (1983) Toxicity of misertoxin and its aglycone (3-nitropropanol) to rats, *Toxicol. Lett.*, 19: 171–178.

Majak, W., Pass, M.A., Muir, A.D., and Rode, L.M. (1984) Absorption of 3-nitropropanol (miserotoxin aglycone) from the compound stomach of cattle, *Toxicol. Lett.*, 23: 9–15.

McDiarmid, R.E., Majak, W., and Yost, G.S. (1986) Conversion of 3-nitropropanol to 3-nitropropionic acid by equine alcohol dehydrogenase, *J. Toxicol Toxin Rev.*, 5: 253.

Ming, L. (1995) Moldy sugar cane poisoning: a case report with a brief review, *Clin. Toxicol.*, 33: 363–367.

Mosher, G.A., Krishnamurti, C.R., and Kitts, W.D. (1971) Metabolism of the toxic principle of *Astragalus miser* var. *serotinus* in ruminants and nonruminants, *Can. J. Animal Sci.*, 51: 475–480.

Moskowitz, G.J. and Cayle, T. (1974) A method for the detection of beta-nitropropionic acid in crude biological extracts, *Cereal Chem.*, 51: 96–105.

Muir, A.D. and Majak, W. (1984) Quantitative determination of 3-nitropropionic acid and 3-nitropropanol in plasma by HPLC, *Toxicol. Lett.*, 20: 133–136.

Muir, A.D., Majak, W., Pass, M.A., and Yost, G.S. (1984) Conversion of 3-nitropropanol (miserotoxin aglycone) to 3-nitropropionic acid in cattle and sheep, *Toxicol Lett.*, 20: 137–141.

Myhr, B.C., Bowers, L.R., and Caspary, W. (1988) Chemical testing with a CHO/HGPRT suspension culture mutation assay, *Environ. Mol. Mutagen.*, 11: 76.

NCI. (1978) *Bioassay of 3-Nitropropionic Acid for Possible Carcinogenicity*, NTIS PB 281102, Carcinogenesis Testing Program, Division of Cancer Cause and Prevention, National Cancer Institute, Bethesda, MD, p. 127.

Nishino, H., Kumazaki, M., Fukuda, A., Fujimoto, I., Shimano, Y., Hida, H., Sakurai, T., Deshpande, S.B., Shimizu, H., Morikawa, H., and Inubushi, T. (1997) Acute 3-nitropropionic acid intoxication induces striatal astrocytic cell death and dysfunction of the blood–brain barrier: involvement of dopamine toxicity, *Neurosci. Res.*, 27: 343–355.

Nishino, H., Nakajima, K., Kumazaki, M., Fukuda, A., Muramatsu, K., and Deshpande, S. (1998) Estrogen protects against while testosterone exacerbates vulnerability of the lateral striatal artery to chemical hypoxia by 3-nitropropionic acid, *Neurosci. Res.*, 30: 303–312.

Nishino, H., Hida, H., Kumazaki, M., Shimano, M., Nakajima, K., Shimizu, H., Ooiwa, T., and Baba, H. (2000) The striatum is the most vulnerable region in the brain to mitochondrial energy compromise: a hypothesis to explain its specific vulnerability, *J. Neurotrauma*, 17: 251–260.

Nony, P.A., Scallet, A.C., Roundtree, R.L., Ye, X., and Biniendra, Z. (1999) 3-Nitropropionic acid (3-NPA) produces hypothermia and inhibits histochemical labelling of succinate dehydrogenase (SDH) in rat brain, *Metab. Brain Dis.*, 14: 83–94.

Olsen, C., Rustad, A., Fonnum, F., Paulsen, R.E., and Hassel, B. (1999) 3-Nitropropionic acid: an astrocyte-sparing neurotoxin *in vitro*, *Brain Res.*, 850: 144–149.

Orth, R. (1977) Mycotoxins of *Aspergillus oryzae* strains used in the food industry as starters and enzyme producing molds, *Ann. Nutr. Aliment.*, 31: 617–624.

Oshiro, Y., Piper, C.E., Balwierz, P.S., and Soelter, S.G. (1991) Chinese hamster ovary cell assays for mutation and chromosome damage: data from non-carcinogens, *J. Appl. Toxicol.*, 11: 167–177.

Ouary, S., Bizat, S., Altairac, H., Menetrat, H., Mittoux, V., Conde, F., Hantraye, P., and Brouillet, E. (2000) Major strain differences in response to chronic systemic administration of the mitochondrial toxin 3-nitropropionic acid in rats: implications for neuroprotection studies, *Neuroscience*, 97: 521–530.

Page, K.J., Besret, L., Jain, M., Monaghan, E.M., Dunnett, S.B., and Everitt, B.J. (2000) Effects of systemic 3-nitropropionic acid-induced lesions of the dorsal striatum on cannabinoid and μ-opioid receptor binding in the basal ganglia, *Exp. Brain Res.*, 130: 142–150.

Palfi, S., Ferrante, R.J., Brouillet, E., Beal, M.F., Dolan, R., Guyot, M.C., Peschanski, M., and Hantraye, P. (1996) Chronic 3-nitropropionic acid treatment in baboons replicates the cognitive and motor deficits of Huntington's disease, *J. Neurosci.*, 16: 3019–3025.

Pang, Z. and Geddes, J.W. (1997) Mechanism of cell death induced by the mitochondrial toxin 3-nitropropionic acid: acute excitotoxic necrosis and delayed apoptosis, *J. Neurosci.*, 17: 3064–3073.

Panigrahi, S. (1993) Bioassay of mycotoxins using terrestrial and aquatic, animal and plant species, *Food Chem. Toxicol.*, 31: 767–790.

Pass, M.A., Majak, W., Muir, A.D., and Yost, G.S. (1984) Absorption of 3-nitropropanol and 3-nitroproionic acid from the digestive system of sheep, *Toxicol. Lett.*, 23: 1–7.

Pass, M.A., Muir, A.D., Majak, W., and Yost, G.S. (1985) Effect of alcohol and aldehyde dehydrogenase inhibitors on the toxicity of 3-nitropropanol in rats, *Toxicol. Appl. Pharmacol.*, 78: 310–315.

Pass, M.A., Majak, W., and Yost, G.S. (1988) Lack of a protective effect of thiamine on the toxicity of 3-nitropropanol and 3-nitropropionic acid in rats, *Can. J. Animal Sci.*, 68: 315–320.

Pasteels, J.M., Rowell-Rahier, M., Braekman, J.C., Daloze, D., and Duffey, S. (1989) Evolution of exocrine chemical defense in leaf beetles *Coleoptera chrysomelidae*, *Experientia*, 45: 295–300.

Paterson, R.R.M. (1986) Standardized one- and two-dimensional thin layer chromatographic methods for the identification of secondary metabolites in *Penicillium* and other fungi, *J. Chromatog.*, 386: 249–264.

Penel, A.J. (1977) *beta-Nitropropionic Acid in Foods with Reference to* Aspergillus oryzae (ATCC 12892), 78–2053, UMI Dissertation Services, Ann Arbor, MI.

Penel, A.J. and Kosikowski, F.V. (1990) Beta-nitropropionic acid production by *Aspergillus oryzae* in selected high protein and carbohydrate-rich food, *J. Food Prot.*, 53: 321–323.

Peraica, M., Radic, B., Lucic, A., and Pavlovic, M. (1999) Toxic effects of mycotoxins in humans, *Bull. World Health Org.*, 77: 754–766.

Porter, D.J. and Bright, H.J. (1987) Propionate-3-nitronate oxidase from *Penicillium atrovenetum* is a flavoprotein which initiates the autooxidation of its substrate by O_2, *J. Biol. Chem.*, 262: 14428–14434.

Randoux, T., Braekman, J.C., Daloza, D., and Pasteels, J.M. (1991) *De novo* biosynthesis of delta-isoxazolin-5-one and 3-nitropropanoic acid derivatives: defensive secretions in *Chrysomela tremulae* (*C. tremula*), *Nautrwissenschaften*, 78: 313–314.

Riepe, M., Hori, N., Ludolph, A.C., Carpenter, D.O., Spencer, P.S., and Allen, C.N. (1992) Inhibition of energy metabolism by 3-nitropropionic acid activates ATP-sensitive potassium channels, *Brain Res.*, 586: 61–66.

RTECS (1994) Registry of Toxic Effects of Chemical Substances, National Laboratory of Medicine database, Bethesda, MD.

Sato, S., Gebbel, G.T., Honkaniemi, J., Li., Y., Kondo, T., Murakami, K., Sato, M., Copin, J.-C., and Chan, P.H. (1997) Apoptosis in the striatum of rats following intraperitoneal injection of 3-nitropropionic acid, *Brain Res.*, 745: 343–347.

Schafer, E.W., Jr. and Bowles, W.A., Jr. (1985) Acute oral toxicity and repellency of 933 chemicals to house and deer mice, *Arch. Environ. Contam. Toxicol.*, 14: 111–129.

Shaw, P.D. (1967) Biosynthesis of nitro compounds. III. Enzymic reduction of beta-nitroacrylic acid to beta-nitropropionic acid, *Biochemistry*, 6: 2243–2260.

Shaw, P.D. and DeAngelo, A.B. (1969) Role of ammonium ion in the biosynthesis of beta-nitropropionic acid, *J. Bacteriol.*, 99: 463–468.

Shaw, P.D. and McCloskey, J.A. (1967) Biosynthesis of nitro compounds. II. Studies on potential precursors for the nitro group of beta-nitropropionic acid, *Biochemistry*, 6: 2247–2252.

Shenk, J.S., Wangness, P.J., Leach, R.M., Gustine, D.L., Gobble, J.L., and Barnes, R.F. (1976) Relationship between beta-nitropropionic acid content of crownvetch and toxicity in nonruminant animals, *J. Animal Sci.*, 42: 616–621.

Siedel, B., Jiang, L., and Wolf, G. (2000) Differential displayed genes in neuroblastoma cells treated with a mitochondrial toxin: evidence for possible involvement of ICAM-1 in 3-nitropropionic acid-mediated neurodegeneration, *Toxicol. Lett.*, 115: 213–222.

Spencer, P.S., Ludolph, A.C., and Kisby, G.E. (1993) Neurologic diseases associated with use of plant components with toxic potential, *Environ. Res.*, 62: 106–113.

Stermitz, F.R., Norris, F.A., and Williams, M.C. (1969) Miserotoxin, a new naturally occurring nitro compound, *J. Am. Chem. Soc.*, 91: 4599–4600.

Sun, Z., Xie, J., and Reiner, A. (2002) The differential vulnerability of striatal projection neurons in 3-nitropropionic-acid-treated rats does not match that typical of adult-onset Huntington's disease, *Exp. Neurol.*, 176:55–65.

Tan, D.Y., Brooks, B.R., Chu, F.S., Nizamuddin, G.S., and Schutta, H.S. (1989) Chronic oral neurotoxicity of 3-nitropropionic acid in mice: clinical and neuropathological parallels with murine retrovirus-induced spinal cord adaxonal changes, *Neurology*, 39: 204.

Tan, D.Y., Bohlmann, T., Nizamuddin, G.S., Chu, F.S., Sufit, R.L., Brooks, B.R., and Schutta, H.S. (1990) Increased resistance to chronic oral 3-nitropropionic acid neurotoxicity in aged mice EM and histochemical studies, *Neuroscience*, 16: 1115.

Traul, K.A., Takayama, K., Kachevsky, V., Hink, R.J., and Wolff, J.S. (1981) Rapid *in vitro* assay for carcinogenicity of chemical substances in mammalian cells utilizing an attachment-independence endpoint. 2. Assay validation, *J. Appl. Toxicol.*, 1: 190–195.

Uchida, K. (1989) Trends in preparation and uses of fermented and acid-hydrolyzed soy sauce, in *Proceedings of the World Congress on Vegetable Protein Utilization in Human Foods and Animal Feedstuffs*, Applewhite, T.H., Ed., American Oil Chemists' Society, Champaign, IL.

Vecsei, L., Diho, G., and Kiss, C. (1998) Neurotoxins and neurodegenerative disorders, *Neurotoxicology*, 19: 511–514.

Wei, D.-L., Chang, S.-C., Lin, S.-C., Doong, M.-L., and Jong, S.-C. (1994) Production of 3-nitropropionic acid by *Arthrinium* species, *Curr. Microbiol.*, 28: 1–5.

Williams, M.C. (1980) Toxicological investigations of *Astragalus hamosus* and *Astragalus sesameus*, *Austral. J. Exp. Agric. Animal Husb.*, 20: 162–165.

Williams, M.C. (1981) Nitro compounds in foreign species of *Astragalus*, *Weed Sci.*, 29: 261–269.

Williams, M.C. and Davis, A.M. (1982) Nitro compounds in introduced *Astragalus* species, *J. Range Manage.*, 35: 113–115.

Williams, M.C. and Gomez-Sosa, E. (1986) Toxic nitro compounds in species of *Astragalus fabaceae* in Argentina, *J. Range Manage.*, 39: 341–344.

Williams, M.C. and James, L.F. (1976) Poisoning in sheep from Emory milk vetch and nitro compounds, *J. Range Manage.*, 29: 165–167.

Williams, G.M., Mori, H., and McQueen, C.A. (1989) Structure–activity relationships in the rat hepatocyte DNA: repair test for 300 chemicals, *Mutat. Res.*, 221: 263–286.

Wullner, U., Young, A.B., Penney, J.B., and Beal, M.F. (1994) 3-Nitropropionic acid toxicity in the striatum, *J. Neurochem.*, 63: 1772–1781.

Yin, H.Y., Yu, H.B., Chen, F., and Ma, J.Z. (1992) Selection of low toxin crownvetch by irradiation, *Grassland China*, 6: 18–22.

Zeevalk, G.D., Derr-Yellin, E., and Nicklas, W.J. (1995) Relative vulnerability of dopamine and GABA neurons in mesencephatic cultures to inhibition of succinate dehydrogenase by malonate and 3-nitropropionic acid and protection by NMDA receptor blockade, *J. Pharmacol. Exp. Ther.*, 275: 1124–1130.

Zeiger, E. (1987) Carcinogenicity of mutagens: predictive capability of the *Salmonella* mutagenesis assay for rodent carcinogenicity, *Cancer Res.*, 47: 1287–1296.

6 Vibrio parahaemolyticus Infections: Causes, Effects, and Role of the Food Chain

Nicholas A. Daniels

CONTENTS

INTRODUCTION

The objective of this chapter is to describe the epidemiology of *Vibrio parahaemolyticus*, a common seafood bacterium, to describe its effects on our food chain from the sea to our dining tables, and to identify where preventive measures could be targeted. Recent research has increased our understanding of the multiple factors involved in seafood safety and has provided us with additional science-based data for making policy decisions for safeguarding our seafood. Ecological, environmental, and epidemiological studies have further characterized these organisms through pre- and post-seafood harvesting practice analyses; through environmental surveys that assess factors that influence *Vibrio parahaemolyticus* growth and reservoirs; and through the identification of risk factors for exposure to and infection by these pathogens. The following areas are emphasized in this review: identification of risk factors and possible intervention strategies, levels of microbial contamination in seafood at retail, identification of seafood harvesting-based solutions that may contribute to decreasing the incidence of *Vibrio parahaemolyticus* infections, and identification of potential sites of organism control in the processing, transportation, retail setting, and consumer consumption of seafood.

0-8493-2757-1/05/$0.00+$1.50

EPIDEMIOLOGY OF *VIBRIO PARAHAEMOLYTICUS*

THE BACTERIA

Vibrio parahaemolyticus is a major gastroenteritis-causing bacteria worldwide that is frequently associated with consumption of raw or undercooked seafood. *Vibrio parahaemolyticus* is a free-living marine bacteria that was first recognized in 1950 in Japan as being an important cause of gastroenteritis related to consumption of semi-dried sardines (Fujino et al., 1953). Subsequently, it has become the leading cause of seafood-borne morbidity in the United States and in many other countries. Twelve *Vibrio* species are known to be pathogenic in humans, and 23 *Vibrio* species are non-pathogenic. *Vibrio parahaemolyticus* synthesizes the major antigens, which include identical H flagellar antigens, 11 distinct O group antigens, and 71 K capsular antigens, which are used for serotype classification (Table 6.1) (Iguchi et al., 1995; Zen-Yoji et al., 1970). Recently, several dominant serotypes have emerged globally. For instance, the *V. parahaemolyticus* O3:K6 serovar accounted for 50 to 80% of the *V. parahaemolyticus* outbreaks in India and Japan in 1996 and 80% of the *V. parahaemolyticus* outbreaks in Taiwan in 1997 (Chiou et al., 2000; Chowdhury et al., 2000; Okuda et al., 1997; Wong et al., 1999a,b). In 1997 and 1998, it and other serotypes emerged in the United States (CDC, 1998, 1999; Daniels et al., 2000a). Over 50% of foodborne bacterial infections in Taiwan and Japan, where seafood is widely consumed, are secondary to *V. parahaemolyticus* (Arakawa et al., 1999; Osawa et al., 1996; Pan et al., 1997). The increased incidence of associated outbreaks and pandemic spread of *V. parahaemolyticus* serotype O3:K6 may illustrate the increased capacity of this serotype to cause human infection. Until recently, no correlation was observed between serotype and virulence.

Because *Vibrio* species are naturally occurring marine bacteria, they are present in many types of seafood, including fish, crustaceans, and molluscan shellfish, and are ubiquitous in estuarine and marine environments, their presence having nothing to do with environmental pollution. *Vibrio* species are incorporated into shellfish through filter feeding; bivalve mollusks concentrate *Vibrio* in their tissues by being very efficient filter feeders of surrounding water (they may filter up to 40 L/hr) (Canesi et al., 2002). Some types of *Vibrio* use transferrin-bound iron for growth (Dai et al., 1992; O'Malley et al., 1999; Wong et al., 1996a,b); the ability of *Vibrio* species to use iron may enhance their survival and proliferation in the human body.

Human infection from *V. parahaemolyticus* occurs in two primary ways: ingestion of contaminated seafood or inoculation of organism through abraded skin. Raw oysters are the most common seafood source of the infection in all published series, and all reported foodborne outbreaks have been attributed to consumption of seafood (Baker, 1974; Barker and Gangarosa, 1978; Barrow and Miller, 1969; CDC, 1998, 1999; Daniels et al., 2000a,b; Dowell et al., 1995; Hlady and Klontz, 1996; Nolan et al., 1984).

Vibrio parahaemolyticus is recognized as an important seafood pathogen worldwide. The first confirmed report in Britain of *V. parahaemolyticus* as a marine bacterium in oysters and as a sporadic cause of foodborne outbreaks was released in 1969 (Barrow and Miller, 1969, 1972). Moreover, *V. parahaemolyticus* infections

TABLE 6.1
Antigenic Schema of *Vibrio parahaemolyticus*

O Group	K Antigen																
1	1	25	26	32	38	41	56	58	64	69	—	—	—	—	—	—	—
2	3	28	—	—	—	—	—	—	—	—	—	—	—	—	—	—	—
3	4	5	6	7	29	30	31	33	37	43	45	48	54	57	58	59	65
4	4	8	9	10	11	12	13	34	42	49	53	55	63	67	—	—	—
5	15	17	30	47	60	61	68	—	—	—	—	—	—	—	—	—	—
6	18	46	—	—	—	—	—	—	—	—	—	—	—	—	—	—	—
7	19	52	—	—	—	—	—	—	—	—	—	—	—	—	—	—	—
8	20	21	22	39	70	—	—	—	—	—	—	—	—	—	—	—	—
9	23	44	—	—	—	—	—	—	—	—	—	—	—	—	—	—	—
10	19	24	52	66	71	—	—	—	—	—	—	—	—	—	—	—	—
11	36	40	50	51	61	—	—	—	—	—	—	—	—	—	—	—	—

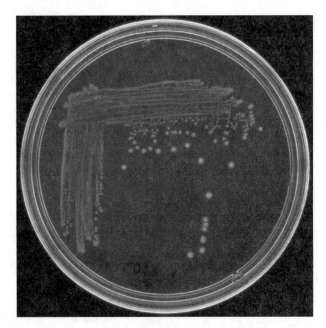

FIGURE 6.1 *Vibrio parahaemolyticus* colonies on TCBS (colonies are darker in color; *Vibrio cholerae* and other sucrose-fermenting *Vibrio* species are lighter).

have been reported worldwide, with infections occurring in Europe, Australia, New Zealand, India, Bangladesh, China, Taiwan, Vietnam, Laos, Indonesia, Malaysia, Japan, Korea, and Peru, Togo (West Africa), among many other countries (Bockemuhl et al., 1975; Department of Health Republic of China, 1996, 1998; Lesmana et al., 2001; Sircar et al., 1976). *Vibrio parahaemolyticus* is widely distributed throughout the world, especially in warm coastal waters, and the principal reservoirs of the bacteria are coastal waters and seafood.

CLINICAL PRESENTATION

Vibrio parahaemolyticus is a Gram-negative, curved, rod-shaped bacteria (Figure 6.1 and Table 6.2). *Vibrio*-associated illness tends to occur in coastal areas in the summer and fall, when the water is warmer and *Vibrio* counts are higher. Infections are seasonal; over 80% occur between April and October in temperate climates, with the median month of occurrence being July (Barker, 1974; Daniels et al., 2000a). The infectious dose of *V. parahaemolyticus* gastroenteritis is between 10^5 and 10^7 organisms (Sanyal and Sen, 1974). The occurrence of *V. parahaemolyticus* infections depends on certain bacterial factors and, to a lesser degree, on host factors. The U.S. Centers for Disease Control and Prevention (CDC) estimate that 8028 *Vibrio* infections and 57 deaths occur annually in the United States, with *V. parahaemolyticus* being the most commonly cited *Vibrio* species (Mead et al., 1999). Although *V. parahaemolyticus* is a relatively common infection, it is likely under-reported, as

TABLE 6.2
Characteristics of *Vibrio parahaemolyticus*

Feature	Observation	Consequence
Infectious dose	10^5 to 10^7 organisms	No person-to-person spread
Environmental stability	Thrives in warm marine waters	Increased infection during warmer months
Strain diversity	Strains vary in pathogenicity	Pathogenic and non-pathogenic strains
Host factors	Invasive in persons with co-morbidities	Persons at risk should avoid raw or undercooked seafood

most patients with acute gastroenteritis, the most commonly reported syndrome, do not routinely seek medical care and are not captured by disease surveillance systems.

Vibrio parahaemolyticus produces a self-limiting gastroenteritis and wound infections and, on rare occasions, can cause septicemia. The median incidence of clinical features of *V. parahaemolyticus* gastroenteritis includes the following: diarrhea (98%), abdominal cramps (82%), nausea (71%), vomiting (52%), headache (42%), fever (27%), and chills (24%) (Barker, 1974; Barker and Gangarosa, 1978; Daniels et al., 2000a). In addition to gastroenteritis, *V. parahaemolyticus* commonly causes soft-tissue infections. The principal vehicles of transmission are seafood and seawater. Among the 345 culture-confirmed *V. parahaemolyticus* infections reported to the CDC between 1988 and 1997 through the *Vibrio* surveillance system, 59% were classified as gastroenteritis, 34% as wound infections, 5% as septicemia, and 2% other or unknown sites of infection (Daniels et al., 2000a). The median patient age was 36 years, the majority of infections occurred in men, 34% of patients had at least one preexisting medical illness, and 45% were hospitalized. Of the patients for whom information on the outcome is available, 12 patients died of their infection (Daniels et al., 2000a). The median incubation period (e.g., time of exposure to onset of illness) is usually less than 24 hours after the ingestion of contaminated seafood (Barker, 1974; Daniels et al., 2000a).

The only well-established host risk factor for *V. parahaemolyticus* infection is a pre-existing wound that predisposes to soft tissue infections. Primary septicemia refers to bloodstream infections that are acquired through ingestion of the organism through the gastrointestinal tract. Persons with known liver disease, particularly those patients with cirrhosis, are likely at high risk for *V. parahaemolyticus* primary septicemia (Daniels et al., 2000a; Hally et al., 1995). *Vibrio parahaemolyticus* bloodstream infections are rare; however, fulminating *V. parahaemolyticus* septicemia has been reported (Zide et al., 1974). *Vibrio parahaemolyticus* wound infection and cellulitis can occur from exposure of abraded skin to warm seawater or brackish inland water; these skin infections may progress to ulceration, necrotizing fasciitis requiring limb amputation, and sepsis. Leg gangrene and endotoxin shock due to *V. parahaemolyticus* have been reported from infection acquired in Northeastern coastal waters (Roland, 1976).

The severity of *V. parahaemolyticus* infections depends on a variety of bacterial and host factors. Persons with elevated transferrin-bound iron saturation, including persons with hemochromatosis, thalassemia, or liver disease, are at increased risk of invasive *Vibrio* infections. Patients with septicemia often have underlying medical conditions (Klontz, 1990). At risk for *V. parahaemolyticus* septicemia are those who have alcoholic liver disease, diabetes, hemochromatosis, thalassemia, chronic hepatitis B and C, cancer, or depressed immune systems. The majority of cases of septicemia have occurred in consumers with alcoholic liver disease (Hally et al., 1995). *Vibrio parahaemolyticus* has also been associated with a cholera-like diarrhea among patients in Indonesia (Lesmana et al., 2001).

In addition to wound infections, septicemias, and gastroenteritis, *V. parahaemolyticus* has been associated with other clinical syndromes, including pneumonia, osteomyelitis, spontaneous bacterial peritonitis, eye and ear infections, reactive arthritis, and meningitis (Klontz, 1990; Steinkuller et al., 1972; Tamura et al., 1993; Tay and Yu, 1978; Yu and Uy-Yu, 1984).

PATHOPHYSIOLOGY

In vitro hemolytic characteristics of *V. parahaemolyticus* are closely correlated with human pathogenicity (Joseph et al., 1982; Miyamoto et al., 1969). *V. parahaemolyticus* strains carry thermo-stable direct hemolysin (TDH) or TDH-related hemolysin (TRH) genes, or both. TDH and TRH are considered major virulence factors as they can cause illness in a human host. The hemolytic action of the TDH toxin on Wagatsuma blood agar plates is referred to as the Kanagawa phenomenon (KP). Strains of *V. parahaemolyticus* from patients are generally KP positive. KP induced by the TDH gene of *V. parahaemolyticus* is almost always associated with clinical specimens; therefore, TDH is an indicator of enteropathogenic strains and an important virulence factor. The results of an extensive survey revealed that 96% of 2720 strains isolated from patients with diarrhea were positive when tested for the Kanagawa hemolysin, whereas only 1% of the 650 strains from seafood and environmental samples were positive (Sakazaki et al., 1968). Kanagawa-positive *V. parahaemolyticus* strains are considered to be human pathogens most commonly associated with diarrheal illness, whereas Kanagawa-negative strains are most frequently isolated from the marine environment and used to be generally considered to be non-pathogenic strains. Recent studies, however, have also shown that Kanagawa-negative *V. parahaemolyticus* strains, which produce TRH, may cause diarrhea indistinguishable from Kanagawa-positive *V. parahaemolyticus* infection (Honda et al., 1987, 1988). Additionally, wound infections caused by Kanagawa-negative *V. parahaemolyticus* strains have also been reported (Johnson et al., 1984). Other strain characteristics, such as invasion of enterocytes or production of enterotoxin or urease, may also be important to pathogenicity (Akeda et al., 1997; Honda et al., 1976; Kelly and Stroh, 1989).

DIAGNOSIS AND TREATMENT

Although some nonselective media may support the growth of *V. parahaemolyticus*, isolation from stool cultures usually requires the use of a selective medium such as

TCBS (thiosulfate, citrate, bile salts, and sucrose agar). A survey of clinical laboratories in the U.S. Gulf Coast, an area highly endemic with *Vibrio* infections, revealed that less than 25% of laboratories routinely used TCBS for evaluation of stool specimens (Marano et al., 2000). Because most cases of gastroenteritis are self-limiting, antimicrobial therapy is generally not required. *V. parahaemolyticus* wound and primary septicemia infections require antimicrobial treatment to improve the course of illness and to prevent complications. Antimicrobial agents most effective against *V. parahaemolyticus* infections include tetracycline, fluoroquinolones, third-generation cephalosporins, and aminoglycosides (French, 1990).

FOOD CHAIN

By virtue of their ability to concentrate *Vibrio* in their tissues, molluscan shellfish such as oysters, mussels, and clams become actively contaminated by filter-feeding seawater and subsequently become good vehicles of transmission. Bivalve molluscan shellfish may rapidly become contaminated with pathogenic *Vibrio* when filter feeding. *Vibrio parahaemolyticus* becomes part of the natural intestinal flora of most seafood. *Vibrio parahaemolyticus* gastroenteritis is associated with seafood that is consumed raw, inadequately cooked, or cooked but recontaminated. Raw seafood, particularly shellfish, has often been associated with *V. parahaemolyticus* enteric infections (Barker, 1974; Barker and Gangarosa, 1978; Barrow and Miller, 1969; CDC, 1998, 1999; Daniels et al., 2000a,b; Dowell et al., 1995). Raw shellfish is consumed by approximately 8% of the U.S. population at least once during a year (Altekruse et al., 1999; Yang et al., 1998). Mean consumption is approximately 6 oysters per serving (U.S. Department of Agriculture, 1999). Some authors have suggested that raw shellfish consumption may have become too risky (DuPont, 1986). Because shellfish is often eaten raw or lightly cooked, the risk of illness after their consumption may be high. A clear dose–response relationship between shellfish contaminated with *V. parahaemolyticus* consumption and illness has been demonstrated (Barker, 1974).

In 1973, during the first U.S. outbreak involving steamed crab contaminated with *V. parahaemolyticus*, different serotypes were recovered from stool specimens and from implicated foods during the course of the foodborne outbreak investigation (Dadisman et al., 1973). Other studies have also found that, during a *V. parahaemolyticus* outbreak, it is difficult to match serotypes of *V. parahaemolyticus* isolates found in both patients and in implicated foods (Fishbein et al., 1974). Fishbein isolated *V. parahaemolyticus* from 86% of the seafood tested, including oysters, clams, scallops, lobsters, sardines, shrimp, eel, squid, crab, and other species of fish. The reason for these discrepancies remains unknown. *Vibrio parahaemolyticus* has been isolated from shrimp (Vanderzant and Nickelson, 1969) and has been associated with disease in crabs in Chesapeake Bay, suggesting that these organisms may be pathogenic in invertebrate animals (Krantz et al., 1969). *Vibrio parahaemolyticus* has been isolated from 30 different marine species, including clams, oysters, lobsters, scallops, sardines, shrimp, squid, crab, eel, and various species of fish (Fishbein et al., 1974). A U.S. Food and Drug Administration (FDA) study found that 546 (86%) of 635 seafood samples were positive for *V. parahaemolyticus* (Fishbein et al., 1974).

Shellfish more frequently test positive for *V. parahaemolyticus* contamination than do finfish (Abeyta, 1983). A survey of fresh seafood in North Carolina found that 46% of samples were positive (Hackney et al., 1980). *Vibrio parahaemolyticus* was recovered from 315 (46%) of 686 seafood samples imported to Taiwan from Hong Kong, Indonesia, Thailand, and Vietnam (Wong, 1996). Another survey found that 100% of raw oysters examined harbored *V. parahaemolyticus*, while 50% of the inadequately cooked oysters tested also contained *V. parahaemolyticus* (Lowry et al., 1989).

From June 1998 to July 1999, 370 lots of oysters in the shell were sampled at 275 different establishments (71% from restaurants or oyster bars; 27% from retail seafood markets, and 2% from wholesale seafood markets) in coastal and inland markets throughout the United States. Densities of *V. parahaemolyticus* in market oysters from all harvest regions followed a seasonal distribution, with highest densities occurring in the summer. Highest densities of both organisms were observed in oysters harvested from the Gulf Coast, where densities often exceeded 10,000 MPN/g (the FDA former guideline level). In this study, storage time significantly affected *V. parahaemolyticus*, with a 7% decrease per day in densities in market oysters. The TDH gene associated with *V. parahaemolyticus* virulence was detected in 0.3%, and *V. parahaemolyticus* cultures were positive for 4.0% of the oysters. These data may be used to estimate the exposure of raw oyster consumers to *V. parahaemolyticus* (Cook et al., 2002a).

In 1999, the FDA was petitioned by the Center for Science in the Public Interest (CSPI) to establish a standard of "non-detectable" for *V. parahaemolyticus* in raw molluscan shellfish harvested from waters that have been linked to illness from the marine organism (CSPI, 1999). The petition cites one such post-harvest treatment, from the AmeriPure Company. The process involves a mild heat treatment of in-shell oysters that is capable of killing *V. parahaemolyticus*. The AmeriPure process is a temperature treatment using warm and ice cold waters (AmeriPure Processing Co., 2003) that eliminates *Vibrio* from shellfish. *Vibrio* is not detectable after this pasteurization process. The use of low-temperature pasteurization appeared to be very effective in reducing *Vibrios* to non-detectable levels, although *V. parahaemolyticus* has been found to be very heat resistant in some low-temperature pasteurization studies (Andrews et al., 2000; Johnson and Liston, 1973; Johnston and Brown, 2002; Thomson and Thacker, 1973). Some processing practices, such as heat-shocking of oysters to facilitate opening, have also been found to reduce the number of *Vibrio bacteria* (Hesselman et al., 1999).

Thoroughly cooking oysters kills *V. parahaemolyticus*. The Japanese food custom of raw fish consumption, such as eating *sashimi* or *sushi*, is thought to be the primary cause of the high frequency of *V. parahaemolyticus* foodborne outbreaks in Japan (Arakawa et al., 1999; Obata et al., 2001). Because transmission occurs when seafood is eaten raw or improperly cooked, those who want to reduce their risk of infection should eat oysters that are fully cooked, as cooking kills *V. parahaemolyticus*.

Vibrio parahaemolyticus may be detected in virtually all oysters harvested from the Gulf of Mexico, at least during warm-weather months (Cook et al., 2002b). Increased consumer advisories have been required at points of retail sale in California,

Louisiana, Florida, Massachusetts, and Mississippi. Such warnings have not been effective because they are not adequately displayed and are rarely placed on dining tables or included on menus (Mouzin et al., 1997). Restaurant warnings are good in that they help educate consumers, but they are not sufficient to prevent *V. parahaemolyticus* infections; it has been found that oyster eaters are more likely to be risk takers and smokers, to not wear seatbelts, to drink alcohol, and to have liver disease (Klontz et al., 1991). Other preventive measures, such as thorough cooking or pasteurization, are warranted.

Restriction of oyster harvesting to areas free of fecal contamination has reduced the risk of foodborne illness from many viral and bacterial pathogens, but no known sanitation or public health controls can limit the harvesting of oysters to those areas free of *V. parahaemolyticus*. Therefore, infections from consumption of raw or undercooked oysters continue to occur, even when the oysters have been legally harvested and properly handled.

Vibrio parahaemolyticus has one of the fastest doubling (or generation) times known for bacteria at 37°C (as short as 9 minutes), but reduced *Vibrio* multiplication occurs if shellstock oysters are held below 10°C (shucked shellfish is cooled to a temperature of 7.2°C) (Oliver and Kaper, 1997). *Vibrio* can grow in seafood to enormous numbers when held for short periods under improper refrigeration (Cook, 1994); therefore, it is extremely important for oysters to be maintained on ice or refrigerated at or below 10°C for transport in order to control bacterial growth. Reducing the time from harvest to refrigeration may also reduce enteric infections. Raw seafood and shellfish should be stored at refrigeration temperature and placed on ice immediately after harvesting or processing to prevent multiplication to numbers likely to cause disease. After cooking, oysters should be eaten immediately or refrigerated to prevent multiplication (Bradshaw et al., 1974; Johnston and Brown, 2002).

Cross-contamination of other cooked foods with raw seafood material should be avoided. The organism proliferates at room temperature but is readily killed by boiling and freezing. The infectious dose of *V. parahaemolyticus* can be reached rapidly because of its generation time in optimal conditions of less than 9 minutes, considerably shorter than that of other bacteria. With the generation time being so short, within 3 to 4 hours a starting inoculum of 10 organisms may grow to over a million, thus approaching infectious levels (Johnson et al., 1971). Improper cooking and handling of seafood and shellfish are associated with foodborne outbreaks due to *V. parahaemolyticus*. During a survey of healthy, asymptomatic *sushi* cooks, *V. parahaemolyticus* was isolated in the stool specimens of 14 (7%) of the 200 cooks examined (Zen-Yogi et al., 1965). The safest seafood is well cooked and properly handled.

New strategies are needed in order to prevent *V. parahaemolyticus* infections. The old dictum of avoiding raw oysters during months without an "r" is not sufficient to completely prevent *V. parahaemolyticus* infections, as infections may also occur during cooler months. Over the past decade, the number of *Vibrio* infections has increased (CDC, 1998, 1999; Daniels et al., 2000a). Some attempts have been made to develop technologies such as pasteurization (mild heat treatment), freezing treatment, or irradiation to eliminate *Vibrio* contamination of shellfish, and these efforts should continue. Irradiation of seafood with gamma radiation is an increasingly attractive way to destroy pathogenic *Vibrio species* (Bandekar et al., 1987).

The public should also be informed that steaming shellfish, as it is currently done, is often inadequate to inactivate the viral agents responsible for clinical disease (Kirkland et al., 1996). The shells of shellfish usually open after steaming for about 1 minute, but between 4 and 6 minutes of steaming is necessary for the internal temperature to reach the required level, and patrons should probably verify the practice before consuming shellfish. Physicians and public health officials should inform patients at risk to avoid raw or undercooked seafood in an attempt to prevent this potentially lethal syndrome. Public health officials will have failed as medical educators if people continue to eat raw or undercooked shellfish without understanding the health risks associated with consumption.

PREVENTION OF *VIBRIO PARAHAEMOLYTICUS* INFECTIONS

To reduce the risk of *V. parahaemolyticus* infections, seafood consumers should avoid eating raw or undercooked molluscan shellfish (particularly oysters), should avoid cross-contamination, and should thoroughly cook all shellfish (oysters, clams, and mussels). The advice to steam for at least 5 minutes is sound and applies to all bacterially contaminated shellfish, as 1 to 2 minutes of steaming (light steaming) would be unlikely to eliminate any *Vibrio* species. The U.S. Department of Health and Human Services recommends boiling until shells open and for 5 more minutes; steaming until shells open and then continue cooking for 9 more minutes; using a small pot to boil or steam to ensure that oysters in the middle are thoroughly cooked; and discarding any oysters that do not open during cooking, as they may not have received adequate heat (CDC, 2000). Avoiding exposure of open wounds to seawater or seafood drippings will reduce the likelihood of developing a *V. parahaemolyticus* wound infection. *Vibrio parahaemolyticus* mitigation processes such as mild pasteurization, freezing, and irradiation have been shown to be effective in reducing *V. parahaemolyticus* levels. Pasteurization and irradiation can eliminate *Vibrio* from shellfish. Pasteurization of oysters has been approved by the FDA. Levels of *V. parahaemolyticus* decrease with cold temperatures (Johnson and Liston, 1973). *Vibrio parahaemolyticus* may be relatively heat resistant during low-temperature pasteurization (Cook, 1994).

ECOLOGY OF *VIBRIO PARAHAEMOLYTICUS*

Vibrio parahaemolyticus is associated with a number of higher organisms, notably shellfish (Sakazaki et al., 1968). Major outbreaks have occurred in the United States during the warmer months of the year, as the seasonal cycle of *V. parahaemolyticus* is temperature dependent, with the higher numbers during the warmer summer months coinciding with increases in the ambient water temperature. The seasonal incidence and concentration of *V. parahaemolyticus* in oysters are highest in warm weather, paralleling the temperature of the overlying water (Baross and Liston,

1970). In fact, water temperature appears to be the single most important factor governing the incidence and density of pathogenic *Vibrio* species in natural aquatic environments. As noted for *V. parahaemolyticus*, in particular, pathogenic *Vibrio* species occur in their highest numbers during the warmer months of the year, when water temperature is high enough to allow rapid proliferation of organisms to numbers that approach infective dose.

Vibrio parahaemolyticus is a halophilic (or salt-loving) organism. Relationships of temperature and sodium chloride concentration (or salinities) have been shown to influence the survival of *V. parahaemolyticus* (Covert and Woodburn, 19772; Zhu et al., 1992). Isolation of *V. parahaemolyticus* has been shown to be independent of sodium chloride content in the environment, whereas the organism is rarely isolated when the surface water temperature is less than 15°C.

No significant correlation between pollution indices (such as fecal indicators) and *V. parahaemolyticus* has been observed. Because pathogenic *Vibrio* species occur naturally in aquatic environments, control of sewage contamination will not completely prevent the spread of infection. Ocean-going vessels have helped to disseminate marine organisms (including non-indigenous marine species; see Hallegraeff and Bolch, 1992; Murrison, 1996; Williams et al., 1988) over the past centuries, and ship ballast water may be a potential source of transport for *V. parahaemolyticus* in the marine environment.

FUTURE DIRECTIONS

The recent development of dominant serotypes of *Vibrio parahaemolyticus* and increased surveillance and molecular techniques may help further define the nature and extent of this important seafood-borne infection (Bag et al., 1999; Gooch et al., 2001; Matsumoto et al., 2000). Future directions of research should focus on defining the disease burden to *V. parahaemolyticus*, development of sensitive and specific DNA probes for pathogenic strains of *V. parahaemolyticus* in seafood (Hara-Kudo et al., 2001), and prevention of infections through education of consumers and the use of acceptable technologies to eliminate *Vibrio* species from seafood.

REFERENCES

Abeyta, C. (1983) Bacteriological quality of fresh seafood products from Seattle retail markets, *J. Food Protect.*, 46: 901–909.

Akeda, Y., Nagayama, K., Yamamoto, K., and Honda, T. (1997) Invasive phenotype of *Vibrio parahaemolyticus*, *J. Infect. Dis.*, 176: 822–824.

Altekruse, S.F., Yang, S., Timbo, B.B., and Angulo, F.J. (1999) A multi-state survey of consumer food-handling and food-consumption practices, *Am. J. Prev. Med.*, 16(3): 216–221.

AmeriPure Processing Co. (2003) *Oysters*, AmeriPure Processing Company, Inc., Franklin, LA, http://www.ameripure.com (accessed January 5, 2003).

Andrews, L.S., Park, D.L., and Chen, Y.P. (2000) Low temperature pasteurization to reduce the risk of *Vibrio* infections from raw shell-stock oysters, *Food Add. Contam.*, 17(9): 787–791.

Arakawa, E., Murase, T., Shimada, T., Okitsu, T., Yamai, S., and Watanabe, H. (1999) Emergence and prevalence of a novel *Vibrio parahaemolyticus* O3:K6 clone in Japan, *Jpn. J. Infect. Dis.*, 52: 246–247.

Bag, P.K., Nandi, S., Bhadra, R.K., Ramamurthy, T., Bhattacharya, S.K., Nishibuchi, M., Hamabata, T., Yamasaki, S., Takeda, Y., and Nair, G.B. (1999) Clonal diversity among recently emerged strains of *Vibrio parahaemolyticus* O3:K6 associated with pandemic spread, *J. Clin. Microbiol.*, 7(7): 2354–2357.

Bandekar, J., Chander, R., and Nerkar, D.P. (1987) Radiation control of *Vibrio parahaemolyticus* in shrimp, *J. Food Safety*, 8: 83–88.

Barker, W.H. (1974) *Vibrio parahaemolyticus* outbreaks in the United States, *Lancet*, 3: 551–554.

Barker, W.H. and Gangarosa, E.J. (1978) Food poisoning due to *Vibrio parahaemolyticus*, *Ann. Rev. Med.*, 25: 75–81.

Baross, J. and Liston, J. (1970) Occurrence of *Vibrio parahaemolyticus* and related hemolytic *Vibrio*s in marine environments of Washington State, *Appl. Microbiol.*, 20(2): 179–186.

Barrow, G. and Miller, D.C. (1969) Marine bacteria in oysters purified for human consumption, *Lancet*, 2(7617): 421–432.

Barrow, G. and Miller, D.C. (1972) *Vibrio parahemolyticus*: a potential pathogen from marine sources in Britain, *Lancet*, 1(7748): 485–486.

Begue, R.E., Meza, R., Castellares, G., Cabezas, C., Vasquez, B., Ballardo, A., Cam, J., and Sanchez, J.L. (1995) Outbreaks of diarrhea due to *Vibrio parahaemolyticus* among military personnel in Lima, Peru, *Clin. Infect. Dis.*, 21: 1513–1514.

Bockemuhl, J., Amedone, A., and Triemer, A. (1975) *Vibrio parahaemolyticus* gastroenteritis during the El Tor cholera epidemic in Togo (West Africa), *Am. J. Trop. Med. Hyg.*, 24: 101–104.

Bradshaw, J., Francis, D.W., and Twedt, R.M. (1974) Survival of *Vibrio parahaemolyticus* in cooked seafood at refrigeration temperatures, *Appl. Microbiol.*, 27(4): 657–661.

Canesi, L., Gallo, G., Gavioli, M., and Pruzzo, C. (2002) Bacteria–hemocyte interactions and phagocytosis in marine bivalves, *Micro-Sci. Res. Technol.*, 57(6): 469–476.

CDC. (1998) Outbreak of *Vibrio parahaemolyticus* infections associated with eating raw oysters: Pacific Northwest, *Morbid. Mortal. Wkly. Rep.*, 47(22): 457–462.

CDC. (1999) Outbreak of *Vibrio parahaemolyticus* infections associated with eating raw oysters and clams harvested from Long Island Sound: Connecticut, New Jersey, and New York, 1998, *Morbid. Mortal. Wkly. Rep.*, 48(3): 48–51.

CDC. (2000) *Vibrio vulnificus General Information*, U.S. Department of Health and Human Services, Atlanta, GA, http://www.cdc.gov/ncidod/dbmd/diseaseinfo/vibriovulnificus _g.htm (accessed January 13, 2003).

Chiou, C., Hsu, S.Y., Chiu, S.I., Wang, T.K., and Chao, C.S. (2000) *Vibrio parahaemolyticus* serovar O3:K6 as cause of unusually high incidence of food-borne disease outbreaks in Taiwan from, 1996 to, 1999, *J. Clin. Microbiol.*, 38(12): 4621–4625.

Chowdhury, N.R., Chakraborty, S., Ramamurthy, T., Nishibuchi, M., Yamasaki, S., Takeda, Y., and Nair, G.B. (2000) Molecular evidence of clonal *Vibrio parahaemolyticus* pandemic strains, *Emerg. Infect. Dis.*, 6(6): 631–636.

Cook, D.W. (1994) Effect of time and temperature on multiplication of *Vibrio vulnificus* in post-harvest Gulf Coast shell-stock oysters, *Appl. Environ. Microbiol.*, 60(9): 3483–3484.

Cook, D.W. and Ruple, A.D. (1989) Indicator bacteria and *Vibrionaceae* multiplication in post-harvest shellstock oysters, *J. Food Protect.*, 52: 343–349.

Cook, D.W., Oleary, P., Hunsucker, J.C., Sloan, E.M., Bowers, J.C., Blodgett, R.J., and Depaola, A. (2002a) *Vibrio vulnificus* and *Vibrio parahaemolyticus* in U.S. retail shell oysters: a national survey from June, 1998 to July, 1999, *J. Food Protect.*, 65(1): 79–87.

Cook, D.W., Oleary, P., Hunsucker, J.C., Sloan, E.M., Bowers, J.C., Blodgett, R.J., and Depaola, A. (2002b) *Vibrio vulnificus* and *Vibrio parahaemolyticus* in U.S. retail shell oysters: a national survey from June, 1998 to July, 1999, *J. Food Protect.*, 65(3): 445.

Covert, D. and Woodburn, M. (1972) Relationships of temperature and sodium chloride concentration to the survival of *Vibrio parahaemolyticus* in broth and fish homogenate, *Appl. Microbiol.*, 23(2): 321–325.

CSPI. (1999) Citizen petition, Center for Science in the Public Interest, HFA-305, Division of Dockets Management, Aquaculture Technology, Inc., Honolulu, HI, http://www.fda.gov/ohrms/dockets/dailys (no longer accessible).

Dadisman, T., Nelson, R., Molenda, J.R., and Garber, H.J. (1973) *Vibrio parahaemolyticus* gastroenteritis in Maryland, *Am. J. Epidemiol.*, 96: 414–426.

Dai, J.H., Lee, Y.S., and Wong, H.C. (1992) Effects of iron limitation on production of a siderophore, outer membrane proteins, and hemolysin and on hydrophobicity, cell adherence, and lethality for mice of *Vibrio parahaemolyticus*, *Infect. Immun.*, 60(7): 2952–2956.

Daniels, N.A., MacKinnon, L., Bishop, R., Altekruse, S., Ray, B., Hammond, R.M., Thompson, S., Wilson, S., Bean, N.H., Griffin, P.M., and Slutsker, L. (2000) *Vibrio parahaemolyticus* infections in the United States, 1973–1998, *J. Infect. Dis.*, 181(5): 1661–1666.

Daniels, N.A., Ray, B., Easton, A., Marano, N., Kahn, E., McShan, A.L., 2nd, Del Rosario, L., Baldwin, T., Kingsley, M.A., Puhr, N.D., Wells, J.G., and Angulo, F.J. (2000) Emergence of a new *Vibrio parahaemolyticus* serotype in raw oysters: a prevention quandary, *J. Am. Med. Assoc.*, 284(12): 1541–1545.

Department of Health, Republic of China. (1996) A large-scale *Vibrio parahaemolyticus* food poisoning outbreak, Vol. 12, Department of Health, Republic of China, pp. 145–157.

Department of Health, Republic of China. (1998) Yuanli Township: investigation of a *Vibrio parahaemolyticus* poisoning at an elementary school in Yuanli township, Miaoli County, Department of Health, Republic of China, pp. 169–187.

Dowell, S.F., Groves, C., Kirkland, K.B., Cicirello, H.G., Ando, T., Jin, Q., Gentsch, J.R., Monroe, S.S., Humphrey, C.D., Slemp, C. et al. (1995) A multi-state outbreak of oyster-associated gastroenteritis: implications for interstate tracing of contaminated shellfish, *J. Infect. Dis.*, 171(6): 1497–1503.

DuPont, H. (1986) Consumption of raw shellfish: is the risk now unacceptable?, *N. Engl. J. Med.*, 314(11): 707–708.

Fishbein, M., Wentz, B., Landry, W.L., and MacEachern, B. (1974) *Vibrio parahaemolyticus* isolates in the U.S.: 1969–1972, in *Int. Symp.* Vibrio parahaemolyticus, Fujino, T., Sakaguchi, G., Sakazaki, R., and Takeda, Y., Eds., Saikon Publishing, Tokyo, pp. 53–58.

French, G.L. (1990) Antibiotics for marine *Vibrios*, *Lancet*, 336(8714): 568–569.

Fujino, T., Oxuno, Y., Nakada, D., Aoyama, A., Fukai, K., Mukai, T., and Ueho, T. (1953) On the bacteriological examination of Shirasu food poisoning, *Med. J. Osaka Univ.*, 4: 299–304.

Gooch, J.A., DePaola, A., Kaysner, C.A., and Marshall, D.L. (2001) Evaluation of two direct plating methods using non-radioactive probes for enumeration of *Vibrio parahaemolyticus* in oysters, *Appl. Environ. Microbiol.*, 67(2): 721–724.

Hackney, C., Bay, B., and Speck, M.L. (1980) Incidence of *Vibrio parahaemolyticus* in and the microbiological quality of seafood in North Carolina, *J. Food Protect.*, 43(10): 769–773.

Hallegraeff, G. and Bolch, C.J. (1992) Transport of diatom and dinoflagellate resting spores in ships' ballast water: implications for plankton biogeography and aquaculture, *J. Plankton Res.*, 14: 1067–1084.

Hally, R., Rubin, R.A., Fraimow, H.S., and Hoffman-Terry, M.L. (1995) Fatal *Vibrio parahemolyticus* septicemia in a patient with cirrhosis: a case report and review of the literature, *Dig. Dis. Sci.*, 40(6): 1257–1260.

Hara-Kudo, Y., Nishina, T., Nakagawa, H., Konuma, H., Hasegawa, J., and Kumagai, S. (2001) Improved method for detection of *Vibrio parahaemolyticus* in seafood, *Appl. Environ. Microbiol.*, 67(12): 5819–5823.

Hesselman, D.M., Motes, M.L., and Lewis, J.P. (1999) Effects of a commercial heat-shock process on *Vibrio vulnificus* in the American oyster, *Crassostrea virginica*, harvested from the Gulf Coast, *J. Food Protect.*, 62(11): 1266–1269.

Hlady, W. and Klontz, K.C. (1996) The epidemiology of *Vibrio* infections in Florida, 1981–1993, *J. Infect. Dis.*, 173(5): 1176–1183.

Honda, S., Goto, I., Minematsu, I., Ikeda, N., Asano, N., Ishibashi, M., Kinoshita, Y., Nishibuchi, N., Honda, T., and Miwatani, T. (1987) Gastroenteritis due to Kanagawa negative *Vibrio parahaemolyticus*, *Lancet*, 1(8528): 331–332.

Honda, T., Shimizu, M., Takeda, Y., and Iwatani, T. (1976) Isolation of a factor causing morphological changes of Chinese hamster ovary cells from the culture filtrate of *Vibrio parahaemolyticus*, *Infect. Immunol.*, 14(4): 1028–1033.

Honda, T., Ni, Y.X., and Miwatani, T. (1988) Purification and characterization of a hemolysin produced by a clinical isolate of Kanagawa phenomenon-negative *Vibrio parahaemolyticus* and related to the thermostable direct hemolysin, *Infect. Immunol.*, 56(4): 961–965.

Hornstrup, M. and Gahran-Hansen, B. (1993) Extraintestinal infections caused by *Vibrio parahaemolyticus* and *Vibrio alginolyticus* in a Danish county, 1987–1992, *Scand. J. Infect. Dis.*, 25(6): 735–740.

Iguchi, T., Kondo, S., and Hisatsune, K. (1995) *Vibrio parahaemolyticus* O serotypes from O1 to O13 all produce R-type lipopolysaccharide: SDS-PAGE and compositional sugar analysis, *FEMS Microbiol. Lett.*, 130(2–3): 287–292.

Johnson, D., Weinberg, L., Ciarkowski, J., West, P., and Colwell, R.R. (1984) Wound infection caused by Kanagawa-negative *Vibrio parahaemolyticus*, *J. Clin. Microbiol.*, 20(4): 811–812.

Johnson, H.C. and Liston, J. (1973) Sensitivity of *Vibrio parahaemolyticus* to cold in oysters, fish fillets and crabmeat, *J. Food Sci.*, 38: 437–441.

Johnson, H.C., Baross, J.A., and Liston, J. (1971) *Vibrio parahaemolyticus* and its importance in seafood hygiene, *J. Am. Vet. Med. Assoc.*, 159(11): 1470–1473.

Johnston, M.D. and Brown, M.H. (2002) An investigation into the changed physiological state of *Vibrio* bacteria as a survival mechanism in response to cold temperatures and studies on their sensitivity to heating and freezing, *J. Appl. Microbiol.*, 92(6): 1066–1077.

Joseph, S., Colwell, R.R., and Kaper, J.B. (1982) *Vibrio parahaemolyticus* and related halophytic *Vibrios*, *Crit. Rev. Microbiol.*, 10(1): 77–124.

Kelly, M.S. and Stroh, E.M. (1989) Urease-positive, Kanagawa-negative *Vibrio parahaemolyticus* from patients and the environment in the Pacific Northwest, *J. Clin. Microbiol.*, 27(12): 2820–2822.

Kirkland, K.B., Meriwether, R.A., Leiss, J.K., and MacKenzie, W.R. (1996) Steaming oysters does not prevent Norwalk-like gastroenteritis, *Public Health Rep.*, 111(6): 527–530.

Klontz, K.C. (1990) Fatalities associated with *Vibrio parahaemolyticus* and *Vibrio cholerae* non-O1 infections in Florida (1981–1988), *South. Med.*, 83: 500–502.

Klontz, K.C., Desenclos, J.C., Wolfe, L.E., Hoecherl, S.A., Roberts, C., and Gunn, R.A. (1991) The raw oyster consumer — a risk taker? Use of the Behavioral Risk Factor Surveillance System, *Epidemiology*, 2(6): 437–440.

Krantz, G.E., Colwell, R.R., and Lovelace, E. (1969) *Vibrio parahaemolyticus* from the blue crab *Callinectes sapidus* in Chesapeake Bay, *Science*, 164(885): 1286–1287.

Lesmana, M., Subekti, D., Simanjuntak, C.H., Tjaniadi, P., Campbell, J.R., and Oyofo, B.A. (2001) *Vibrio parahaemolyticus* associated with cholera-like diarrhea among patients in North Jakarta, Indonesia, *Diag. Microbiol. Infect. Dis.*, 39(2): 71–75.

Lowry, P.W., McFarland, L.M., Peltier, B.H., Roberts, N.C., Bradford, H.B., Herndon, J.L., Stroup, D.F., Mathison, J.B., Blake, P.A., and Gunn, R.A. (1989) *Vibrio* gastroenteritis in Louisiana: a prospective study among attendees of a scientific congress in New Orleans, *J. Infect. Dis.*, 160(6): 978–984.

Marano N.N., Daniels, N.A., Easton, A.N., McShan, A., Ray, B., Wells, J.G., Griffin, P.M., and Angulo, F.J. (2000) A survey of stool culturing practices for *Vibrio* species at clinical laboratories in Gulf Coast states, *J. Clin. Microbiol.*, 38: 2267–2270.

Matsumoto, C., Okuda, J., Ishibashi, M., Iwanaga, M., Garg, P., Rammamurthy, T., Wong, H.C., Depaola, A., Kim, Y.B., Albert, M.J., and Nishibuchi, M. (2000) Pandemic spread of an O3:K6 clone of *Vibrio parahaemolyticus* and emergence of related strains evidenced by arbitrarily primed PCR and toxRS Sequence Analyses, *J. Clin. Microbiol.*, 38(2): 578–585.

Mead, P.S., Slutsker, L., Dietz, V., McCaig, L.F., Bresee, J.S., Shapiro, C., Griffin, P.M., and Tauxe, R.V. (1999) Food-related illness and death in the United States, *Emerg. Infect. Dis.*, 5(5): 607–625.

Miyamoto, Y., Kato, T., Boar, Y., Akiyama, S., Takizawa, K., and Yam, S.A. (1969) *In vitro* hemolytic characteristic of *Vibrio parahaemolyticus*: its close correlation with human pathogenicity, *J. Bacteriol.*, 100: 1147–1149.

Mouzin, E., Mascola, L., Tormey, M.P., and Dassey, D.E. (1997) Prevention of *Vibrio vulnificus* infections: assessment of regulatory educational strategies, *JAMA*, 278(7): 576–578.

Murrison, A. (1996) Marine hitchhikers: the transport of pathogens in ballast water, *J. Roy. Nav. Med. Serv.*, 82: 40–43.

Nakasone, N., Ikema, M., Higa, N., Yamashiro, T., and Iwanaga, M. (1999) A filamentous phage of *Vibrio parahaemolyticus* O3:K6 isolated in Laos, *Microbiol. Immunol.*, 43: 285–288.

Nolan, C., Ballard, J., Kaysner, C.A., Lilja, J.L., Williams, Jr., L.P., and Tenover, F.C. (1984) *Vibrio parahaemolyticus* gastroenteritis: an outbreak associated with raw oysters in the Pacific Northwest, *Diagn. Microbiol. Infect. Dis.*, 2(2): 119–128.

Obata, H., Kai, A., and Morozumi, S. (2001) The trends of *Vibrio parahaemolyticus* foodborne outbreaks in Tokyo: 1989–2000, *Kansenshogaku Zasshi*, 75(6): 485–489.

Okuda, J., Ishibashi, M., Hayakawa, E., Nishinom, T., Takeda, Y., Mukhopadhyay, A.K., Garg, S., Bhattacharya, S.K., Nair, G.B., and Nishibuchi, M. (1997) Emergence of a unique O3:K6 clone of *V. parahaemolyticus* in Calcutta, India, and isolation of strains from the same clonal group from Southeast Asian travelers arriving in Japan, *J. Clin. Microbiol.*, 35(12): 3150–3155.

Oliver, J.D. and Kaper, J.B. (1997) *Vibrio* species, in *Food Microbiology: Fundamentals and Frontiers*, Doyle, M., Beuchat, L.R., and Montville, T.J., Eds., American Society of Microbiology Press, Washington, D.C., pp. 228–263.

O'Malley, S.M., Mouton, S.L., Occhino, D.A., Deanda, M.T., Rashidi, J.R., Fuson, K.L., Rashidi, C.E., Mora, M.Y., Payne, S.M., and Henderson, D.P. (1999) Comparison of the heme iron utilization systems of pathogenic *Vibrios*, *J. Bacteriol.*, 181(11): 3594–3598.

Osawa, R., Okitus, T., Morozumi, H., and Yamai, S. (1996) Occurrence of urease-positive *Vibrio parahemolyticus* in Kanagawa, Japan, with specific reference to presence of thermo-stable direct hemolysin (TDH) and the TDH-related hemolysin genes, *Appl. Environ. Microbiol.*, 62(2): 725–727.

Pan, T.M., Want, T.K., Lee, C.L., Chien, S.W., and Horng, C.B. (1997) Food-borne disease outbreaks due to bacteria in Taiwan, 1986–1995, *J. Clin. Microbiol.*, 35: 1260–1262.

Roland F. (1976) Leg gangrene and endotoxin shock due to *Vibrio parahaemolyticus*: an infection acquired in New England coastal waters, *N. Engl. J. Med.*, 282: 1306.

Sakazaki, R., Tamura, K., Kato, T., Obara, Y., and Yamai, S. (1968) Studies on the entero-pathogenic, facultatively halophilic bacterium *Vibrio parahaemolyticus*. 3. Entero-pathogenicity, *Jpn. J. Med. Sci. Biol.* 21: 325–331.

Sanyal, S.C. and Sen, P.C. (1974) Human volunteer study on the pathogenicity of *Vibrio parahaemolyticus*, in *Int. Symp. on* Vibrio parahaemolyticus, Fujino, T. et al., Eds., Saikon Publishing, Japan, pp. 227–230.

Sircar, B., Deb, B.C., De, S.P., Ghosh, A., and Pal, S.C. (1976) Clinical and epidemiological studies on *V. parahaemolyticus* infection in Calcutta (1975), *Indian J. Med. Res.*, 64(11): 1576–1580.

Steinkuller, P., Kelly, M.T., Sands, S.J., and Barber, J.C. (1972) *Vibrio parahaemolyticus* endophthalmitis, *J. Pediatr. Infect. Dis.*, 17: 150–153.

Tamura, N., Kobyashi, S., Hashimoto, H., and Hirose, S. (1993) Reactive arthritis induced by *Vibrio parahaemolyticus*, *J. Rheumatol.*, 20(6): 1062–1063.

Tay, L. and Yu, M. (1978) *Vibrio parahaemolyticus* isolated from blood cultures, *Singapore Med. J.*, 19: 89–92.

Thomson, W. and Thacker, C.L. (1973) Effect of temperature on *Vibrio parahaemolyticus* in oysters at refrigerator and deep freeze temperatures, *J. Inst. Can. Sci. Technol. Aliment.*, 6: 156–158.

U.S. Department of Agriculture. (1999) Nutrient Database, Release 11, http://www.nal.usda.gov/fnic/foodcomp/ (accessed January 13, 2003).

U.S. Food and Drug Administration. (2000) National Shellfish Sanitation Program Model Ordinance, Center for Food Safety and Applied Nutrition, Office of Seafood, http://www.cfsan.fda.gov/~dms/qa-top.html.

Vanderzant, C. and Nickelson, R. (1969) Isolation of *Vibrio parahemolyticus* from Gulf Coast Shrimp, Animal Science Department, J.C. Parker Agricultural Extension Service, Texas A&M University, College Station, TX, pp. 161–162.

Williams, R., Griffiths, F.B., Van der Wal, E.J., and Kelly, J. (1988) Cargo vessel ballast water as a vector for the transport of non-indigenous marine species, *Estuarine Coastal Shelf Sci.*, 26: 409–420.

Wong, H.C., Liu, C.C., Yu, C.M., and Lee, Y.S. (1996) Utilization of iron sources and its possible roles in the pathogenesis of *Vibrio parahaemolyticus*, *Microbiol. Immunol.*, 40: 791–798.

Wong, H.C., Chen, M.C., Liu, S.H., and Liu, D.P. (1999a) Incidence of highly genetically diversified *Vibrio parahaemolyticus* in seafood imported from Asian countries, *Int. J. Food Microbiol.*, 52(3): 181–188.

Wong, H.C., Ho, C.Y., Kuo, L.P., Wang, T.K., Lee, C.L., and Shih, D.Y. (1999b) Ribotyping of *Vibrio parahaemolyticus* isolates obtained from food-poisoning outbreaks in Taiwan, *Microbiol. Immunol.*, 43(7): 631–636.

Yang, S., Leff, M.G., McTague, D., Horvath, K.A., Jackson-Thompson, J., Murayi, T., Boeselager, G.K., Melnik, T.A., Gildemaster, M.C., Ridings, D.L., Altekruse, S.F., and Angulo, F.J. (1998) Multistate surveillance for food-handling, preparation, and consumption behaviors associated with foodborne diseases: 1995 and, 1996 BRFSS food-safety questions, *Morbid. Mortal. Wkly. Rep.*, *CDC Surveil. Summ.*, 47(4): 33–57.

Yu, S.L. and Uy-Yu, O. (1984) *Vibrio parahaemolyticus* pneumonia, *Ann. Intern. Med.*, 100(2): 320.

Zen-Yoji, H., Sakai, S., Terayma, T., Kudo, Y., Ito, T., Benoki, M., and Nagasaki, M. (1965) Epidemiology, enteropathogenicity, and classification of *Vibrio parahaemolyticus*, *J. Infect. Dis.*, 115(5): 436–444.

Zen-Yoji, H., Sakai, S., Kudoh, Y., Itoh, T., and Terayama, T. (1970) Antigenic schema and epidemiology of *Vibrio parahaemolyticus*, *Health Lab. Sci.*, 7: 100–108.

Zhu, B.C., Lo, J.Y., Li, Y.T., Li, S.C., Jaynes, J.M., Gildemeister, O.S., Laine, R.A., and Ou, C.Y. (1992) Thermostable, salt tolerant, wide pH range novel chitobase from *Vibrio parahaemolyticus*: isolation, characterization, molecular cloning, and expression, *J. Biochem.*, 112(1): 163–167.

Zide, N., Davis, J., and Ehrenkranz, N.J. (1974) Fulminating *Vibrio parahemolyticus* septicemia: a syndrome of erythemia multiforme, hemolytic anemia, and hypotension, *Arch. Intern. Med.*, 133(3): 479–481.

7 Cellular Effects of Bacterial Toxins: Implications for Foodborne Illness

Rajkumar Rajendram, Ross J. Hunter, and Victor R. Preedy

CONTENTS

Abstract   In bacterial foodborne illness, food acts as a vector for the transmission
of actively growing or non-replicating microbes, toxic products of bacterial metabolism, or stable toxins. This review discusses the cellular effects of toxins implicated
in the pathogenesis of bacterial foodborne illness. Foodborne bacteria can manipulate
many functions and pathways of eukaryotic cells by using toxins. Some toxins are
solely responsible for the clinical syndrome produced by infection, but most are simply
part of the pathogenic cascade resulting from foodborne bacteria infection. The cellular
effects of foodborne bacterial toxins are diverse. Some toxins act at the target cell
surface to irreparably damage the cell membrane or modify cellular signal transduction; however, others act only when the toxin has gained access to the cytoplasm of
the sensitive cell by endocytosis (for example, those with enzyme activity). Other
bacterial toxins inhibit or amplify normal host cell function. Although detrimental to
the susceptible host during an infection, the activities of several bacterial toxins have
been used to investigate cellular pathways and for medicinal applications. Thus,
research on bacterial toxins has provided information not only about the roles of those
toxins in disease but also the properties of host cells affected by the toxin.

Abbreviations   A, active subunit; ADP, adenosine diphosphate; ADPR, adenosine
diphosphate–ribose; B, binding domains; BoNTs, *Clostridium botulinum* neurotoxins;
cAMP, cyclic adenosine monophosphate; DIC, disseminated intravascular coagulation;
EHEC, enterohemorrhagic *Escherichia coli;* ETEC, enterotoxinogenic *Escherichia
coli*; GI, gastrointestinal; GMP, guanosine monophosphate; HUS, hemolytic uremic
syndrome; IL, interleukin; iNOS, inducible NO synthase; LBP, LPS-binding protein,
LOS, lipooligosaccharide; LPS, lipopolysaccharide; MHC, major histocompatibility
complex; NAD, nicotinamide adenine dinucleotide; NO, nitric oxide; PAF, platelet-
activating factor; RNA, ribonucleic acid; rRNA, ribosomal RNA; tRNA, transfer RNA;
STs, heat-stable toxins; Stx, Shiga toxins; SNAP-25, synaptosomal-associated protein
25; TeNT, tetanus neurotoxin; VTEC, verotoxin-producing *Escherichia coli*

INTRODUCTION

Foodborne illnesses are a collection of clinical syndromes, the prevalence of which
is second only to that of respiratory disease (Archer and Young, 1988). In bacterial
foodborne illnesses, food acts as a vector for the transmission of actively growing
or non-replicating bacteria, toxic products of bacterial metabolism, or stable toxins.
The clinical syndromes associated with foodborne illness are usually acute. As the

TABLE 7.1
Bacterial Causes of Various Clinical Presentations of Foodborne Illness

Clinical Presentation	Possible Bacterial Food-Related Pathogens
Gastroenteritis is noted (mainly vomiting, but diarrhea may be present).	Food poisoning due to preformed toxins (e.g., vomitoxin, *Staphylococcus aureus* toxin, *Bacillus cereus* toxin)
Noninflammatory diarrhea generally involves the small intestine. It is characterized by mucosal hypersecretion or decreased absorption without mucosal destruction. Most patients experience minimal dehydration with few physical findings. Severe watery diarrhea may cause dehydration and critical illness in the young and the elderly. Sudden onset and short duration are typical. Fever and systemic symptoms (except those due to fluid loss) are usually absent.	Can be caused by virtually all enteric pathogens but classically is due to: Enterotoxigenic *E. coli* (ETEC) *Vibrio cholerae*
Inflammatory diarrhea generally involves the large intestine and is characterized by mucosal invasion with inflammation due to invasive/cytotoxigenic bacteria. The diarrhea may be bloody and can contain fecal leukocytes. It may be associated with fever and systemic symptoms (abdominal pain and tenderness, headache, nausea, vomiting, malaise, myalgia).	*Shigella* spp. *Campylobacter* spp. *Salmonella* spp. Enteroinvasive *Escherichia coli* Enterohemorrhagic *Escherichia coli* (EHEC) *Vibrio parahaemolyticus*
Traveler's diarrhea is a common condition that affects many travelers, particularly to developing countries, and is usually due to ingestion of contaminated food or water. It is often self-limiting, resolving within a few days. It may be defined as the passage of three unformed stools per day during or after a journey or fever, cramping abdominal pain, or vomiting accompanied by any number of unformed stools, during or after a journey.	*Escherichia coli* (particularly ETEC) *Campylobacter jejuni* *Salmonella* spp. *Shigella* spp.
Neurological manifestations are observed (e.g., paresthesias, respiratory depression, bronchospasm)	*Clostridium botulinum* (botulism)
Systemic illness occurs.	*Listeria monocytogenes* *Vibrio vulnificus*

Source: Adapted from Fang, G. et al., *Infect. Dis. Clin. North Am.*, 5, 681–701, 1991.

causative agent enters the body via the mouth, problems often start in the gastrointestinal (GI) tract. Nausea, vomiting, abdominal cramps, diarrhea and non-specific symptoms of lethargy, weakness, and malaise are therefore common in many foodborne illnesses (see Table 7.1). Although the exact clinical presentation depends on the bacterial pathogen, it is rarely possible to determine the cause of a foodborne illness unless the organism is identified by microbiological means or the illness is part of a recognized outbreak. Bacterial pathogenicity is the ability of a bacterium to cause disease. Components of bacteria that contribute to their pathogenicity are known as *virulence factors*. Bacterial toxins are soluble virulence factors that adversely alter the metabolism of cells. The pathogenesis of bacterial foodborne illness is complex and often involves toxin production. This review discusses some of the bacterial toxins implicated in the pathogenesis of foodborne illness.

CLINICAL SYNDROMES PRODUCED BY FOODBORNE BACTERIAL TOXINS

Patients with foodborne illnesses typically present with GI symptoms (e.g., vomiting, diarrhea, and abdominal pain). Important clues to the etiology of a foodborne disease include:

- Incubation period
- Duration of the resultant illness
- Predominant clinical symptoms
- Population involved in the outbreak

Tables 7.1 and 7.2 highlight the clinical syndromes produced by toxin-producing foodborne pathogens. Although most toxins play a part in the pathogenesis of disease, a few bacterial toxins are entirely responsible for the pattern of clinical illness. The major clinical symptoms associated with infection with *Vibrio cholerae* (cholera), *Bacillus anthracis* (anthrax), *Clostridium botulinum* (botulism), and enterohemorrhagic *Escherichia coli* (bloody diarrhea and hemolytic uremic syndrome) are all related to the toxins produced by these organisms (see Table 7.2).

CLASSIFICATION OF BACTERIAL TOXINS

Bacterial toxins are traditionally classified into two categories:

- Exotoxins
- Endotoxins

Exotoxins are bacterial proteins that are released from bacteria during growth and which are toxic to target cells. While usually secreted by bacteria, in some cases exotoxins are also released by lysis of bacterial cells as a result of immune system activity or antibiotics (Finlay and Falkow, 1997). Endotoxins are cell-associated toxic components of Gram-negative bacteria and primarily consist of the lipopolysaccharide (LPS) component of the outer membrane; however, endotoxins may be released from growing bacterial cells or from lysis of cells (Holzheimer, 2001). Thus, either type of bacterial toxin can act close to the producing bacteria or at tissues distant from the site of bacterial invasion or growth. Please see Figure 7.1 and Table 7.3 for further classification of bacterial toxins.

TABLE 7.2
Classification of Bacterial Toxins

The following are among the numerous ways to classify toxins:
Pattern of release (e.g., endotoxin or exotoxin)
Chemical structure
        Lipopolysaccharide (endotoxin)
        Protein (exotoxin)
Structural model (subunit toxins)
        Enzymatic component (A)
        Binding component (B)
Cellular target
        Cell membrane
        Intracellular
Tissue target (e.g., enterotoxins, neurotoxins, leukotoxins, hemolysins)
Mechanism of action
        Cytolysins
        Receptor modulation
        Inhibition of protein synthesis
        Internalized/enzymatic toxins
        ADP-ribosylating toxins
        Inhibition of neurotransmitter release
        Activation of the host immune response
        Modification of second-messenger systems (e.g., adenylate cyclase toxins)
Major biological effects (e.g., edema, hemolysis, diarrhea)

Foodborne bacteria produce both endotoxins and exotoxins, and this review summarizes a variety of foodborne bacterial toxins categorized according to mode of action (see Figure 7.1).

EXOTOXINS

The two main types of bacterial exotoxins are:

- Exotoxins with intracellular targets
- Exotoxins with cellular targets

EXOTOXINS WITH INTRACELLULAR TARGETS

Exotoxins with intracellular targets generally conform to a structural model characterized by at least two functional subunits. The binding subunit (B) mediates absorption of the toxin onto the target cell surface and transfer of active component (A) across the cell membrane. Uptake and internalization occur via receptor-mediated endocytosis (Hazes and Read, 1997). Once inside a cell, the A subunit enzymatically disrupts cellular functions, such as protein synthesis and second-messenger systems (Endo et al., 1988; Saxena et al., 1989; Giannella, 1995; Halpern and Neale, 1995;

TABLE 7.3
A Summary of the Clinical Manifestations and Sources of Toxins Involved in Some Foodborne Bacterial Illnesses

Organism; Disease	Iᵃ and Dᵇ	Clinical Manifestations	Source	Lab Tests	Toxin and Mode of Action	Target	Toxin Implicated in Disease?
Activation of Second-Messenger Systems							
Enterotoxigenic *Escherichia coli* (ETEC); noninflammatory diarrhea	I: 1–3 days D: 3–7+ days	Watery diarrhea, abdominal cramps, some vomiting	Water or food contaminated with human feces	Stool culture; requires specific lab techniques for identification	LT: ADP-ribosyltransferase ST: stimulates guanylate cyclase EAST: may be like ST	G-proteins Guanylate cyclase receptor Unknown	Yes Yes ?
Bacillus anthracis; anthrax	I: 2 days to weeks D: weeks	Nausea, vomiting, malaise, bloody diarrhea, acute abdominal pain	Undercooked contaminated meat	Blood	Edema factor Adenylate cyclase	ATP	Yes
Clostridium botulinum; botulism	I: 12–72 hr D: variable (days to months)	Vomiting, diarrhea, blurred vision, diplopia, dysphagia, and descending muscle weakness; respiratory failure and death may occur	Badly canned commercial foods, fermented fish, herb-infused oils, baked potatoes in aluminum foil, cheese sauce, bottled garlic, foods kept warm for extended periods of time (e.g., in a warm oven)	Stool, serum, and food can be tested for toxin; stool and food can also be cultured for the organism	C2 toxin C3 toxin Ribosyltransferase	Monomeric G-actin Rho G-protein	?

Vibrio cholerae; cholera	I: 24–72 hr D: 3–7 days	Profuse watery diarrhea and vomiting that can lead to severe dehydration and death within hours	Contaminated water, fish, shellfish, street-vended food	Stool culture; specific media required for V. cholerae	Cholera toxin ADP-ribosyltransferase	G-protein	Yes
Inhibition of Protein Synthesis							
Escherichia coli/Shigella dysenteriae; hemorrhagic colitis and hemolytic uremic syndrome	I: 1–8 days D: 5–10 days	Severe, often bloody, diarrhea with abdominal pain and vomiting; usually little or no fever; more common in children under 4 years of age	Undercooked beef, unpasteurized milk and juice, raw fruits and vegetables (e.g., sprouts), salami, salad dressing, and contaminated water	Stool culture; special media required for E. coli O157:H7; kits available for Shiga toxin testing	Verotoxins and Shiga toxins N-glycosidase	28S rRNA	Yes
Cytolysins							
Bacillus anthracis; anthrax	As above	—	—	—	Lethal factor metalloprotease	MAPKK1/MAPKK2	Yes
Clostridium botulinum; botulism	As above	—	—	—	Neurotoxins A–G Zinc-metalloprotease	VAMP/synaptobrevin SNAP-25 syntaxin	Yes
Activation of Immune System Response							
Staphylococcus aureus; gastroenteritis	I: 1–6 hr D: 24–48 hr	Sudden onset of severe nausea and vomiting; abdominal cramps; diarrhea and fever may be present	Unrefrigerated meats, potato and egg salads, cream pastries	Stool, vomitus, and food can be tested for toxin and cultured	Preformed enterotoxins Superantigen	—	Yes

TABLE 7.3 (cont.)
A Summary of the Clinical Manifestations and Sources of Toxins Involved in Some Foodborne Bacterial Illnesses

Organism; Disease	I[a] and D[b]	Clinical Manifestations	Source	Lab Tests	Toxin and Mode of Action	Target	Toxin Implicated in Disease?
Membrane Damage							
Aeromonas hydrophila; noninflammatory diarrhea, dysentery	I: not defined D: up to 2 weeks	Two types of gastrointestinal disease associated with *A. hydrophila*: (1) watery diarrhea, and (2) dysentery-like diarrheal disease (loose stools containing blood and mucus)	Fish and shellfish, red meats (beef, pork, lamb), and poultry	Cultured from feces or blood by plating onto agar with sheep blood and ampicillin (prevents growth of competing organisms); species detected by biochemical tests; production confirmed by tissue culture assays	Aerolysin Pore-former	Glycophorin	(Yes)

Organism	Incubation/Duration	Symptoms	Foods	Diagnosis	Toxin	Receptor	Enterotoxin
Listeria monocytogenes; foodborne systemic illness meningitis	I: 9–48 hr for gastrointestinal symptoms, 2–6 weeks for invasive disease D: variable	Fever, myalgia, and nausea or diarrhea; pregnant women may have mild flu-like illness and can have premature delivery or stillbirth; elderly or immunosuppressed may have bacteremia or meningitis	Fresh soft cheeses, unpasteurized milk, inadequately pasteurized milk, ready-to-eat meats	Blood or CSF cultures; asymptomatic fecal carriage means stool culture not helpful; can detect antibody to listerolysin O to identify outbreak retrospectively	Listeriolysin O Pore-former	Cholesterol	(Yes)
Staphylococcus aureus	As above	—	—	—	α-Toxin Pore-former	Plasma membrane	(Yes)

[a] Incubation period.
[b] Duration of illness.

Abbreviations: CSF, cerebrospinal fluid; EAST, enteroaggregative *Escherichia coli* heat-stable toxin; *EHEC*, enterohemorrhagic *Escherichia coli*; ETEC, enterotoxigenic *Escherichia coli*; LT, heat-labile toxin; MAPKK, mitogen-activated protein kinase kinase; SNAP-25, synaptosomal-associated protein; ST, heat-stable toxin; VAMP, vesicle-associated membrane protein.

Source: Data from Fang et al. (1991); Boyce et al. (1995); Merritt and Hol (1995); Bhakdi et al. (1996); Aktories (1997); Harrington (1997); Stevens (1997); Lacy and Stevens (1998); Rago and Schlievert (1998).

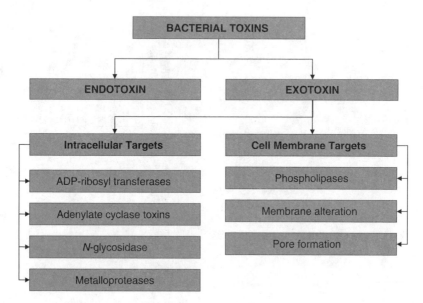

FIGURE 7.1 Classification of bacterial toxins used in this review.

Turton et al., 2002). Exotoxins with intracellular targets can be divided into groups based on mechanism of action:

- Adenosine diphosphate (ADP)–ribosyltransferase activity (e.g., cholera toxin)
- Adenylate cyclase toxins (e.g., *Bacillus anthracis* edema factor)
- Ribonucleic acid *N*-glycosidase toxins (e.g., Shiga toxin)
- Metalloprotease toxins (e.g., botulinum toxin)

Inhibition of Protein Synthesis

Inhibition of protein synthesis usually results in cell death. Verotoxins, also known as Shiga toxins (Stx), are produced by *Shigella dysenteriae* serotype 1 and the verotoxin-producing *Escherichia coli* (VTEC). Shiga toxins inactivate ribosomal RNA so the affected ribosomes are no longer able to interact with elongation factors (see Figure 7.2) (Endo et al., 1988; Saxena et al., 1989). Shiga toxins are potent cytotoxins divided into two antigenically distinct groups that share 50 to 60% homology (Tesh and O'Brien, 1991):

- Stx/Stx1
- Stx2

Stx and Stx1 are produced by *Shigella dysenteriae* serotype 1 and *Escherichia coli*, respectively, but differ by only one amino acid. Stx2-type toxins are produced by *Escherichia coli* alone but are quite diverse. Variants have been found that differ in

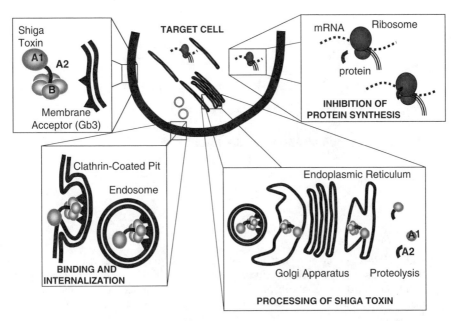

FIGURE 7.2 Shiga toxins are A–B5 toxins consisting of an active subunit (A) and five binding subunits (B). Entry to cells is initiated by binding of the B subunits to globotriasylceramide (Gb3) receptors on cell membranes. After binding, Shiga toxin is interalized via endocytosis of clathrin-coated pits. The endosomes then fuse with liposomes and subsequently pass through the Golgi apparatus and endoplasmic reticulum before their contents are translocated to the cytosol. The enzymatically active A1 fragment is released from the A2 fragment by proteolysis, which may occur within the endosome/Golgi apparatus/ER or within the cytosol. The A1 fragment interacts with the acceptor site on the 60S ribosomal subunit and binds the 28S rRNA. The A1 fragment catalyzes the removal of a single adenine residue from that part of the rRNA that is the binding site for elongation factor 2. Shiga toxin thus inhibits protein synthesis by preventing binding of amino-acyl-tRNA to the 60S ribosomal subunit. (Adapted from Lacy and Stevens, 1998; Sandvig, 2001.)

receptor specificity and activation by intestinal mucus, as well as antigenically. Some of these properties stem from only one or two nucleotide differences between the toxin genes (Tesh and O'Brien, 1991; O'Brien et al., 1992).

Shiga toxins are AB$_5$-toxins (see Figure 7.2), a subset of the A/B toxins characterized by the assembly of five binding domains (B) for each active subunit (A) (Merritt and Hol, 1995). Once internalized, the A domain is cleaved into an active A^1 portion and an A^2 portion. The A^2 portion links the A^1 fragment and the B$_5$ complex. The A^1 subunit, which has *N*-glycosidase activity, cleaves a single adenine residue from 28S ribosomal RNA (Endo et al., 1988; Saxena et al., 1989). Prokaryotic ribosomes are as sensitive to the *N*-glycosidase activity of the A^1 subunit of Stx as eukaryotic ribosomes (Suh et al., 1998). This results in inhibition of protein synthesis (Figure 7.3) and ultimately cell death.

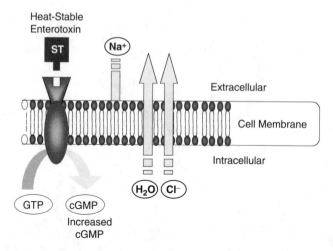

FIGURE 7.3 Mechanism of heat-stable enterotoxins. Binding of heat-stable enterotoxins (STs) to guanylate cyclase results in activation and increased cyclic guanosine monophosphate (cGMP) in intestinal epithelial cells. Increased cGMP results in reduced sodium absorption and increased chloride and bicarbonate secretion, causing secretory diarrhea as water passively follows the ions out of the cells. (Adapted from Gianella, 1995.)

The Role of Shiga Toxins in the Hemolytic Uremic Syndrome

Enterohemorrhagic *Escherichia coli* (EHEC) were first described in 1983 when an outbreak of hemorrhagic colitis was associated with undercooked hamburgers (Riley et al., 1983). *Escherichia coli* O157:H7 is an EHEC that causes hemolytic uremic syndrome (HUS), a life-threatening illness resulting in acute renal failure, hemolytic anemia, thrombocytopenia, and hemorrhagic colitis (Kaplan et al., 1990; Zoja et al., 2001). Around 20,000 cases of hemorrhagic colitis, 1000 cases of HUS, and 100 deaths are attributed each year to *Escherichia coli* O157:H7 in the United States (Boyce et al., 1995). Histologically, HUS is characterized by thrombotic microangiopathy, which consists of vessel wall thickening with swelling and detachment of endothelial cells from the basement membrane. The development of the microangiopathy of HUS is initiated by damage to the vascular endothelium. Shiga toxins are extremely important in the development of this damage (Zoja et al., 2001). After ingestion, *Escherichia coli* binds specific receptors on the colonic mucosa, multiplies, and causes cell death, usually resulting in diarrhea; however, *Escherichia coli* O157:H7, which produces Stx, prevents regeneration of the mucosal vascular endothelium by inhibition of protein synthesis. The resultant damage to the mucosal vasculature causes hemorrhagic colitis. Microvascular damage develops at target organs such as the kidney when the toxin gains access to the systemic circulation.

Modification of Second-Messenger Pathways

Modification of second messengers can dramatically alter signal transduction pathways involved in a variety of cellular functions. Bacterial toxins can thus influence several cellular functions without directly causing cell death. Toxins in this category include the heat-stable enterotoxins. Two families of diarrhea-inducing heat-stable toxins (STs) have been described: STa (or STI) and STb (or STII). Distinct STa are produced by a variety of enteropathogenic organisms: enterotoxinogenic *E. coli* (ETEC), *Vibrio cholerae*, *Vibrio mimicus*, *Yersinia enterocolitica*, and *Klebsiella*. Strains of ETEC associated with human disease produce either STa or heat-labile toxin I, or both. The STa from ETEC isolates are related but distinct toxins (Nair and Takeda, 1998). Binding of STa to its cellular receptor stimulates membrane-bound guanylate cyclase, thus increasing intracellular cyclic guanosine monophosphate (Figure 7.3) (Giannella, 1995). The increase in cGMP inhibits sodium absorption and stimulates chloride secretion, resulting in secretory diarrhea. Enterotoxinogenic *E. coli* is a common cause of traveler's diarrhea (see Table 7.1 for definition) and is a major cause of childhood diarrhea in many parts of the world.

Neurotoxins Produced by Foodborne Bacteria

The *Clostridium botulinum* neurotoxins (BoNTs, serotypes A–G) are metalloproteinases that target proteins in the motor neurons of the nervous system (Figure 7.4). Botulinum neurotoxins are most commonly associated with infant and foodborne botulism (Turton et al., 2002). Although botulinum and tetanus neurotoxins share virtually identical modes of action and a strong amino acid sequence homology, the two differ in that only botulism is a foodborne illness. The difference seems to result from an additional group of proteins produced by *Clostridium botulinum* that complex with the neurotoxin. These complexing proteins may protect and stabilize the botulinum neurotoxin in the GI tract. No such protein is produced by *Clostridium tetani*, suggesting that the lack of complexing proteins results in breakdown of tetanus neurotoxin (TeNT) in the GI tract, preventing foodborne transmission of tetanus (Jahn et al., 1995; Singh et al., 1995).

The BoNTs are A/B toxins consisting of a heavy (100-kDa) and light (50-kDa) chain linked by a single disulfide bond (Singh et al., 1995; Schiavo and Montecucco, 1997). The heavy chains of the BoNTs contain two domains: a region necessary for toxin translocation located in the N-terminal half of the molecule and a cell-binding domain located within the C-terminus of the heavy chain (Kessler and Benecke, 1997; Schiavo and Montecucco, 1997). The light chains of both the BoNTs contain zinc-binding motifs required for their zinc-dependent protease activities (Kessler and Benecke, 1997; Schiavo and Montecucco, 1997).

The cellular target of the BoNTs is a group of proteins required for docking and fusion of synaptic vesicles to presynaptic plasma membranes and therefore essential for the release of neurotransmitters. The BoNTs bind to receptors on the presynaptic membrane of motor neurons associated with the peripheral nervous system. Proteolysis of target proteins in these neurons inhibits the release of acetylcholine, thereby preventing muscle contraction (Halpern and Neale, 1995; Turton et al., 2002). This manifests clinically as flaccid paralysis of skeletal muscle. BoNTs B, D, F, and G cleave the vesicle-associated membrane protein and synaptobrevin, BoNTs A and E target the synaptosomal-associated protein 25 (SNAP-25), and BoNT C hydrolyzes syntaxin and SNAP-25 (Singh et al., 1995; Kessler and Benecke, 1997; Schiavo and Montecucco, 1997).

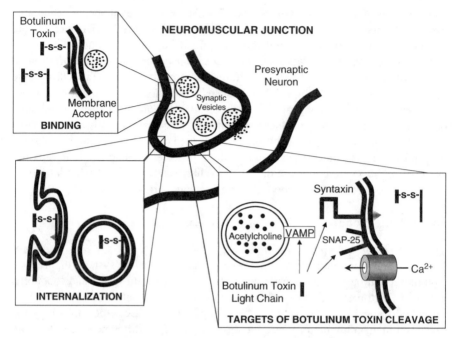

FIGURE 7.4 Cellular effects of botulinum toxin. *Clostridium botulinum* produces seven serotypes (A–G) of botulinum toxin. They are metalloproteinases that cause muscle paralysis by blocking the release of acetylcholine from the neuromuscular junction (NMJ). Botulinum toxin is an A–B toxin composed of light and heavy chains linked by a disulfide bond. The purified toxin is surrounded by five proteins believed to stabilize it and facilitate its passage through the gastrointestinal tract. These proteins are shed before internalization at the NMJ. The three stages of the pathogenesis of botulism are (1) binding and internalization, (2) translocation, and (3) proteolysis. Botulinum toxin binds specific receptors on the neuronal cell membrane at the NMJ, which triggers internalizatioin by endocytosis. Acidification of the endocytic vesicle induces structural changes, resulting in translocation of the light chain across the vesicle membrane into the cytosol of the cell. The targets of the botulinum toxins are proteins involved in the fusion of acetylcholine vesicles at the presynaptic membrane. Vesicle fusion requires the interaction of vesicle-associated membrane protein (VAMP), 25-kDa synaptosomal-associated protein (SNAP-25), and syntaxin, among other proteins, to form the SNAP receptor (SNARE) complex. Each serotype (A–G) of botulinum toxin has a unique target site. For example, both A and E cleave the C-terminus of SNAP-25; however, A removes 9 amino acids and E removes 26. This difference affects the duration of action of each toxin. The effects of toxin A last up to 4 months, while the effects of E wear off within 2 weeks. (Adapted from Halpern and Neal, 1995; Jahn et al., 1995; Turton et al., 2002.)

Bacterial Superantigens

Some bacterial toxins directly affect the function of T cells and antigen-presenting cells of the immune system. For example, the pyrogenic toxin superantigens massively stimulate the immune system, causing release of inflammatory mediators and promoting septic shock (Lee and Schlievert, 1991; Schlievert, 1997; Rago and

Schlievert, 1998). These stable, secreted toxins include the staphylococcal entero-toxin serotypes A to E, G, and H. The pyrogenic toxin superantigens generally act by binding major histocompatibility complex (MHC) class II molecules on the surface of antigen-presenting cells and to the T-cell receptor. This results in a massive proliferation of peripheral T cells, which greatly skews the T-cell receptor repertoire (Papageorgiou and Acharya, 2000; Stevens, 1997); however, the T cells produced do not function normally and exist in a state of anergy or undergo apoptosis (Stevens, 1997). Concomitant with the T-cell proliferation is a massive release of both lymphocyte-derived cytokines, such as interleukin-2 (IL-2), tumor necrosis factor β (TNF-β), and gamma-interferon (γ-INF), and monocyte-derived cytokines, such as IL-1, IL-6, and TNF-α (Schlievert 1997; Stevens 1997). These cytokines mediate the hypotension, high fever, and diffuse erythematous rash that are characteristic of the septic-shock syndrome.

Exotoxins with Cellular Targets

Exotoxins with cellular targets are either cytolytic exotoxins (usually degradative enzymes) or cytolysins that induce hemolysis and tissue necrosis and may be lethal when administered intravenously.

Membrane-Damaging Toxins (Cytolysins)

Cytolysins damage the extracellular matrix or the plasma membrane of cells. The resulting lysis of cells also facilitates the spread of bacteria through tissues. Cytoly-sins can be divided into groups based on the mechanism of action:

- Pore formation (e.g., *Staphylococcus aureus* α-toxin)
- Alteration of membrane permeability, thiol(-SH)-activated cytolysins (oxygen-labile) (e.g., streptolysin O of *Streptococcus*)
- Phospholipases, hydrolyse membrane phospholipids (e.g., *Clostridium*, *Staphylococcus*)

Bacterial hyaluronidases, collagenases, and phospholipases have the capacity to degrade cellular membranes or matrices. Examples of these types of toxins include the α-toxin of *Clostridium perfringens*, which has phospholipase C activity, and the clostridial collagenases (Lottenberg et al., 1994; Harrington, 1996; Songer, 1997).

Pore-forming toxins insert transmembrane pores into cell membranes, disrupting the influx and efflux of ions and resulting in cytolysis. The *Staphylococcus aureus* α-toxin is able to lyse a variety of cell lines, including human monocytes, lympho-cytes, erythrocytes, platelets, and endothelial cells (Bhakdi and Tranum-Jensen, 1991; Bhakdi et al., 1996). The crystallographic structure of the fully assembled α-toxin pore has been elucidated (Song et al., 1996). Seven toxin protomers assemble on the cell membrane, forming a mushroom-shaped heptamer (Figure 7.5) (Song et al., 1996; Lesieur et al., 1997). The cap of the heptamer rests on the cell membrane, while the stem domain traverses the membrane to form the transmembrane channel (Song et al., 1996; Lesieur et al., 1997; Lacy and Stevens, 1998).

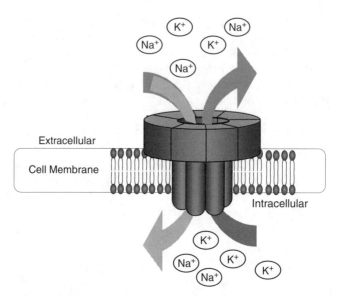

FIGURE 7.5 The mechanism of cytolysis of the *Staphylococcus aureus* α-toxin. After binding membrane receptors and oligomerization, the stem of α-toxin heptamer inserts into the target cell membrane. The resulting pore permits unregulated traffic of ions into and out of the cell, eventually resulting in swelling and death. (Adapted from Bhakdi et al., 1996; Lacy and Stevens, 1998.)

Three sequential events occur during α-toxin pore formation (see Figure 7.5):

1. Toxin protomers bind to target membranes by either unidentified high-affinity receptors or through nonspecific absorption to substances such as phosphatidylcholine or cholesterol on the lipid bilayer (Bhakdi and Tranum-Jensen, 1991; Bhakdi et al., 1996; Tomita and Kamio, 1997).
2. Membrane-bound protomers oligomerize into a nonlytic prepore heptamer complex.
3. The heptamer undergoes a series of conformational changes, creating a stem domain that is then inserted into the membrane (Song et al., 1996; Lesieur et al., 1997).

The pore formed by the α-toxin allows the influx and efflux of small molecules and ions that eventually result in the swelling and death of nucleated cells and the osmotic lysis of erythrocytes. Pore formation has also been shown to trigger secondary events that could promote development of pathologic sequelae. These events include endonuclease activation, increased platelet exocytosis, release of cytokines and inflammatory mediators, and production of eicosanoids (Bhakdi and Tranum-Jensen 1991; Bhakdi et al., 1996). The α-toxin is required for *Staphylococcus aureus* virulence in these systems in animal models (Bhakdi and Tranum-Jensen, 1991; Bhakdi et al., 1996); however, the precise role of α-toxin in staphylococcal diseases in humans remains unclear.

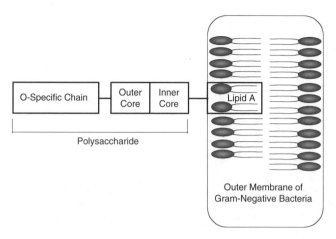

FIGURE 7.6 Endotoxin components: polysaccharide (including an O-specific side chain and an in inner and outer core region) and lipid A, the toxic, hydrophobic component.

ENDOTOXINS

Endotoxins are present in the outer membrane of all Gram-negative bacteria, including *Salmonella* and *E. coli* (Glauser et al., 1991; Remick, 1995; Ulevitch and Tobias, 1995; Rietschel et al., 1996). The endotoxins of foodborne Gram-negative bacteria are causal or complicating factors in many foodborne illnesses. Endotoxin consists of two distinct components (see Figure 7.6) (Glauser et al., 1991; Rietschel et al., 1996):

- Polysaccharide (including an O-specific side chain and an inner and outer core region)
- Lipid A (toxic, hydrophobic component)

O-SPECIFIC CHAINS OF ENDOTOXIN

Although, the general structure of O-specific chains is highly conserved among Gram-negative bacteria, considerable structural diversity occurs between species. The O-specific chain is constructed by the sequential addition of oligosaccharides. As a result, at any given time the endotoxin of a bacterium is a mixture of molecules with short (lipooligosaccharide [LOS]), intermediate, and long O-specific chains (lipopolysaccharide [LPS]) (Remick, 1995; Rietschel et al., 1996).

The structural variance of O-specific side chains produces two distinct types of Gram-negative bacterial growth in culture:

- "Rough" (short O-specific-chain-containing LPS)
- "Smooth" (long O-specific-chain-containing LPS)

This variation determines the virulence of the organism. Experimentally, "smooth" bacteria (i.e., bacteria with long O-specific-chain-containing LPS) are more resistant to complement-mediated killing (McCallum et al., 1989). "Smooth" *Salmonella* strains demonstrate accelerated rates of proliferation and mortality in mouse models of infection (Lyman et al., 1976). In addition, anti-endotoxin antibodies have greater binding affinity for "rough" Gram-negative bacteria than do smooth strains (Siegel et al., 1993). These characteristics have obvious therapeutic implications.

LIPID A COMPONENTS OF ENDOTOXIN

Lipid A is responsible for the biological effects of endotoxin and is highly conserved between bacterial families (Rietschel et al., 1996).

EFFECTS OF ENDOTOXIN

Endotoxin interacts with many interconnected cellular and plasma mediators to cause local and systemic inflammation. These elements routinely mediate the normal host response to infection. These may be self-limiting, but if the host's normal homeostatic mechanisms break down the inflammatory response is manifested clinically as fever, tachycardia, tachypnea myocardial depression, and ultimately septic shock, organ failure, and death. (Glauser et al., 1991; Remick, 1995; Ulevitch and Tobias, 1995; Rietschel et al., 1996). Currently, therapy is limited to supportive medical care and antibiotics, but when bacteria are killed residual endotoxin continues to drive the inflammatory response.

Endotoxin interacts with most of the cellular immune system (Glauser et al., 1991; Rietschel et al., 1996). It is taken up by and activates neutrophils, thus enhancing phagocytosis. Endotoxin may also activate neutrophils to express adhesion molecules that mediate neutrophil-to-neutrophil, neutrophil-to-vascular endothelial cell, and neutrophil-to-tissue binding, thus inducing local inflammation and vascular leakage. LPS also appears to affect various populations of lymphocytes, stimulating B-cell proliferation and antibody production, activating T cells to secrete cytokines, and downregulating T-suppressor cells (Glauser et al., 1991; Rietschel et al., 1996).

The most widely studied and probably the most significant cellular effects of endotoxin involve the interaction with monocytes and macrophages, which express the principal cellular receptor of endotoxin, CD14. Circulating LPS binds LPS-binding protein (LBP), a glycoprotein that facilitates the binding of LPS to CD14 (Glauser et al., 1991; Remick 1995; Ulevitch and Tobias, 1995; Rietschel et al., 1996).

The effects of the interaction between LPS and monocytes and macrophages include:

- Production of cytokines
- Production of nitric oxide
- Activation of the complement cascade
- Activation of the coagulation cascade

Production of Cytokines

Endotoxin induces the production and release of several cytokines, including IL-1, IL-6, IL-8, tumor necrosis factor, and platelet-activating factor (PAF), which in turn stimulate production of prostaglandins and leukotrienes. These are powerful mediators of inflammation. Endotoxin enhances macrophage phagocytosis and cytotoxicity (Remick, 1995; Ulevitch and Tobias, 1995; Rietschel et al., 1996).

Production of Nitric Oxide

Nitric oxide (NO) is a vasodilator produced by macrophages and endothelial cells. When released, the resulting vasodilation, if extensive, can result in hypotension. Endotoxin induces the production of inducible NO synthase (iNOS) in macrophages, thus NO release from macrophages occurs after several hours. However, NO is produced by constitutive NOS (cNOS) in endothelial cells, so NO release occurs within minutes and may be responsible for the hypotension associated with septic shock (Vane et al., 1990).

Activation of the Complement Cascade

Endotoxin activates complement through two separate pathways: (1) bacteria and bacterial cell wall components complexed with antibodies activate the classical (antibody-dependent) complement pathway intended to kill the bacteria, and (2) endotoxin directly activates the alternative (antibody-independent) pathway (Glauser et al., 1991). The resulting complement cascade induced by LPS produces, among other mediators, the anaphylotoxins C3a and C5a, which contribute to vasodilatation, increased vascular permeability, and circulatory collapse (Glauser et al., 1991). In addition, complement components induce adhesion and activation of platelets and neutrophils, stimulating the secondary events of platelet aggregation, release of lysosomal enzymes and arachidonic acid metabolites, and microvascular injury. The effects of complement activation are interlinked with those of the overproduction of cytokines (Glauser et al., 1991).

Coagulation

When activated by LPS, Factor XII activates the intrinsic coagulation pathway, which subsequently activates the extrinsic pathway. Pathological activation by endotoxin thus converts the usually beneficial coagulation cascade into a pathological process, culminating in the development of disseminated intravascular coagulation (DIC) (Glauser et al., 1991).

ROLE OF ENDOTOXIN IN DISEASE

Sepsis and septic shock are the syndromes most commonly associated with endotoxin. It has been suggested that antibiotic therapy increases endotoxin release via bacterial lysis, exacerbating the inflammatory response (Prins, 1996). Antibiotic-associated endotoxin release remains unproven, and its clinical significance is uncertain; however, the sensible use of specific rather than broad-spectrum antibiotics may reduce the release of endotoxins from non-pathogenic Gram-negative commensals (Prins, 1996). Endotoxin has also been associated with numerous other clinical syndromes involving documented infection by exogenous Gram-negative bacteria, such as hemolytic uremic syndrome due to EHEC (Kaplan et al., 1990); however, the role of endotoxin in these diseases is less clear than its role in sepsis.

ROLE OF ENDOTOXIN IN THE HEMOLYTIC UREMIC SYNDROME

Antibodies against *Escherichia coli* LPS are present in over 70% of patients with HUS (Greatorex and Thorne, 1994). Animal models have shown that LPS, in addition to the Shiga-like toxins produced by *Escherichia coli*, may contribute to O157:H7 nephropathology, gastrointestinal abnormalities, and death (Karpman et al., 1997). Intragastric inoculation of mice with *Escherichia coli* O157:H7 resulted in GI tract, neurological, and systemic symptoms. Histology revealed necrotic foci in the colon, lesions in the glomeruli and tubules of the kidneys, and fragmented erythrocytes. Disease in LPS-responder mice is characterized by a combination of neurological and systemic symptoms; however, mutant non-responder mice develop disease with a biphasic course. Systemic symptoms occur first, followed by severe neurological symptoms. Mice inoculated with Shiga-like toxin-II-positive strains develop disease characterized by severe neurological symptoms and a higher frequency of systemic symptoms and glomerular pathology than disease due to Shiga-like toxin-II-negative strains. Anti-Shiga-like toxin-II antibodies protect against these symptoms and pathology. These results suggest that both LPS and Shiga-like toxin are required for the development of HUS (Karpman et al., 1997). Additional research is needed to clarify the clinical significance of these findings, as HUS and other Gram-negative bacterial foodborne illnesses may present opportunities for intervention directed against endotoxin-related disease.

USES OF BACTERIAL TOXINS

BASIC SCIENCE RESEARCH

Some of these powerful disease-causing toxins have been exploited to further our basic knowledge of cell biology and for medical purposes. For example, cholera toxin and the related labile-toxin of *Escherichia coli* have been used as biologic tools to understand the mechanism of adenylate cyclase activation and the role of cyclic adenosine monophosphate (cAMP) as a second messenger in the eukaryotic cell (Bokoch et al., 1983; Harnett, 1994; Neer, 1995).

BIOLOGICAL WARFARE

The September 11, 2001, attacks on America have raised concerns about biological threats to society, such as warfare with engineered bacteria such as *Bacillus anthracis*. The cutaneous form of anthrax results from *Bacillus anthracis* infection through the skin. The skin forms a pustule around the germinating spores of *Bacillus anthracis* 3 to 5 days after infection. This causes little pain or discomfort, and the majority of cutaneous anthrax victims survive (Spencer, 2002). Fortunately, anthrax is rarely foodborne, but if the infection spreads to the lymphatic system from the GI tract it can be more severe than the cutaneous form. *Bacillus anthracis* can enter the blood from the lymph nodes and begin secreting toxins systemically. From the first onset of symptoms to the time of death is usually only 3 days. Sadly, by the time the disease has been diagnosed, the toxin load is usually so great that death is inevitable (Spencer, 2002).

CLINICAL MEDICINE

The toxins produced by foodborne bacteria may be used to help diagnose diseases caused by the bacteria and help guide therapy. For example, the introduction of new techniques to rapidly detect Stx and *Escherichia coli* in stool samples may allow the early diagnosis of HUS and the differentiation of EHEC from other *Escherichia coli* not associated with HUS (Trachtman and Christen, 1999).

As toxins can disrupt normal cellular function, it is possible that they could be utilized to therapeutically disrupt the function of abnormal cells such as cancers. Cancers are caused by the development of genetic mutations, resulting in the immortalization of cell lines. The immortalized cells then proliferate at the expense of normal tissues. The activities of several potent cellular toxins have been considered as potential therapies for certain cancers. Such toxins can either be used directly in treatment or as components of immunotoxins (Ghetie et al., 1997; Pastan, 1997; Winkler et al., 1997). Immunotoxins are hybrids of the enzymatically active portion of a toxin molecule and monoclonal antibodies (or a receptor). For example, Stx binds to the cell surface glycolipid CD77, which is expressed by B cells in certain B-cell lymphomas (Murray et al., 1985; Taga et al., 1995). Subsequently, it was found that Stx can purge murine (and, therefore, potentially human) bone marrow of malignant CD77+ B cells before autologous bone marrow transplant (LaCasse et al., 1996). Other toxins that inhibit protein synthesis are frequently engineered as the cell-killing component of immunotoxins. Immunotoxins are in clinical trials for the treatment of B-cell lymphomas, leukemia, and bone marrow transplants (Ghetie et al., 1997; Pastan, 1997; Winkler et al., 1998).

Several clinical applications have also been found for the powerful botulinum neurotoxin type A (BoNT/A) (Kessler and Benecke, 1997; Wheeler, 1997). Disorders that respond to BoNT/A involve muscle hyperactivity. A tiny amount of purified toxin injected into specific sites stops the muscle spasm by paralysis of the target muscle. As the effect lasts for no more than a few months, Botox® therapy must be continuous. The first maladies treated with BoNT/A were eye movement abnormalities (Averbuch-Heller and Leigh, 1997); however, the therapeutic value of BoNT/A has been shown for many other disorders, including cervical and laryngeal dystonia, writer's cramp, hemifacial spasm, tremors, and tics (Kessler and Benecke, 1997; Wheeler, 1997). BoNT/A is also used cosmetically to reduce deep wrinkles caused by the contraction of facial muscles (Carter and Seiff, 1997). Derivatives of some of these toxins (e.g., cholera toxin) have been incorporated into human vaccines (Holmgren et al., 1993; Snider, 1995).

THE USE OF TOXOIDS FOR VACCINATION AGAINST FOODBORNE ILLNESS

Exotoxins are solely responsible for or play a major role in the pathogenesis of many diseases; therefore, producing neutralizing antibodies against these exotoxins can provide effective protection against the disease. Antitoxins against diphtheria, tetanus, and botulinum toxoids are in clinical use for the treatment of seriously ill patients (Farthing et al., 1998). The anthrax vaccine contains the protective antigen and small amounts of the lethal factor and edema factor toxins (Schmitt et al., 1999). Antitoxins designed to bind verotoxins produced by *Escherichia coli* O157:H7 and other VTECs are under development for the treatment and prevention of hemolytic uremic syndrome, a life-threatening consequence of these infections (Trachtman and Christen, 1999).

Most toxoid vaccines consist of partially purified toxin preparations obtained from cultures of bacteria such as *Clostridium diphtheriae* or *Bacillus anthracis*. Formaldehyde treatment inactivates the diphtheria and tetanus toxins for vaccine formulation. New vaccines aimed at toxins are in various stages of development. The next generation of toxoid vaccines falls into four general categories:

- Purified inactivated toxoid
- Live, attenuated strains of the causative agent producing genetically modified toxoid
- Live, attenuated unrelated bacterial vector strains that produce the target toxoid
- Chemically synthesized antigens and artificial vaccines

Advances in the development of specific toxoid vaccines are published annually by the National Institutes of Health in *The Jordan Report* (NIAID and NIH, 2001).

The rational development of toxoid vaccines has been facilitated by advances in the understanding of toxin structure and function. For example, in A/B toxins, while the B domain is required for the delivery of the toxic A domain, the B domain is not toxic; therefore, the B portions of toxins should make ideal vaccines. Several bacterial toxins bind membrane receptors to initiate their uptake into cells. Some toxins have an affinity for the sugars that are associated with either glycolipids or glycoproteins on their target membrane; however, the receptors for many of the bacterial toxins are still unknown. Advances in the understanding of toxin–receptor binding interactions could lead to the development of receptor antagonists to prevent entry of bacterial toxins into cells (Lacy and Stephens, 1998).

SUMMARY

Bacteria in general, and foodborne bacteria in particular, have evolved toxins capable of interrupting or hyperstimulating essential functions and pathways of eukaryotic cells. These toxins presumably confer some benefit to the bacterium, either during a stage of the host–parasite interaction or perhaps in the environment encountered by the bacterium. The effects of foodborne bacterial toxins are as varied as the bacteria that produce them. Some toxins act at the target cell surface to irreparably damage the cell membrane or modify normal cellular signal transduction. Others, however, act only when the toxin has gained access to the cytoplasm of the sensitive cell by endocytosis (for example, those with enzyme activity). Still other bacterial toxins act by inhibiting or amplifying normal host cell function. Some toxins are solely responsible for the clinical syndrome produced by infection with the foodborne bacteria, but most are simply part of the pathogenic-cascade-induced infection. Although detrimental to the susceptible host during an infection, the activities of several bacterial toxins have been exploited as probes of eukaryotic cellular pathways and for medicinal applications. Thus, research on bacterial toxins has provided information not only about the roles of those toxins in disease but also the properties of host cells affected by the toxin.

REFERENCES

Aktories, K. (1997) Rho proteins: targets for bacterial toxins, *Trends Microbiol.*, 5: 282–288.

Archer, D.L. and Young, F.E. (1988) Contemporary issues: diseases with a food vector, *Clin. Microbiol. Rev.*, 1: 377–398.

Averbuch-Heller, L. and Leigh, R.J. (1997) Medical treatments for abnormal eye movements: pharmacological, optical and immunological strategies, *Austr. N. Zeal. J. Ophthal.*, 25: 7–13.

Bhakdi, S. and Tranum-Jensen, J. (1991) Alpha-toxin of *Staphylococcus aureus*, *Microbiol. Rev.*, 55: 733–751.

Bhakdi, S., Bayley, H., Valeva, A., Walev, I., Walker, B., Kehoe, M., and Palmer, M. (1996) Staphylococcal alpha-toxin, streptolysin-O and *Escherichia coli* hemolysin: prototypes of pore-forming bacterial cytolysins, *Arch. Microbiol.*, 165: 73–79.

Bokoch, G.M., Katada, T., Northup, J.K., Hewlett, E.L., and Gilman, A.G. (1983) Identification of the predominant substrate for ADP-ribosylation by islet activating protein, *J. Biol. Chem.*, 258: 2072–2075.

Boyce T.G., Swerdlow D.L., and Griffin P.M. (1995) *Escherichia coli* O157:H7 and the hemolytic-uraemic syndrome, *N. Engl. J. Med.*, 333: 364–368.

Carter, S.R. and Seiff, S.R. (1997) Cosmetic botulinum toxin injections, *Int. Ophthalmol. Clin.*, 37: 69–79.

Endo, Y., Tsurugi, K., Yutsudo, T., Takeda, Y., Ogasawara, T., and Igarashi K. (1988) Site of action of a Vero toxin (VT2) from *Escherichia coli* O157:H7 and of Shiga toxin on eucaryotic ribosomes, *Eur. J. Biochem.*, 171: 45–50.

Fang, G., Araujo, V., and Guerrant R.L. (1991) Enteric infections associated with exposure to animals or animal products, *Infect. Dis. Clin. North Am.*, 5: 681–701.

Farthing, M.G.J., Jeffries, D.J., and Anderson J, (1998) Infectious diseases, tropical medicine and sexually transmitted diseases, in *Clinical Medicine*, 4th ed., Kumar, P. and Clark, M., Eds., W.B. Saunders, London, pp. 1–124.

Finlay, B.B. and Falkow, S. (1997) Common themes in microbial pathogenicity revisited, *Microbiol. Mol. Biol. Rev.*, 16: 136–169.

Ghetie, M.A., Ghetie, V., and Vitetta, E.S. (1997) Immunotoxins for the treatment of B-cell lymphomas, *Mol. Med.*, 3: 420–427.

Giannella, R.A. (1995) *Escherichia coli* heat-stable enterotoxins, guanylins, and their receptors: what are they and what do they do?, *J. Lab. Clin. Med.*, 125: 173–181.

Glauser, M., Zanetti, G., Baumgartner, J., and Cohen, J. (1991) Septic shock: pathogenesis, *Lancet*, 338: 732–736.

Greatorex, J. and Thorne, G. (1994) Humoral immune responses to shigalike toxins and *Escherichia coli* O157 lipopolysaccharide in hemolytic–uremic syndrome patients and health subjects, *J. Clin. Microbiol.*, 32: 1172–1178.

Halpern, J.L. and Neale, E.A. (1995) Neurospecific binding, internalization and retrograde axonal transport, *Curr. Top. Microbiol. Immunol.*, 195: 221–241.

Harnett, M.M. (1994) Analysis of G-proteins regulating signal transduction pathways, *Meth. Mol. Biol.*, 27: 199–211.

Harrington, D.J. (1996) Bacterial collagenases and collagen-degrading enzymes and their potential role in human disease, *Infect. Immun.*, 64: 1885–1891.

Hazes, B. and Read, R.J. (1997) Accumulating evidence suggests that several AB-toxins subvert the endoplasmic reticulum-associated protein degradation pathway to enter target cells, *Biochemistry*, 36: 11051–11054.

Holmgren, J., Lycke, N., and Czerkinsky, C. (1993) Cholera toxin and cholera-B subunit as oral mucosal adjuvant and antigen vector systems, *Vaccine*, 11: 1179–1184.

Holzheimer, R.G. (2001) Antibiotic-induced endotoxin release and clinical sepsis: a review, *J. Chemother.*, 13: 159–172.

Jahn, R., Hanson, P.I., Otto, H., and Ahnert-Hilger, G. (1995) Botulinum and tetanus neurotoxins: emerging tools for the study of membrane fusion, *Cold Spring Harbor Symp. Quant. Biol.*, 60: 329–335.

Kaplan, B.S., Cleary, T.G., and Obrig, T.G. (1990) Recent advances in understanding the pathogenesis of the hemolytic uraemic syndromes, *Pediatr. Nephrol.*, 4: 276–283.

Karpman, D., Connell, H., Svensson, M., Scheutz, F., Alm, P., and Svanborg, C. (1997). The role of lipopolysaccharide and Shiga-like toxin in a mouse model of *Escherichia coli* O157:H7 infection, *J. Infect. Dis.*, 175: 611–620.

Kessler, K.R. and Benecke R. (1997) Botulinum toxin: from poison to remedy, *Neurotoxicology*, 18: 761–770.

LaCasse, E.C., Saleh, M.T., Patterson, B., Minden, M.D., and Gariepy, J. (1996) Shiga-like toxin purges human lymphoma from bone marrow of severe combined immunodeficient mice, *Blood*, 88: 1551–1567.

Lacy, D.B. and Stevens, R.C. (1998) Unraveling the structures and modes of action of bacterial toxins, *Curr. Opin. Struct. Biol.*, 8: 778–784.

Lee, P.K. and Schlievert, P.M. (1991) Molecular genetics of pyrogenic exotoxin "superantigens" of group A streptococci and *Staphylococcus*, *Curr. Top. Microbiol. Immunol.*, 174: 1–19.

Lesieur, C., Vecsey-Semjen, B., Abrami, L., Fivaz, M., and Gisou van der Goot, F. (1997) Membrane insertion: the strategies of toxins, *Mol. Membrane Biol.*, 14: 45–64.

Lottenberg, R., Minning-Wenz, D., and Boyle, M.D. (1994) Capturing host plasmin(ogen): a common mechanism for invasive pathogens?, *Trends Microbiol.*, 2: 20–24.

Lyman, M., Steward, J., and Roantree, R. (1976) Characterization of the virulence and antigenic structure of *Salmonella typhimurium* strains with lipopolysaccharide core defects, *Infect. Immun.*, 13: 1539–1542.

McCallum, K., Schoenhals, G., Laakso, D., Clarke, B., and Whitfield, C. (1989) A high-molecular-weight fraction of smooth lipopolysaccharide in *Klebsiella* serotype O1:K20 contains a unique O-antigen epitope and determines resistance to nonspecific serum killing, *Infect. Immun.*, 57: 3816–3822.

Merritt, E.A. and Hol, W.G.J. (1995) AB-5 toxins, *Curr. Opin. Struct. Biol.*, 5: 165–171.

Murray, L.J., Habeshaw, J.A., Wiels, J., and Greaves, M.F. (1985) Expression of Burkitt lymphoma-associated antigen (defined by the monoclonal antibody 38.13) on both normal and malignant germinal-centre B cells, *Int. J. Cancer*, 36: 561–565.

Nair, G.B. and Takeda, Y. (1998) The heat-stable enterotoxins, *Microb. Pathogen.*, 24: 123–131.

Neer, E.J. (1995) Heterotrimeric G proteins: organizers of transmembrane signals, *Cell*, 80: 249–257.

NIAID and NIH. (2000) *The Jordan Report: Accelerated Development of Vaccines*, National Institutes of Allergy and Infectious Disease, National Institutes of Health, U.S. Government Printing Office, Washington, D.C.

O'Brien, A.D., Tesh, V.L., Donohue-Rolfe, A., Jackson, M.P., Olsnes, S., Sandvig, K., Lindberg, A.A., and Keusch, G.T. (1992) Shiga toxin: biochemistry, genetics, mode of action, and role in pathogenesis, *Curr. Top. Microbiol. Immunol.*, 180: 65–94.

Papageorgious, A.C. and Acharya, K.R. (2000) Microbial superantigens: from structure to function, *Trends Microbiol.*, 8: 369–375.

Pastan, I. (1997) Targeted therapy of cancer with recombinant immunotoxins, *Biochim. Biophys. Acta*, 1333: C1–C6.

Prins, J. (1996) Antibiotic induced release of endotoxin: clinical data and human studies, *J. Endotoxin Res.*, 3: 269–273.

Rago, J.V. and Schlievert, P.M. (1998) Mechanisms of pathogenesis of staphylococcal and streptococcal superantigens, *Curr. Top. Microbiol. Immunol.*, 225: 81–97.

Remick, D. (1995) Applied molecular biology of sepsis, *J. Crit. Care*, 10: 198–212.

Rietschel, E.T., Brade, H., Holst, O., Brade, L., Muller-Loennies, S., Mamat, U., Zahringer, U., Beckmann, F., Seydel, U., Brandenburg, K., Ulmer, A.J., Mattern, T., Heine, H., Schletter, J., Loppnow, H., Schonbeck, U., Flad, H.D., Hauschildt, S., Schade, U.F., Di Padova, F., Kusumoto, S., and Schumann, R.R. (1996) Bacterial endotoxin: chemical constitution, biological recognition, host response, and immunological detoxification, *Curr. Top. Microbiol. Immunol.*, 216: 39–81.

Riley, L.W., Remis, R.S., Helgerson, S.D., McGee, H.B., Wells, J.G., Davis, B.R., Hebert, R.J., Olcott, E.S., Johnson, L.M., Hargrett, N.T., Blake, P.A., and Cohen, M.L. (1983) Hemorrhagic colitis associated with a rare *Escherichia coli* serotype, *N. Engl. J. Med.* 308: 681–685.

Sandvig K. (2001) Shiga toxins, *Toxicon*, 39: 1629–1635.

Saxena, S.K., O'Brien, A.D., and Ackerman, E.J. (1989) Shiga toxin, Shiga-like toxin II variant, and ricin are all single-site RNA N-glycosidases of 28 S RNA when microinjected into *Xenopus* oocytes, *J. Biol. Chem.*, 264: 596–601.

Schiavo G. and Montecucco, C. (1997) The structure and mode of action of botulinum and tetanus toxins, in *The Clostridia: Molecular Biology and Pathogenesis*, Rood, J.I., McClane, B.A., Songer, J.G., and Titball, R.W., Eds., Academic Press, San Diego, CA, pp. 295–322.

Schlievert P.M. (1997) Searching for superantigens, *Immunol. Invest.*, 26: 283–290.

Schmitt, C.K., Meysick, K.C., and O'Brien A.D. (1999) Bacterial toxins: friends or foes?, *Emerg. Infect. Dis.*, 5: 224–234.

Siegel, S., Evans, M., Pollack, M., Leone, A.O., Kinney, C.S., Tam, S.H., and Daddona, P.E. (1993) Antibiotics enhance binding by human lipid A-reactive monoclonal antibody HA-1A to smooth Gram-negative bacteria, *Infect. Immun.*, 61: 512–519.

Singh, B.R., Li, B., and Read, D. (1995) Botulinum versus tetanus neurotoxins: why is botulinum neurotoxin but not tetanus neurotoxin a food poison?, *Toxicon*, 33: 1541–1547.

Snider, D.P. (1995) The mucosal adjuvant activities of ADP-ribosylating bacterial enterotoxins, *CRC Crit. Rev. Immunol.*, 15: 317–348.

Song, L., Hobaugh, M.R., Shustak, C., Cheley, S., Bayley, H., and Gouaux, J.E. (1996) Structure of staphylococcal alpha-hemolysin, a heptameric transmembrane pore, *Science* 274: 1859–1866.

Songer, J.G. (1997) Bacterial phospholipases and their role in virulence, *Trends Microbiol.*, 5: 156–161.

Spencer, R.C. (2002) Bacillus anthracis, *J. Clin. Pathol.*, 56: 182–187.

Stevens, D.L. (1997) Superantigens: their role in infectious diseases, *Immunol. Invest.*, 26: 275–281.

Suh, J.-K., Hovde, C.J., and Robertus, J.D. (1998) Shiga toxin attacks bacterial ribosomes as effectively as eukaryotic ribosomes, *Biochemistry*, 37: 9394–9398.

Taga S., Mangeney, M., Tursz, T., and Wiels, J. (1995) Differential regulation of glycosphingolipid biosynthesis in phenotypically distinct Burkitt's lymphoma cell lines, *Int. J. Cancer*, 61: 261–267.

Tesh, V.L. and O'Brien, A.D. (1991) The pathogenic mechanisms of Shiga toxin and the Shiga-like toxins, *Mol. Microbiol.*, 5: 1817–1822.

Tomita, T. and Kamio, Y. (1997) Molecular biology of the pore-forming cytolysins from *Staphylococcus aureus*, alpha- and gamma-hemolysins and leukocidin, *Biosci. Biotechnol. Biochem.*, 61: 565–572.

Trachtman, H. and Christen, E. (1999) Pathogenesis, treatment, and therapeutic trials in hemolytic uremic syndrome, *Curr. Opin. Pediatr.*, 11: 162–168.

Turton, K., Chaddock, J.A., and Acharya, K.R. (2002) Botulinum and tetanus neurotoxins: structure, function, and therapeutic utility, *Trends Biochem. Sci.*, 27: 552–558.

Ulevitch, R. and Tobias, P. (1995) Receptor-dependent mechanisms of cell stimulation by bacterial endotoxin, *Ann. Rev. Immunol.*, 13: 437–457.

Vane, J., Änggard, E., and Botting, R. (1990) Regulatory functions of the vascular endothelium, *N. Engl. J. Med.*, 323: 27–36.

Wheeler, A.H. (1997) Therapeutic uses of botulinum toxin, *Am. Family Phys.*, 55: 541–548.

Winkler, U., Barth, S., Schnell, R., Diehl, V., and Engert, A. (1997) The emerging role of immunotoxins in leukemia and lymphoma, *Ann. Oncol.*, 8: 139–146.

Zoja, C., Morigi, M., and Remuzzi, G. (2001) The role of the endothelium in hemolytic uremic syndrome, *J. Nephrol.*, 14: S58–S62.

8 Pesticide Toxicology: Mode of Action, Residues in Fruit Crops, and Risk Assessment

Noubar John Bostanian

CONTENTS

Abstract   A review of the published residue levels of 71 different pesticides in 23 different crops from 19 different countries shows us that, with few exceptions, residue levels are within internationally acceptable levels. The review also shows us that no generalizations can be made regarding the effects of processing fresh fruit on pesticide residues. In some instances, residues increase; in others, residues decrease or remain at the same level as in unprocessed fruit. The first step in the risk-assessment process for pesticide residues is establishment of the theoretical maximum residue contribution (TMRC). This parameter overestimates the risk because it assumes that the entire crop is treated with the pesticide at the highest allowable dose. The next step in the process is to compare human exposure estimates with the results from animal toxicological studies so as to provide an estimate of the risks associated with exposure. Two key assumptions are made. The first assumes that the effects from chemical exposures in experimental animals can be used to predict adverse effects in humans. The second assumes that effects observed at high doses can be mathematically related to effects at low doses. When animal studies indicate that the chemical is a non-carcinogen, then uncertainty factors are introduced to compensate for the uncertainties and assumptions made. On the other hand, when animal studies indicate that the chemical is a potential carcinogen, then conservative mathematical models of tumor formation along with statistical corrections are used. Currently, the public is very much concerned about pesticide residues in foods, particularly vegetables and fruit. This concern is mostly based on misinterpretation and misunderstanding of the risk-assessment process.

INTRODUCTION

In addition to their beneficial effects, pesticides may cause both human illness and human death. Another effect, the human body burden of pesticide residues as a result of long-term exposure, may or may not be associated with illnesses. This uncertainty reflects, in part, questions about the contribution of pesticide residues to chronic disease. This chapter, without claiming completeness, examines pesticide residues in fruit crops. Because of constraints of space and the vastness of the scientific information made available in recent years, this chapter attempts to provide the reader with a basic understanding of the subject. It also hopes to generate enough interest in the reader to pursue additional in-depth information currently available in the literature. To retain some form of brevity in a subject that can easily become overwhelming, an overview of residues in different fruit crops published in international journals is reported in table format at the end of the chapter. Pesticides are discussed by their mode of action, and detailed toxicological information is provided for a selected few examples. Finally, the highlights of risk assessment and interpretation of residue data are presented.

INSECTICIDES

NERVE INHIBITORS

Interference with Synaptic Transmission

This group includes inhibitors of the enzyme acetylcholinesterase, agonists and antagonists of gamma-aminobutyric acid (GABA) inhibitors, and mimics of acetylcholine.

Inhibition of acetylcholinesterase: organophosphates and carbamate insecticides

Organophosphates cover a very large group of toxic compounds containing phosphorus. It is possible to have wide variations in structure around the active phosphorus center so as to give it a wide range of physical and biological properties, chemical stability, and selectivity. Organophosphates can be synthesized with the exact lipophilic–hydrophilic balance required for movement within plants (e.g., dimethoate and demeton methyl). Organophosphates have a very specific mode of action, and their biological activity is easily destroyed by the simplest chemical or biochemical modification. They are also relatively unstable in biological systems. Most organophosphates can be considered as esters of alcohols with a phosphorus acid or as anhydrides of a phosphorus acid with some other acid.

Organophosphates are divided into three groups of derivatives: aliphatic, phenyl, and heterocyclic. Unless specified to the contrary, the figures within parentheses following the common name of a pesticide in this review are the acute oral LD_{50} for the rat (Meister, 2002).

Aliphatic derivatives include disulfoton (2–12 mg kg^{-1}), mevinphos (3–12 mg kg^{-1}), oxydemeton-methyl (50 mg kg^{-1}), dimethoate (235 mg kg^{-1}), acephate (1447 mg kg⁻¹), methamidophos (21 mg kg⁻¹), and malathion (5500 mg kg⁻¹). The aliphatic organophosphate insecticides are the simplest in structure and have a wide range of toxicities. Among the examples mentioned here, the first five compounds are systemic, and only methamidophos and malathion are not systemic.

Examples of phenyl derivatives used in horticulture include ethyl parathion (2 mg kg⁻¹), methyl parathion (6 mg kg⁻¹), isofenphos (20 mg kg⁻¹), sulprofos (200 mg kg⁻¹), fenitrothion (250 mg kg⁻¹), fenthion (250 mg kg⁻¹), and profenofos (358 mg kg⁻¹). The phenyl derivatives are generally more stable than the aliphatic derivatives. Again, a wide range in mammalian toxicity exists.

Heterocyclic derivatives are still more complex in structure, and one or more of the carbon atoms in the ring are displaced by oxygen, nitrogen, or sulfur. Their residual toxicity is longer than the previously mentioned derivatives, and they often have several metabolites, which makes their analysis complicated. Azinphos-methyl (4 mg kg⁻¹), methidathion (44 mg kg⁻¹), chlorpyrifos (96–270 mg kg⁻¹), phosalone (120 mg kg⁻¹), phosmet (113–160 mg kg⁻¹) (Kidd and James, 1991), and diazinon (1250 mg kg⁻¹) are examples of this group.

An essential characteristic of organophosphates is the electrophilic phosphorus atom, which is brought about partly by the polarization of the P=O bond and partly by the electron-withdrawal properties of the other groups in the molecule. The two most important non-enzymatic features of organophosphates are hydrolysis and isomerization. The speed of hydrolysis is directly related to the concentration of the alkaline medium, because it is the OH⁻ ion that causes the hydrolysis, and it attacks the partially charged positive P moiety. The conversion of P=S to P=O is isomerization, and it is termed *desulfuration*. The process is hastened by heat and light and usually increases the rate of hydrolysis and anticholinesterase activity. All compounds containing =S are *latent inhibitors* and become *direct inhibitors* after desulfuration. Most organophosphates would be poor toxicants if they were not activated in living systems. The reactions are desulfuration, hydroxylation (found in phosphoramidates), thioether oxidation, and cyclization, all four of which take place in vertebrates and insects. In vertebrates, the catalytic systems are the microsomes of the liver.

Carbamates are another very important class of anticholinesterases in wide use at the present time. They are derivatives of carbamic acid (HOOCNH₂). Today, three groups describe most of the carbamates: (1) aryl *N*-methylcarbamate, represented by carbaryl; (2) dimethylcarbamyl ester of a heterocyclic hydroxy compound, represented by pirimicarb; and (3) *N*-methylcarbamyl ester of an oxime, also called oxime carbamates and represented by methomyl and thiodicarb. As a class they tend to be rapid acting and degrade fairly rapidly.

When compared to organophosphates, a greater percentage of carbamates are systemically active in plants, indicating that they have high water solubility. Carbamates are *direct inhibitors*, and bioactivation is not an important phenomenon. The following carbamates used on horticultural crops are presented in descending order of toxicity: Aldicarb (1 mg kg⁻¹), oxamyl (5.4 mg kg⁻¹), carbofuran (8 mg kg⁻¹), methomyl (17–24 mg kg⁻¹), methiocarb (20 mg kg⁻¹), propoxur (50 mg kg⁻¹), and carbaryl (246–286 mg kg⁻¹).

Modes of action

Organophosphates and carbamates exert their toxic action by inhibition of cholinesterase. Following the transmission of an impulse and the release of acetylcholine, a
return to normality is brought about by hydrolysis of the acetylcholine by acetylcholinesterase to acetic acid and choline. In the presence of organophosphates and
carbamates, this hydrolysis is inhibited, resulting in the accumulation of acetylcholine. The inhibition can be explained in three steps. The first step is the formation
of a complex (E–OH.AZ). The second step involves phosphorylation, acetylation,
or carbamylation (E–OA) of the enzyme at the esteratic site of the amino acid serine
in the acetylcholinesterase, while the remainder of the molecule is attached to the
anionic site. The third and last step involves hydrolysis (i.e., dephosphorylation,
deacetylation, or decarbamylation) to yield the original enzyme (E–OH). These
events are summarized by Corbett et al. (1984) in the following scheme:

$$E\text{–}OH + AZ \underset{k_{-1}}{\overset{k_1}{\rightleftharpoons}} E\text{–}OH \cdot AZ \xrightarrow{k_2} E\text{–}OA \xrightarrow{k_3} E\text{–}OH + AOH$$

$$\searrow ZH$$

where A is a symbol for the acetyl group, the dialkyl phosphoryl group, or the
methylcarbamyl group, and Z represents the leaving group (i.e., choline in uninhibited
acetylcholine, *p*-nitrophenol in paraoxon, or 1-naphthol in carbaryl). Kinetic studies
have shown the following: With organophosphates, k_2 is moderately fast and k_3 is
extremely slow; therefore, E–OA accumulates. The values of k_1, k_{-1}, and k_2 are such
that under normal conditions no E–OH.AZ is ever present. With carbamates, k_2 is
much slower and k_3 is even slower, so that under normal conditions low concentrations
of the complex E–OH.AZ and high concentrations of the carbamylated enzyme E–OA
(half life of a few minutes) have been noted. With organophosphates, then, the
inhibitory reaction is reversed very slowly; with carbamates, decarbamylation takes
place within a few hours, and the inhibition is readily reversible. The build-up of
acetylcholine in the synapses of insects and of vertebrates leads to repetitive firing
followed by blockage of nerve transmission. In mammals, this inhibition takes place
at the neuromuscular junction, and death is brought about by paralysis of the inter-
costal muscles, which results in asphyxiation. Organophosphates may also cause
neuropathology of the visual system or effects on cognitive functions (i.e., learning
and memory). Among the organophosphates used in fruit, induced delayed toxicity
has also been reported with chlorpyrifos, methamidophos, and methyl parathion.

Profile of vertebrate toxicology for phosmet

Phosmet is a moderately toxic organophosphate when administered orally; the acute
oral LD_{50} ranges from 113 to 160 mg kg^{-1} in rats. It is slightly toxic dermally; the
dermal LD_{50} ranges from 3160 to over 4640 mg in rabbits (Kidd and James, 1991;
Smith, 1993). It is a mild eye and skin irritant, and it also has a low toxicity via
inhalation. The LC_{50} for 1 hour of inhalation is 2.76 mg L^{-1}. Symptoms of acute
intoxication occur within 30 minutes of exposure and are typical of inhibition of

cholinesterase by organophosphate pesticides. The following have been noted: numbness, tingling sensations, incoordination, headache, dizziness, tremor, nausea, abdominal cramps, sweating, blurred vision, difficulty in breathing or respiratory depression, and slow heartbeat. High doses may result in unconsciousness, incontinence, and convulsions or death. Rats fed 22.5 to 300 mg kg^{-1} of phosmet for 16 weeks suffered mortality and exhibited a number of toxic effects (USEPA, 1983–1985). A dose of 1 mg kg^{-1} day^{-1} in a 2-year feeding study with rats produced no observable chronic effects (USEPA, 1983–1985; PHS, 1995). In dermal toxicity studies, rabbits suffered high mortality when phosmet at 300 to 600 mg kg^{-1} day^{-1} was applied to their skin for 5 days a week for 3 weeks. At 50 mg kg^{-1} day^{-1}, significant depression of brain cholinesterase was observed. No reproductive effects were noted in a three-generation study with rats fed phosmet at 2.0 mg kg^{-1} day^{-1} during gestation days of the first generation and a dose of 4 mg kg^{-1} day^{-1} for the second and third generations (PHS, 1995). Female rabbits given phosmet both dermally and orally (10 to 60 mg kg^{-1} day^{-1}) for 3 weeks prior to mating and for 189 consecutive days of gestation showed no undesirable effects on reproduction (USFDA, 1986). Teratogenic effects were negative with rats fed 10 to 30 mg kg^{-1} day^{-1} on days 6 through 15 of gestation; however, doses of 30 mg kg^{-1} day^{-1} administered to rats between days 9 and 13 of gestation resulted in a dose-dependent hydrocephaly (USFDA, 1986). Mutagenic tests with bacteria were negative; however, workers producing phosmet showed some changes in their chromosomes (PHS, 1995). Rats fed diets with phosmet at a rate of 1 to 20 mg kg^{-1} day^{-1} for 2 years showed no increase in cancer; however, a 2-year mouse study showed that phosmet acted as a liver and stomach tumor promoter (USEPA, 1983–1985). Studies with rats also indicated that phosmet crosses the placenta (PHS, 1995).

Profile of vertebrate toxicology for methomyl

Methomyl is a highly toxic carbamate when administered orally; the oral LD$_{50}$ in rats ranges from 17 to 24 mg kg^{-1} (Kidd and James, 1991), while the LD$_{50}$ is 10 mg kg^{-1} in mice. Symptoms of exposure are typical of cholinesterase inhibitors (Baron, 1991). The LC$_{50}$ via inhalation in male rats is 0.3 mg L^{-1}. Inhalation of dust or aerosol may cause irritation and lung and eye problems, with symptoms of chest tightness, blurred vision, tearing, wheezing, and headache following exposure. Other symptoms of cholinesterase inhibition may appear after a few minutes to several hours of exposure (USEPA, 1987a). It is slightly toxic via the dermal route. The dermal LD$_{50}$ in rabbits is 5880 mg kg^{-1} (Kidd and James, 1991). It is not readily absorbed through the skin. When absorbed, symptoms similar to those induced by ingestion or inhalation will be experienced (Baron, 1991). It is a mild eye irritant. In rabbits, pain, shortsightedness, blurring of distant vision, tearing, and other eye disturbances may occur within a few minutes of eye contact with methomyl. Chronic toxicity studies have shown that prolonged or repeated exposure to methomyl may cause symptoms similar to exposure to acute doses (Baron, 1991). Repeated exposure to small doses may cause an unsuspected inhibition of cholinesterase, resulting in flu-like symptoms, such as weakness, lack of appetite, and muscle aches. Cholinesterase inhibition may persist for 2 to 6 weeks. This condition is reversible if exposure is discontinued. In a 24-month study with rats fed doses of 2.5, 5, or 20 mg kg^{-1} day^{-1}, effects were only observed at the highest dose tested. At the high dose, red blood cell counts and hemoglobin levels were significantly reduced in female rats (USEPA, 1987a). It is unlikely that chronic effects would be seen in humans unless exposures were unexpectedly high, as in chronic misuse. A three-generation feeding study with rats at doses of 2.5 or 5 mg kg^{-1} caused no effect. No fetal toxicity was noted in the progeny of pregnant rats fed 33.9 mg kg^{-1} day^{-1} on days 6 to 21 of gestation (Baron, 1991). No teratogenic effects were demonstrated in rats administered 34 mg kg^{-1} day^{-1} (Baron, 1991). Mutagenicity studies have demonstrated that methomyl is not mutagenic (USEPA, 1987a; NLM, 1995). Similarly carcinogenic studies were negative in rats and dogs fed high doses of methomyl for 2 years. In humans and other vertebrates, methomyl is quickly absorbed through the skin, lungs, and gastrointestinal tract and is metabolized in the liver. Metabolites are excreted via respiration and urine (Kidd and James, 1991).

Agonists and antagonists of GABA inhibitors

γ-Aminobutyric acid is an inhibitory transmitter that suppresses nerve activities in both the post- and presynaptic terminals. It induces these inhibitory actions by its ability to increase chloride ion permeability of the nerve membrane. Control of chloride channels has been described as a revolving tap mechanism. GABA activation (agonists) rotates the tap to the open position, whereas receptor antagonists oppose this activation. Avermectins are a mixture of macrocyclic lactone antibiotics isolated from *Streptomyces avermitilis*. They bind with high affinity to sites in the head and muscle neuronal membranes of various arthropod species (Deng and Casida, 1992), thereby acting as agonists for GABA-gated chloride channels (Albrecht and Sherman, 1987). In susceptible organisms, avermectins may cause loss of motor function and paralysis. Abamectin is very toxic to phytophagous mites, whereas it is less toxic to some lepidopteran and homopteran species (Lasota and Dybas, 1991). It decomposes rapidly but provides residual toxicity through its translaminar activity.

Profile of vertebrate toxicology for abamectin

Abamectin is a mixture of avermectins containing more than 80% avermectin B_1a and less than 20% avermectin B_1b. These two components have similar biological and toxicological properties (Lankas and Gordon, 1989). At high doses, it may penetrate the mammalian blood–brain barrier, causing symptoms of central nervous system (CNS) depression such as incoordination, tremors, lethargy, excitation, and pupil dilation. Very high doses have caused death from respiratory failure (Ray, 1991). Abamectin is not readily absorbed through the skin. Tests with monkeys indicate that less than 1% of dermally applied abamectin is absorbed into the bloodstream (Lankas and Gordon, 1989). The acute oral LD_{50} in rats is 10 mg kg^{-1} and in mice it is 14 to 80 mg kg^{-1}. The acute dermal LD_{50} for technical abamectin in rabbits is over 333 mg kg^{-1}. It is very irritating to eyes and leads to corneal opacity, conjunctivitis, and iritis. Skin irritation is minimal, and dermal sensitization results are negative. A 14-week subchronic oral toxicity study with rats yielded negative results. A 1-year chronic toxicity study with dogs fed 0.5 and 1 mg kg^{-1} day^{-1} showed pupil dilation, weight loss, lethargy, tremors, and recumbency (Lankas and Gordon, 1989). Rats fed 0.40 mg kg^{-1} day^{-1} of abamectin had fewer pups, which had decreased weights; decreased lactation; and increased stillbirths (USEPA, 1990b). Mutagenicity studies showed that abamectin was not mutagenic in microbial systems nor was it carcinogenic in rats fed dietary doses of 0.75, 1.5, or 2.0 mg kg^{-1} day^{-1} for 24 months or in mice fed 2, 4, or 8 mg kg^{-1} day^{-1} for 22 months.

Mimics of acetylcholine: nicotine and the neonicotinoids

Once released into the synapse, the neurotransmitter acetylcholine cannot exert any effect unless it binds to the receptors in the postsynaptic membrane. Nicotine, its sulfate, and neonicotinoids, also known as chloronicotinyl insecticides (synthetic compounds), mimic the transmitter acetylcholine in mammals. At low concentrations, they bind to the transmitter's receptor at the neuromuscular junction and at the ganglion. The molecular geometry of these compounds resembles acetylcholine in dimension and distribution of electrical charges; hence, the receptor is unable to distinguish either of them, and the result is stimulation of voluntary muscles, ganglia, and glands followed by paralysis (Sone et al., 1994; Nauen, 1995). They do not inhibit or bind with cholinesterase. All of the neonicotinoids already on the market, along with those that will be available in the foreseeable future, are potent agonists on nicotinic acetylcholine receptors (nAChRs) (Nauen et al., 1999).

Profile of vertebrate toxicology for imidacloprid

Imidacloprid is a neonicotinoid with an oral LD$_{50}$ of 450 mg kg^{-1} for rats and 131 mg kg^{-1} for mice. The dermal LD$_{50}$ is over 5000 mg kg^{-1}. It is non-irritating to the eyes and skin of rabbits, and an aerosol formulation has a LC$_{50}$ of >69 mg m^{-3} for airborne imidacloprid and over 5323 mg m^{-3} for dust formulations (Kidd and James, 1991). The no-observed-adverse-effect level (NOAEL) is 100 ppm (5.7 mg kg^{-1} in male rats and 7.6 mg kg^{-1} for female rats) after feeding rats up to 1800 ppm for 2 years. At 300 ppm, thyroid lesions were noted in male rats, and reduced weight gain was observed in females. Thyroid lesions in females appeared at 900 ppm. In the dog, a 1-year feeding study resulted in a NOAEL of 1250 ppm. Undesirable effects included increased cholesterol levels in the blood and elevated P-450 in the liver (USEPA, 1995a). A three-generation reproduction study with rats fed up to 700 ppm of imidacloprid resulted in a NOAEL of 100 ppm, which was estimated based on decreased pup weight observed at the 250-ppm dose level. A developmental toxicity study in rats administered up to 100 ppm of imidacloprid by gavage on days 6 to 16 of gestation resulted in a NOAEL of 30 mg kg^{-1} day^{-1} (USEPA, 1995a). A similar study with rabbits given doses by gavage during days 6 to 19 of gestation resulted in a NOAEL of 24 mg kg^{-1} day^{-1} based on decreased body weight, and skeletal abnormalities were noted at 72 mg kg^{-1} day^{-1}. Imidacloprid may be weakly mutagenic, as changes in human lymphocytes and Chinese hamster ovary cells have been noted. It is considered to be of minimal cancer risk. Imidacloprid is quickly absorbed from the gastrointestinal tract; 70 to 80% is eliminated in the urine and the remainder in feces. The most important metabolic step is degradation of the active ingredient to 6-chloronicotinic acid, which acts on the nervous system; therefore, signs of intoxication would be similar to nicotine, and the symptoms would be fatigue, twitching, cramps, and muscle weakness, including those muscles necessary for breathing (Doull et al., 1991).

Interference with Axonic Transmission

Pyrethrins and pyrethroids

The pyrethrin and pyrethroid group includes compounds that interfere with normal functioning of the sodium channels in the axon. Pyrethrins are a mixture of insecticidal esters obtained by grinding the flowers of *Chrysanthemum cinerariaefolium*. The composition of pyrethrins is complex. Synthetic analogs of pyrethrins, known as pyrethroids, emerged from systematic research efforts begun in 1940 and the first photostable pyrethroid was synthesized in 1973 (Elliot et al., 1973). Currently, pyrethroids are recognized as the fourth major class of synthetic organic insecticides. Examples include permethrin (430–4000 mg kg^{-1}), fenvalerate (451 mg kg^{-1}), cypermethrin (250 mg kg^{-1}), deltamethrin (128.5 mg kg^{-1}), esfenvalerate (458 mg kg^{-1}), λ-cyhalothrin (56–79 mg kg^{-1}), fenpropathrin (70.6–164 mg kg^{-1}), fluvalinate (261–282 mg kg^{-1}), prallethrin (640 mg kg^{-1}), tralomethrin (1250 mg kg^{-1}), and tefluthrin (1531–3091 mg kg^{-1}).

Modes of action

The nervous system is the primary target of pyrethroids. In this respect, they differ from organophosphates and carbamates as they do not appear to react covalently with the target, but, similar to DDT, shape and lipophilic properties are central to chemical reactivity. Nerve preparations from squid (Lund and Narahashi, 1981) and frogs (Vijverberg et al., 1982) have suggested that pyrethroids delay the closing of a small percentage of the sodium channels, which open on depolarization; meanwhile, the majority of the channels behave normally. The delay of the closure of axonal sodium channels causes the membrane potential to remain above the threshold for a longer period. As a result, a number of spike potentials are triggered, a process known as repetitive spiking. These repeated action potentials lead to a greater release of transmitter and hence to postsynaptic hyperstimulation. The time required to close the modified channels depends on the pyrethroid in question (Vijverberg et al., 1982). It is particularly slow with α-cyano pyrethroids. Gray and Rickard (1982a,b) reported two distinct intoxication syndromes in mammals. One syndrome is characterized by whole body tremors and is produced by early pyrethroids and permethrin. The other syndrome is characterized by sinuous, writhing convulsions accompanied by profuse salivation and is produced by pyrethroids containing the α-cyano 3-phenoxybenzyl alcohol moiety (deltamethrin). Gammon et al. (1981) classified pyrethroids causing only tremors as type I and those causing convulsions with salivation as type II. Another interesting difference between these two types is the effect of temperature. The toxicity of type I pyrethroids is inversely related to temperature; in other words, they are more toxic when the temperature is lowered. In contrast, the toxicity of type II pyrethroids is directly related to temperature.

Metabolism

Pyrethroids possess two or three chiral centers, which result in four or eight optical and geometrical isomers that differ in toxicity and metabolism; therefore, to avoid misunderstanding, the pyrethroid structure should be described as specifically as possible. Because the nomenclature is complicated and beyond the scope of this review, the reader is referred to Elliott et al. (1974). Pyrethroid metabolism is dependent on the cleavage of the central ester bond by carboxylesterases found in large quantities in mammalian tissue (Casida and Ruzo, 1980; Chambers, 1980). It may also be catalyzed at several sites by oxidative mechanisms to produce primary and secondary metabolites of little or no neurotoxicity (Hutson, 1979). This second mechanism is more important in *cis*-isomers than *trans*-isomers. In mammals, pyrethroid toxicity is generally low because mammals readily hydrolyze the *trans*-isomers. The cleavage of ester bonds produces products that conjugate to form glycosides. Some of these glycosides may have very complex structures (Leahey, 1985).

User risks

The very low rates necessary for insecticidal action along with the generally low mammalian toxicity of pyrethroids when administered orally or by dermal routes decreases the probability of systemic poisoning during spraying or by consumption of contaminated foodstuffs. Poisoning by inhalation is also less likely to occur, as the droplets produced by sprayers may be too large to be inhaled. Nevertheless, pyrethroids are neurotoxins, and misuse or abuse can result in poisoning. Today, the major problem to workers exposed to pyrethroids is associated with local irritation of the face and upper respiratory tract. This is more pronounced with α-cyano-substituted compounds (Tucker and Flannigan, 1983). The irritation is initiated by direct contact with the pyrethroid as a solution, a fine powder (Le Quesne et al., 1980), or a dried residue on crops (Kolmodin-Hedman et al., 1982). The regions affected are the areas around the eyes, lips, mouth, cheeks, and nose. The symptoms have been described as episodes of hot and cold irritation with a prickling, tingling, or burning sensation. These symptoms, referred to as paresthesia by the medical profession, become more painful if the skin is in contact with water or if the person is perspiring. Kolmodin-Hedman et al. (1982) also reported lacrimation following exposure to deltamethrin or fenvalerate. Le Quesne et al. (1980) have concluded that these effects are due to direct action of the pyrethroids on sensory nerves in the face, as no abnormal neurological signs were noted elsewhere. Paresthesia causes considerable discomfort; however, it is unlikely to result in permanent damage. Actually, paresthesia is an excellent indicator of overexposure to the pyrethroid concerned.

Profile of vertebrate toxicology for esfenvalerate

Esfenvalerate is a moderately toxic compound via the oral route. The oral LD_{50} in the rat is 458 mg kg^{-1}. It is slightly toxic via the dermal route; the dermal LD_{50} in rabbits is 2500 mg kg^{-1}. It is almost non-toxic via inhalation; the LC_{50} is greater than 2.93 mg L^{-1} in rats (Ray, 1991; Kidd and James, 1991). Symptoms of acute poisoning are dizziness, burning, and itching. In rats, high doses produce muscle incoordination, tremors, convulsions, nerve damage, and weight loss. In humans, acute exposures may produce nausea, vomiting, headache, and temporary nervous system effects such as weakness and tremors. Esfenvalerate is a strong eye irritant that causes tears and blurred vision. Two-year feeding studies in rats at 12.5 mg kg^{-1} showed no effect in the blood and urine. A three-generation rat study at low doses increasing to 12.5 mg kg^{-1} day^{-1} had no effect on the fetus. At the higher dose, some maternal toxicity was noted in the second generation. When pregnant mice and rabbits were dosed with 2.5 mg kg^{-1} day^{-1} on days 6 to 15 of gestation, maternal toxicity was noted in both species. It seems that, during pregnancy, the females are more sensitive than the fetus. Teratogenic and mutagenic studies were negative. It is unlikely that esfenvalerate would pose a risk in humans. Similarly, extensive studies with rats over a wide range of doses of up to 7 mg kg^{-1} for 2 years produced no carcinogenic effects. It is rapidly metabolized in the rat and was almost completely eliminated within a few days.

METABOLIC INHIBITORS

Inhibitors of Mitochondrial Electron Transport

The production of energy from the oxidation of carbohydrates, fats, and proteins takes place in the mitochondria of a cell. Certain insecticides such as rotenone (132–1500 mg kg^{-1}) and pyridaben (820–1350 mg kg^{-1}) interfere with the normal function of coenzyme Q (a respiratory enzyme responsible for carrying electrons in some electron transport chains) and result in failure of the respiratory functions and eventual death of the cell.

Inhibition of Insect Development

Insect growth regulators (IGRs) alter the growth and development of insects. These compounds disrupt insect growth and development in three ways: as juvenile hormones, as precocenes, and as chitin synthesis inhibitors. The juvenile hormones (JHs) and their analogs (JHAs), including the molting hormone ecdysone, interfere with the development and emergence of insects as adults. The resultant insects have juvenile and adult characteristics, cannot feed or reproduce, and soon die. These compounds act as agonists. Methoprene (over 36,600 mg kg^{-1}) and fenoxycarb (16,800 mg kg^{-1}) are examples of JHAs. Mosquito larvae exposed to methoprene develop until the last larval stage, and then they die. It has no activity against pupae and adults. Similarly, fenoxycarb causes ovicidal effects, inhibits metamorphosis, and interferes with molting of early instars of several caterpillars in fruit crops.

Precocenes interfere with the normal functioning of the glands that produce the juvenile hormones. They act as antagonists by activating enzymes in the corpus allatum, which then begins to produce compounds cytotoxic to itself (Bowers, 1984). Chitin synthesis inhibitors inhibit the production of new exoskeletons when insects are molting. Diflubenzuron (over 4640 mg kg^{-1}), teflubenzuron (over 5000 mg kg^{-1}), and tebufenozide (over 5000 mg kg^{-1}) are examples of this group.

The molecular mode of action of these compounds is not fully established. A working hypothesis is that juvenile hormone enters a cell, combines with a cytoplasmic receptor protein, and is allowed into the nucleus, where it interferes with the pattern of messengers being transcribed from the DNA. In conjunction with other hormones, the juvenile phase of development is maintained and adult genes are not expressed.

The IGRs are effective in small doses and have no adverse effects on humans; however, they are non-specific and especially the chitin inhibitors may adversely affect non-target organisms, such as crustacea, that contain chitin in their exoskeletons. Nevertheless, there is some specificity among IGRs; thus, tebufenozide is very effective on most *Lepidoptera* species but ineffective on members of most other orders of insects. Finally, IGRs differ from other pesticides in that they are toxic to an entire population of insects rather than to individuals.

The following compounds in ascending order of rat toxicity are effective in minute amounts: methoprene (34,600 mg kg^{-1}), fenoxycarb (16,800 mg kg^{-1}), chlorfluazuron (>8500 mg kg^{-1}), hexafluron (>5000 mg kg^{-1}), teflubenzuron (>5000 mg kg^{-1}), flucycloxuron (>5000 mg kg^{-1}), novaluron (>5000 mg kg^{-1}), tebufenozide (>5000 mg kg^{-1}), diflubenzuron (4640 mg kg^{-1}), cyromazine (3387 mg kg^{-1}), and flufenoxuron (>3000 mg kg^{-1}). To date, none of these compounds has been shown to be toxic to humans.

Profile of vertebrate toxicity for tebufenozide

Acute toxicity studies with the technical material have shown the LD$_{50}$ as well as the dermal toxicity for male and female rats to be over 5 g kg^{-1}. The inhalation LD$_{50}$ in the rat is over 4.5 mg L^{-1}. Primary eye irritation studies in the rabbit show that it is not an irritant and does not sensitize skin. Several mutagenicity studies were all negative. Reproductive and developmental studies with Sprague–Dawley rats were all negative. The NOAEL was 1 g^{-1} day^{-1}. A 1-year dog feeding study established the lowest-observed-adverse-effect level (LOAEL) at 250 ppm (9 mg^{-1} kg^{-1} day^{-1}). The NOAEL for both sexes was 50 ppm (1.9 mg^{-1} kg^{-1} day). A 2-year carcinogenicity study showed no development of cancer at rates as high as 97 mg^{-1} kg^{-1} day^{-1} and 125 mg^{-1} kg^{-1} day^{-1} for males and females, respectively. Animal metabolic studies showed that the majority of the material was eliminated in the feces within 48 hours. A negligible amount (1 to 7%) was eliminated in the urine. In the feces, 96 to 99% of the material was the parent compound; the remaining were 11 metabolites. No parent compound was ever found in the urine. In the bile, 13 metabolites have been reported. The metabolism takes place primarily by oxidation of the benzylic carbons to alcohols, aldehydes, or acids.

FUNGICIDES

Fungicides may be classified according to their mode of action as preventative or curative, or both. Preventative fungicides prevent the establishment and development of a pathogen on the plant surface. By this property, preventive fungicides are insurance against an infection. Curative or eradicant fungicides, on the other hand, are systemic and will move to where an infection has occurred and prevent further development of the pathogen. The preventive fungicides commonly used in fruit production include dithiocarbamates, ethylenebisdithiocarbamates (EBDCs), phthalimides, benzothiazole, and dicarboximides, The curative fungicides include anilinopyrimidines, benzimidazoles, phosphonates, sterol inhibitors (pyrimidines and triazoles), and strobilurins. Often, systemic fungicides have preventive properties in addition to curative properties.

PREVENTIVE FUNGICIDES

Dithiocarbamates

Dithiocarbamates include broad-spectrum compounds that interfere with oxygen uptake and inhibition of sulfur-containing enzymes. They have multiple sites of action. Examples include thiram and ziram (1400 mg kg^{-1}).

Profile of vertebrate toxicology for thiram

Thiram is a dimethyl dithiocarbamate that is slightly toxic by ingestion and inhalation. It is moderately toxic by dermal absorption. The 4-hour inhalation LC$_{50}$ is over 500 mg L^{-1} in rats. The oral LD$_{50}$ in rats is 620 to, 1900 mg kg^{-1}, and in mice it is 1500 to 2000 mg kg^{-1}. The dermal LD$_{50}$ is over 1000 mg kg^{-1} in rats (Edwards et al., 1991; Kidd and James, 1991) and rabbits (NLM, 1995). Acute exposure in humans may cause headaches, dizziness, fatigue, nausea, diarrhea, and other gastrointestinal discomforts. It is irritating to the eyes, skin, and respiratory tract and is a skin sensitizer. Chronic toxicity studies have shown thiram to cause drowsiness, confusion, loss of sex drive, incoordination, and slurred speech in humans, in addition to the symptoms manifested by acute exposure. In rats, a dietary dose of 125 mg kg^{-1} day^{-1} was fatal to all the animals within 17 weeks of intoxication. Two-year feeding studies at 49 mg kg^{-1} day^{-1} produced weakness, muscle incoordination, and paralysis of the hind legs. Symptoms of muscle incoordination and paralysis have been shown to be associated with degeneration of nerves in the lower lumber and pelvic regions. In rabbits, at doses of about 10% of the oral LD$_{50}$, blood platelet and white blood cell counts were reduced, blood formation was suppressed, and blood coagulation slowed (Edwards et al., 1991). Reproductive studies have shown that oral doses of 1200 mg kg^{-1} day^{-1} given to mice on days 6 to 17 of pregnancy caused resorption of embryos and retarded fetal development. Edwards et al. (1991) also reported that dietary intake of 132 mg kg^{-1} day^{-1} for 13 weeks produced infertility in male mice, whereas doses of 96 mg kg^{-1} day^{-1} for 14 days delayed the estrous cycle in females. They have also shown that feeding mice 50 mg kg^{-1} day^{-1} from day 16 of pregnancy to 21 days after birth caused reduced growth and survival of pups. Pups that were transferred to untreated dams recovered, whereas pups transferred from untreated to treated dams showed signs of toxic effect. Teratogenic studies showed that mice fed thiram (1200 mg kg^{-1} day^{-1}) on days 6 to 17 of gestation produced progeny with cleft palate, wavy ribs, and curved long legs. Maternal doses of 125 mg kg^{-1} day^{-1} were teratogenic in hamsters, causing incomplete formation of the skull and spine, fused ribs, and abnormalities of the legs, heart, great vessels, and kidneys. These findings show that at high doses of thiram may cause teratogenic effects. Thiram was found to be mutagenic in some test organisms but not to others; hence, the evidence is inconclusive (Edwards et al., 1991). At the highest possible dose that could be administered to mice it was not carcinogenic. Rats fed 125 mg kg^{-1} day^{-1} for 2 years did not develop tumors. In humans, metabolism of thiram produces carbon disulfide, which is toxic to the liver. It is not an ethylenebisdithiocarbamate, and its metabolism does not generate ethylene thiourea, which is an oncogen (Edwards et al., 1991).

Ethylenebisdithiocarbamates (EBDCs)

Ethylenebisdithiocarbamates are broad-spectrum compounds that break down to cyanide, which reacts with thiol compounds in the cell and interferes with sulfhydryl groups. Examples include mancozeb, maneb (7990 mg kg^{-1}), metiram (6810 mg kg^{-1}), and zineb (5200 mg kg^{-1}).

Profile of vertebrate toxicology for mancozeb

Mancozeb is almost a non-toxic compound to mammals. The oral LD$_{50}$ for rats ranges from 5000 mg kg^{-1} to over 11,200 mg kg^{-1} (Edwards et al., 1991). The dermal toxicity is just as low, with LD$_{50}$ values exceeding 10,000 mg kg^{-1} in rats and greater than 5000 mg kg^{-1} in mice (NLM, 1995). It is a mild skin irritant and sensitizer and a mild to moderate eye irritant in rabbits. When inhaled, it is irritating to the skin and respiratory mucous membranes. Morgan (1982) states that symptoms of poisoning from EBDCs include itching, scratchy throat, sneezing, coughing, inflammation of the nose or throat, and bronchitis. In chronic toxicity studies, dogs fed 0.625, 2.5, and 25 mg kg^{-1} of mancozeb for 24 months showed impaired thyroid function at the highest and second highest doses and no effect at 0.625 mg kg^{-1}. A serious toxicological concern for chronic exposure is the presence of ethylenethiourea (ETU) as a contaminant, as well as a breakdown product of mancozeb and other EBDCs. In experimental animals, ETUs administered orally at appropriate doses for various time periods caused goiter, cancer, and birth defects (USEPA, 1987b). ETUs may also be produced when EBDCs are applied to stored produce and during cooking (Ripley et al., 1978). A three-generation rat reproductive study with 50 mg kg^{-1} day^{-1} of mancozeb in the diet reduced fertility but had no adverse effects on the embryo (EPA, 1987b; Edwards et al., 1991). When it was inhaled by pregnant rats, toxic symptoms were seen on the dams and pups at doses of 55 mg m^{-3}. No teratogenic effects were observed in a three-generation rat study with rats fed 50 mg kg^{-1} day^{-1} of mancozeb (Edwards et al., 1991).

In another study, the offspring of pregnant rats fed 5 mg kg^{-1} day^{-1} showed signs of delayed hardening of skull bones (USEPA, 1987b). When a very high dose of 1320 mg kg^{-1} was fed to rats on the 11th day of gestation, developmental abnormalities of the body wall, central nervous system, eye, ear, and musculosketal system were noted (NIOSH, 1995). New studies are required to resolve these conflicting results to establish the teratogenicity of mancozeb. Mutagenic studies with mancozeb are also inconclusive; in one study, it was mutagenic but it did not cause mutations in another. To date, no conclusive work has been carried out to measure the carcinogenic effects of mancozeb; nevertheless, it must be recognized that mancozeb contains ETU as an impurity, and ETU is a carcinogen at high doses (USEPA, 1987b, 1988). ETU is also the major metabolite resulting from the breakdown of mancozeb *in vivo* and *in vitro*.

The main target organ is the thyroid gland, which develops a goiter, probably caused by the ETU metabolite (USEPA, 1987b, 1988). Mancozeb is rapidly absorbed from the gastrointestinal tract into the body and almost completely excreted in 96 hours. ETU is the major metabolite, whereas carbon disulfide, which is also toxic, is the minor metabolite.

Phthalimides

Compounds of this group are broad spectrum with multiple sites of action. Phthalimides degrade to thiophosgene, which inhibits a number of fungal enzymes. Captan is an example.

Profile of vertebrate toxicology for captan

The acute oral LD_{50} of captan for rats ranges from 8400 to 15,000 mg kg^{-1}, indicating very low acute toxicity. The mouse LD_{50} is 7000 mg kg^{-1}. The inhalation LC_{50} (2-hour) in mice is 5.0 mg L^{-1} (NLM, 1995). Captan caused little or no skin sensitization in rabbits, while guinea pigs were moderately sensitive (NLM, 1995). Workers exposed to 6 mg m^{-3} of captan in the air experienced eye irritation, including burning, itching, and tearing. Skin irritation also occurred in a number of cases. Chronic toxicity studies showed that rats fed up to 750 mg kg^{-1} day^{-1} of the formulated material for 4 weeks had decreased food intake and body weights. No deaths occurred in pigs given as much as 420 to 4000 mg kg^{-1} day^{-1} in the diet for 12 to 25 weeks. Mice fed 50 mg kg^{-1} day^{-1} over three generations reproduced normally. Meanwhile, pregnant mice exposed by inhalation to high doses of captan for 4 hours a day during days 6 to 15 of gestation showed significant mortality or weight loss. These events were accompanied by fetal mortality. Teratogenicity studies with rats, rabbits, hamsters, and dogs were contradictory. Currently, the weight of evidence suggests that captan does not produce birth defects (USEPA, 1989). In some laboratory studies with isolated tissue cultures, captan was mutagenic; however, the weight of evidence indicates that captan is non-mutagenic (USEPA, 1989). Carcinogenicity studies show that high doses of captan caused cancer in female mice and in male rats. Tumors appeared in the gastrointestinal tract and to a lesser degree in the kidneys of test animals at doses of about 300 mg kg^{-1} day^{-1} (NLM, 1995) Most organ-specific toxic effects were noted in the kidneys of rats at and above 100 mg kg^{-1} day^{-1}. Studies in several animal species have shown that captan is rapidly absorbed from the gastrointestinal tract and is rapidly metabolized. Residues are excreted primarily in the urine. Rats fed with captan in their diets excreted, within 24 hours, 33% of the captan in their feces and 50% in their urine.

Dicarboximides

Compounds of this group are mainly preventive with some curative properties. The mode of action is not clear; nevertheless, they inhibit spore germination. Examples include iprodione and vinclozolin (>15,000 mg kg^{-1}).

Profile of vertebrate toxicology for iprodione

Iprodione is a slightly toxic compound by ingestion, with acute oral LD_{50} values of 3500 mg kg^{-1} in rats and 4000 mg kg^{-1} in mice (Kidd and James, 1991). Slight dermal toxicity was noted at doses of over 2500 mg kg^{-1} in the rat and at 1000 mg kg^{-1} in the rabbit (Kidd and James, 1991; NLM, 1995). Toxicity caused by inhalation was low, and the 4-hour inhalation LC_{50} is over 3.3 mg L^{-1} in the rat (NLM, 1995). Rats given dietary doses of approximately 60 mg kg^{-1} day^{-1} over 18 months in chronic toxicity studies suffered no ill effects (Kidd and James, 1991; NLM, 1995).

Dogs fed approximately 60 mg kg^{-1} day^{-1} over 18 months also showed no adverse effects (Kidd and James, 1991; NLM, 1995). In another study, beagle dogs fed dietary doses of about 2.3 mg kg^{-1} day^{-1} for 1 year showed liver and kidney weight increases. At doses starting at about 1.5 mg kg^{-1} day^{-1}, the dogs had decreased prostrate weights and showed damage to the hemoglobin molecules in the red blood cells. Females also had slight decreases in uterus weights. No effects were noted below a dose of 0.5 mg kg^{-1} day^{-1} (USEPA, 1990a). In reproductive studies, female rats fed iprodione over three successive generations showed no effects on reproduction at doses at and below 1.25 mg kg^{-1} day^{-1} (USEPA, 1990a). Reductions in fertility and fecundity were not observed at doses of 5 mg kg^{-1} day^{-1} (USEPA, 1990a). Based on these data, iprodione is not likely to cause reproductive effects. Similarly, no teratogenic effects were noted in the offspring of pregnant rats receiving dietary doses of about 5.4 mg kg^{-1} day^{-1} (USEPA, 1990a); however, at about 120 mg kg^{-1} day^{-1}, it caused unspecified developmental toxicity in rats (USEPA, 1990a). Rabbits did not develop any dose-related toxicity at or below 2.7 mg kg^{-1} day^{-1} of iprodione but did develop toxicity at 6 mg kg^{-1} day^{-1} (USEPA, 1990a). It appears that iprodione is not likely to cause teratogenic effects at expected exposure levels. Current evidence on the carcinogenicity of iprodione is inconclusive. A 2-year feeding study with rats showed no increases in tumor formation or neoplastic foci at dietary doses of about 2.5 mg kg^{-1} day^{-1} (USEPA, 1990a). An 18-month study in mice revealed cancer-related effects at doses up to approximately 22 mg kg^{-1} day^{-1} (USEPA, 1990a). Target organs identified in animal studies include the reproductive system (prostate gland and uterus), liver, and kidneys.

CURATIVE FUNGICIDES

Benzimidazoles

Benzimidazoles are broad-spectrum compounds with a single site of action. They prevent polymerization of β-tubulin and thus inhibit mitosis. Benomyl is an example.

Profile of vertebrate toxicology for benomyl

The acute toxicity of benomyl to mammals is so low that it has been impossible to administer doses large enough to firmly establish an LD$_{50}$. Using the formulated material, the LD$_{50}$ is over 10,000 mg kg^{-1} in rats and over 3400 mg kg^{-1} in rabbits. Skin irritation may be noted among workers exposed to benomyl. Skin reactions have also been seen in rats and guinea pigs. Benomyl is readily absorbed into the body by inhaling the dust, but there are no reports of toxic effects to humans by this route of exposure. The inhalation LC$_{50}$ in rats is over 2 mg L^{-1} (NLM, 1995). Chronic toxicity studies with rats fed 150 mg kg^{-1} day^{-1} for 2 years showed no toxic effects (Edwards et al., 1991). Dogs fed benomyl in their diets for 3 months had no major toxic effects but did show proof of altered liver function at the highest dose (150 mg kg^{-1}). The damage progressed, and after 2 years developed into cirrhosis of the liver. A three-generation reproductive study with rats fed 150 mg kg^{-1} day^{-1} showed no reproductive or lactational differences. In another study with rats, the testes were the most affected sites at relatively low doses of about 15 mg kg^{-1} day^{-1}. Male rats had decreased sperm counts, decreased testicular weight, and lower fertility rates. The animals recovered from these effects 70 days after dietary intake of the pesticide was discontinued (Edwards et al., 1991). Reproductive effects in humans are unlikely at expected exposure levels. Teratogenic studies showed that very high doses of benomyl could cause birth defects in test animals (Cummings et al., 1992). Rats fed 150 mg kg^{-1} day^{-1} in the diet for three generations showed no birth defects. No teratogenicity was observed in another study of rats given 300 mg kg^{-1} day^{-1} on days 6 to 15 of gestation (Cummings et al., 1992). At higher doses, some birth defects were noted, but they were accompanied by toxicity to the fetus (Cummings et al., 1992). These data suggest that benomyl is not likely to cause teratogenic effects under normal circumstances. Mutagenicity studies have produced conflicting negative and positive results; hence, no conclusions about the mutagenicity of benomyl can be drawn (Edwards et al., 1991). Carcinogenicity studies have shown tumors in the livers of both male and female mice in lifetime studies at benomyl doses of 40 to 400 mg kg^{-1} day^{-1}. In a 2-year dietary study, benomyl fed to albino rats at a rate of 2500 mg kg^{-1} day^{-1} produced no significant adverse effects (Kidd and James, 1991). Based on these data, it is not possible to determine the carcinogenicity of benomyl (NRC, 1987). The target organs identified in animal studies are the liver and testes. In mammals, benomyl is rapidly broken down to carbendazim and then to other compounds, such as 5-hydroxy-2-benzimidazole carbamate (5-HBC), and then eliminated. In a rat study, the urine contained about 40 to 70% of the dose, and the feces 20 to 45%. No residues were found in muscle or fat.

Sterol Inhibitors

This group is comprised of five different chemical families. In fruit culture, the most important chemical families are the pyrimidines, for which fenarimol (2500 mg kg^{-1}) is an example, and the triazoles, for which myclobutanil (1600–2290 mg kg^{-1}) is an example. They are broad spectrum with a single site of action. They arrest sterol biosynthesis via inhibition of 14-demethylase. They are often referred to as demethylation inhibitors (DMIs) or inhibitors of ergosterol biosynthesis (EBIs).

Strobilurins

This group is comprised of the β-methoxyacrylates; azoxystrobin (>5000 mg kg^{-1}), trifloxystrobin (>4000 mg kg^{-1}), and kresoxim-methyl (7500 mg kg^{-1}) are examples. These compounds are broad spectrum with a single mode of action. They disrupt the electron transport in cytochrome bc$_1$ complex. These compounds have preventive and limited curative properties.

RISK ASSESSMENT

The preceding pages provided us with a bird's-eye view of the mode of action of several groups of pesticides and summaries of vertebrate toxicology for a selected few compounds. Table 8.1 (see end of chapter) is self explanatory; most of the analyses are from planned residue trials, while a few of the examples are from market basket analyses. The effects of processing on pesticide residues on certain fruits such as prunes are also reported and discussed. Residue levels from 65 studies are summarized in Table 8.1. These studies were carried out in 19 different countries on 23 different fruit crops. The residues of 71 different pesticides are reported. Approximately 42% of the data is from Europe, 32% from North America, 18% from Asia, 3% from the South Pacific, 3% from South America, and 2% from Africa.

An issue that has been much discussed and hotly debated is whether or not these residues pose a health hazard. In order to provide an answer, we must first determine how much of a particular fruit is consumed by the population (different age groups and different ethnic groups within multicultural societies) in question, then we must relate human exposure to results of animal toxicology studies to predict human risk. Fruit consumption can be determined relatively easily from statistical records, but to carry out the second step we must rely on assumptions, many of which may not be amenable to scientific verification. For example, in the absence of epidemiological data linking pesticide residues to human cancer, the only source of information for assessing potential risk to humans has been the use of results from high-dose rodent studies. Use of these data requires two sorts of extrapolation: a quantitative extrapolation from high to low dose and a qualitative extrapolation from rodents to humans. In each extrapolation, assumptions are made that may not be verifiable scientifically; therefore, considerable uncertainty is introduced, and to overcome this uncertainty "uncertainty factors" are introduced. The first uncertainty factor assumes that humans are tenfold more sensitive than test animals (interspecies differences). The second uncertainty factor, again tenfold, accounts for differences among human populations (intraspecies differences).

In the United States, a third uncertainty factor, anywhere between 1 and 10, is now included in the calculations since passage of the Food Quality Protection Act (FQPA) in 1996. Following residue studies carried out by the manufacturer, the maximum residue level (MRL), also known as the tolerance level, that provides a satisfactory control of a pest on a particular crop is established. Thus, uses of a pesticide on various crops may have different MRL values. The MRL multiplied by the mean food consumption estimate for a particular crop yields the theoretical maximum residue contribution (TMRC). The TMRC is expressed in milligrams of pesticide per kilogram of body weight per day. In calculating the TMRC, it is assumed that the pesticide has been applied to the entire crop at the highest allowable level in the field. This parameter is an overestimate and may be readjusted following residue data obtained from market basket samples and other residue monitoring programs initiated by regulatory agencies.

Theoretical maximum residue contribution values from all crops treated with the pesticide are added together and compared with the acute reference dose (RfD). To obtain the RfD, the first step is to establish the no-observed-effect level (NOEL). The NOEL is established from acute and chronic studies with appropriate animals. Because all measured effects may not be adverse health effects, a no-observed-adverse-effect level (NOAEL) may also be established and used in the analyses. The NOEL is then usually divided by 100, and the quotient is considered the RfD. The RfD is a level at or below which daily aggregate exposure over a lifetime will not pose adverse risks to human health. If an exposure is below the RfD, the risks associated with exposure to the chemical are considered insignificant. For additional details, the reader is referred to Chaisson et al. (1989), Winter (1992), and Goodman (1994).

If toxicological studies with laboratory animals indicate the potential for carcinogenicity, then all relevant toxicological data, including short- and long-term mutagenicity studies, as well as structure–activity relationships, are evaluated. This is because, for non-carcinogenic effects, it is assumed that a toxicity threshold (NOAEL) exists, and exposure at levels below this threshold should not cause any effects. For carcinogens, such a threshold does not exist, and current practices of carcinogen risk assessment use one theoretical cancer case per million members of a population as a threshold. Risks below this level are considered "insignificant." To carry out the risk assessment, strains of animals sensitive to carcinogens are exposed in a variety of ways to the pesticide at various doses, sacrificed, and evaluated by pathologists. Evaluations are to some extent subjective, and all tumors (benign and malignant) are usually counted in the determination of a chemical as a carcinogen. Benign tumors are not differentiated from malignant ones, and they are all counted together. Chemicals are labeled oncogens based on this tumor count (NRC, 1987). The highest dose used (maximum tolerataed dose, or MTD) is usually high enough to cause some form of general toxicity. Because experimental data do not exist to relate ultra-low doses of suspected carcinogens to increases in cancer incidence, several mathematical models are used that make assumptions about the manner in which cancer may develop in the human body. The linearized, multistage mathematical model is currently the most popular. It simulates the development of cancer as a result of multiple events in the body and some approximate threshold dose for the carcinogen. Statistical corrections are carried out, and the cancer risk is expressed on the basis of the upper 95% confidence interval of the slope of the dose–response curve. Doing so adds an additional element of conservatism to the risks. The slope of the curve is calculated and expressed as the cancer potency factor, or Q^* (mg kg^{-1} day^{-1}). Multiplication of the exposure estimate (mg kg^{-1} day^{-1}) by Q^* yields the carcinogenic or, more accurately, the oncogenic risk, expressed as the probability of excess cancer occurrence (NRC, 1987). For details, the reader is referred to Peto et al. (1984), Sawyer et al. (1984), Bernstein et al. (1985), USEPA (1986, 1995b, 1996), Ames and Gold (1990), Krewski et al. (1990), Gold and Stone (1993), and Goodman (1994).

The brief review provided here demonstrates that estimated cancer risks include uncertainties and are therefore poor indicators of actual human cancer incidence. It is generally agreed that the uncertainty corrections built into the risk assessment may greatly exaggerate the risks. This is most relevant when exposure estimates are based on the tTMRC. Nevertheless, the exercise is important in identifying and prioritizing risks and developing risk mitigation strategies.

CONCLUSION

As mentioned in the introduction, agricultural uses of pesticides result in residues in food. This is a complex topic involving scientific, legal, and public policies that are often misunderstood. Pesticide use in agriculture often attracts the attention of environmental and consumer advocacy groups that argue against what they claim to be the unrestricted use of pesticides in agriculture which are harmful to both the environment and consumers. In recent years, this concern has particularly focused on fruit and vegetables because consumption of these commodities is being encouraged for nutritional reasons. This negative attitude toward pesticide residues and to a certain extent toward regulatory agencies has partly been brought about by journalistic sensationalism based on inappropriate interpretations of valid scientific data and partly by the inability of regulatory agencies to explain satisfactorily complex toxicological interpretations to advocacy groups. Thus, Kilham (1991) reported that, "The National Academy of Sciences estimates approximately 1.4 million cancer deaths due to the consumption of pesticide residues in foods." Along the same lines, Mott and Snyder (1987) claimed that an additional one million cancer cases would occur in the U.S. population because of cancer-causing pesticides in the food. On the other hand, epidemiologists tell us that the major preventable causes of cancer are tobacco, dietary imbalances, chronic inflammation from chronic infections, and hormones. It is hoped that this review elucidates the low level of residues in different fruit crops and at the same time shows us the limitations of the risk-assessment process, including the uncertainties of the process, so that interpretations of residue data can be carried out objectively and in a responsible manner.

ACKNOWLEDGMENTS

I wish to thank Dr. J.M. Hardman for commenting on an earlier draft of this manuscript and Mr. Gaétan Racette, M.Sc., for proofreading and formatting the text.

REFERENCES

Ahmed, M.T. and Ismail, M.M.S. (1995) Residues of methomyl in strawberries, tomatoes and cucumbers, *Pest. Sci.*, 44:, 197–199.

Albrecht, C.P. and Sherman, M. (1987) Lethal and sublethal effect of avermectin B1 on three fruit fly species (Diptera: Tephritidae), *J. Econ. Entomol.*, 80: 344–347.

Ames, B.N. and Gold, L.S. (1990) Chemical carcinogenesis: too many rodent carcinogens, *Proc. Natl. Acad. Sci. USA*, 87: 7772–7776.

Archer, T.E., Stokes, J.D., and Bringhurst, R.S. (1977) Fate of carbofuran and its metabolites on strawberries in the environment, *J. Agric. Food Chem.*, 25: 536–541.

Awasthi, M.D. (1988) Persistence of synthetic pyrethroid residues on mango fruits, *Acta Hort.*, 231: 612–615.

Barba, A., Camara, M.A., Garcia, S.N., Sanchez-Fresneda, C., Lopez de Hierro, N., and Acebes, A. (1991) Disappearance of bromopropylate residues in artichokes, strawberries and beans, *J. Environ. Sci. Health*, B26: 323–332.

Barba, A., Garcia, S.N., Camara, M.A., Molina, R., and Buendia, J. (1995) Disappearance of carbosulfan residues in peaches, *Pest. Sci.*, 43: 317–320.

Barbé, L. (1983) Étude de résidus de quelques pesticides sur les raisins, *Arboriculture Fruitière*, 348: 46–47.

Baron, R.L. (1991) Carbamate insecticides, in *Handbook of Pesticide Toxicology*, Hayes, W.J., Jr. and Laws, E.R., Jr., Eds., Academic Press, San Diego, CA, pp. 1125–1189.

Bélanger, A., Bostanian, N.J., and Rivard I. (1985) Apple maggot (Diptera: Trypetidae) control with insecticides and their residues in and on apples, *J. Econ. Entomol.*, 78: 463–466.

Berstein, L., Gold, L.S., Ames, B.N., Pike, M.C., and Hoel, D.G. (1985) Some tautologous aspects of the comparison of carcinogenic potency in rats and mice, *Fund. Appl. Toxicol.*, 5: 79–86.

Bicchi, C., D'Amato, A., and Balbo, C. (1997) Multiresidue method for quantitive gas chromatographic determination of pesticide residues in sweet cherries, *J. AOAC Int.*, 80: 1281–1286.

Bowers W. S. (1984) insect-plant interactions: endocrine defences, *Ciba Found. Symp.*, 119–137.

Cabras, P., Garau, V.L., Melis, M., Pirisi, F.M., Spanedda, L., Cabitza, F., and Cubeddu, M. (1995a) Persistence of some organophosphorus insecticides in orange fruit, *Ital. J. Food Sci.*, 7: 291–298.

Cabras, P., Melis, M., Cabitza, F., Cubeddu, M., and Spanedda, L. (1995b) Persistence of pirimicarb in peaches and nectarines, *J. Agric. Food Chem.*, 43: 2279–2282.

Cabras, P., Angioni, A., Garau, V.L, Minelli, E.V., Cabitza, F., and Cubeddu, M. (1997) Residues of some pesticides in fresh and dried apricots, *J. Agric. Food Chem.*, 45: 3221–3222.

Cabras, P., Angioni, A., Garau, V.L., Melis, M., Pirisi, F.M., Cabitza, F., and Cubeddu, M. (1998a) Pesticide residues on field-sprayed apricots and in apricots drying processes, *J. Agric. Food Chem.*, 46: 2306–2308.

Cabras, P., Angioni, A., Garau, V.L., Melis, M., Pirisi, F.M., Cabitza, F., and Pala, M. (1998b) Pesticide residues in raisin processing, *J. Agric. Food Chem.*, 46: 2309–2311.

Cabras, P., Angioni., A., Garau, V.L., Minelli, E.V., Cabitza, F., and Cubbedu, M. (1998c) Pesticide residues in plums from fields treatment to the drying process, *Ital. J. Food Sci.*, 10: 81–85.

Cabras, P., Angioni, A., Garau, V.L., Pirisi, F.M., Brandolini, V., Cabitza, F., and Cubeddu, M. (1998d) Pesticide residues in prune processing, *J. Agric. Food Chem.*, 46: 3772–3774.

Casida, J.E. and Ruzo, L.O. (1980) Metabolic chemistry of pyrethroid insecticides, *Pest. Sci.*, 11: 257–269.

Chaisson, C.F., Petersen, B.J., Eickhoff, J.C., and Slesinki, R.S. (1989) *Pesticides in Our Foods: Facts, Issues, Debates, Perceptions*, Technical Assessment Systems, Washington, D.C.

Chambers, J. (1980) An introduction to the metabolism of pyrethroids, *Residues Rev.*, 73: 101–124.

Chrisholm, D. and Specht, H.B. (1978) Residues and control of aphids on strawberries with banded surface applications of disulfoton, *J. Econ. Entomol.*, 71: 469–472.

Corbett, J.R., Wright, K., and Baillie, A.C. (1984) *The Biochemical Mode of Action of Pesticides*, 2nd ed., Academic Press, London.

Cummings, A.M., Ebron, McCoy, M.T., Rogers, J.M., Barbee, B.D., and Harris, S.T. (1992) Developmental effects of methyl benzimidazole carbamate following exposure during early pregnancy, *Fund. Appl. Toxicol.*, 18: 288–293.

Deng, Y. and Casida, J.E. (1992) Housefly head GABA-gated chloride channel: toxicological relevant binding site for avermectins coupled to site for ethynyl-bicylo orthobenzoate, *Pest. Biochem. Physiol.*, 43: 116–122.

Doull, J., Klassen, C.D., and Amdur, M.O., Eds. (1991) *Cassarett and Doull's Toxicology: The Basic Science of Poisons*, 4th ed., Pergamon Press, Elmsford, NY.

Dumas, T. and Bond, E.J. (1975) Bromide residues in apples fumigated with ethylene dibromide, *J. Agric. Food Chem.*, 23: 95–98.

Edwards, I.R., Ferry, D.G., and Temple, W.A. (1991) Fungicides and related compounds, in *Handbook of Pesticide Toxicology*, Hayes, W.J., Jr., and Laws, E.R., Jr., Eds., Academic Press, San Diego, CA, pp. 1409–1470.

Elkins, E.R., Farrow, R.P., and Kim, E.S. (1972) The effect of heat processing and storage on pesticide residues in spinach and apricots, *J. Agric. Food Chem.*, 20: 286–291.

Elliot, M., Farham, A.W., James, N.F., Needham, P.H., Pulman, D.A., and Stevenson, J.H. (1973) A photostable pyrethroid, *Nature*, 246: 169–170.

Elliot, M., Farnham, A.W., James, N.F., Needham, P.H., and Pulman, D.A. (1974) Synthetic insecticide with a new order of activity, *Nature*, 248: 710–711.

FAO. (1981) *1980 Evaluations: FAO: Pesticide Residues in Food*, Food and Agriculture Organization of the United Nations, Rome, pp. 254–256.

Ferreira, J.R., Falcão, M.M., and Tainha, A. (1987) Residues of dimethoate and omethoate in peaches and apples following repeated applications of dimethoate, *J. Agric. Food Chem.*, 35: 506–508.

Gammon, D.W., Brown, M.A., and Casida, J.E. (1981) Two classes of pyrethroid action in the cockroach, *Pest. Biochem. Physiol.*, 15: 181–191.

Gold, L.S. and Stone, T.H. (1993) Predictions of carcinogenicity from 2 vs. 4 sex-species groups in the carcinogenic potency database, *J. Toxicol. Environ. Health*, 39: 147–161.

Gonzalez, R.H. and Curkovic, S.T. (1994) Manejo de plagas y degracion de residuos de pesticidas en kiwi, *Revista Fruticola*, 15: 5–20.

Goodman, J.I. (1994) A rational approach to risk assessment requires the use of biological information: an analysis of the national toxicology program (NTP), final report of the advisory review by the NTP board of scientific couselors, *Regul. Toxicol. Pharmacol.*, 19: 51–59.

Goodwin, S., Ahmad, N., and Newell, G. (1985) Dimethoate spray residues in strawberries, *Pest. Sci.*, 16: 143–146.

Gray, A.J. and Rickard, J. (1982a) The toxicokinetics of deltamethrin in rats after intravenous administration of a toxic dose, *Pest. Biochem. Physiol.*, 18: 205–215.

Gray, A.J. and Rickard, J. (1982b) Toxicity of pyrethroids to cats after direct injection into central nervous systems, *Neurotoxicology*, 3: 25–35.

Greenberg, R.S. (1981) Determination of fenvalerate, a synthetic pyrethroid, in grapes, peppers, apples, and cottonseeds by gas–liquid chromatography, *J. Agric. Food Chem.*, 29: 856–860.

Guindani, C.M.A. and Ungaro, M.T.S. (1988) Avaliacão de resíduos de dicifol e endosulfan em morangos comercializados, *Biologico*, 54: 53–54.

Hameed, S.F. and Allen, J.G. (1976) Toxicity and persistence of some organophosphorus insecticides and permethrin on apple fruits for the control of colding moth, *Laspeyresia pomonella* (L.), *J. Hort. Sci.*, 51: 105–115.

Hutson, D.H. (1979) The metabolic fate of synthetic pyrethroid insecticides in mammals, in *Progress in Drug Metabolism*, Vol. 3, Bridges, J.W. and Chassaud, L.F., Eds., Wiley, Chichester, pp. 215–252.

Iwata, Y., Westlake, W.E., Barkley, J.H., Carman, G.E., and Gunther, F.A. (1977) Behavior of phenthoate (Cidial) deposits and residues on and in grapefruits, lemons and lemon leaves, oranges and orange leaves, and in the soil beneath orange trees, *J. Agric. Food Chem.*, 25: 362–368.

Iwata, Y., Düsch, M.E., Carman, G.E., and Gunther, F.A. (1979) Worker environment research: residues from carbaryl, chlorobenzilate, dimethoate, and trichlorfon applied to citrus trees, *J. Agric. Food Chem.*, 27: 1141–1145.

Iwata, Y., MacConnell, J.G., Flor, J.E., Putter, I., and Dinoff, T.M. (1985a) Residues of avermectin B_1a on and in citrus fruits and foliage, *J. Agric. Food Chem.*, 33: 467–471.

Iwata, Y., Walker, G.P., O'Neal, J.R., and Barkley, J.H. (1985b) Residues of acephate, amitraz, chlorpyrifos and formetanate hydrochloride on and in fruits after low-volume applications to orange trees, *Pest. Sci.*, 16: 172–178.

Johnson, G.D., Geronimo, J., and Hughes, D.L. (1997) Diphenylamine residues in apples (*Malus domestica* Borkh.), cider, and pomace following commercial controlled atmosphere storage, *J. Agric. Food Chem.*, 45: 976–979.

Kidd, H. and James, D.R., Eds. (1991) *The Agrochemicals Handbook*, 3rd ed., Royal Society of Chemistry Information Services, Cambridge, U.K.

Kilham, C.S. (1991) *The Bread and Circus Whole Food Bible*, Addison-Wesley, Reading, MA.

King, J.R. and Benschoter, C.A. (1991) Comparative methyl bromide residues in Florida citrus: a basis for proposing quarantine treatments against the caribbean fruit fly, *J. Agric. Food Chem.*, 39: 1307–1309.

King, J.R., Benschoter, C.A., and Burditt, A.K., Jr. (1981) Residues of methyl bromide in fumigated grapefruit determined by a rapid, headspace assay, *J. Agric. Food Chem.*, 29: 1003–1005.

Kolmodin-Hedman, B., Swensson, A., and Akevblom, M. (1982) Occupational exposure to some synthetic pyrethroids (permethrin and fenvalerate), *Arch. Toxicol.*, 50: 27–33.

Königer, M. and Wallnöfer, P.R. (1993) Untersuchungen über das Verhalten von Thiabendazol bei Bananen, *Deutshe Lebensmittel-Rundschau*, 89: 384–385.

Krewski, F., Szyszkowicz, M., and Rosenkranz, H. (1990) Quantitative factors in chemical carcinogenesis: variations in carcinogenic potency, *Regul. Toxicol. Pharmacol.*, 12: 13–29.

Lankas, G.R. and Gordon, L.R. (1989) Toxicology, in *Ivermectin and Abamectin*, Campbell, W.C., Ed., Springer-Verlag, New York.

Lasota, J.A. and Dybas, R.A. (1991) Avermectin, a novel class of compounds: implications for use in arthropod pest control, *Annu. Rev. Entomol.*, 36: 96–117.

Le Quesne, P.M., Maxwell, I.C., and Butterworth, S.T.G. (1980) Transient facial sensory symptoms following exposure to synthetic pyrethroids: a clinical and electrophysiological assessment, *Neurotoxicology*, 2: 1–11.

Leahey, J.P. (1985) Metabolism and environmental degradation, in *The Pyrethroid Insecticides*, Leahey J.P., Ed., Taylor & Francis, London, pp. 263–342.

Lentza-Rizos, Ch. (1995) Residues of iprodione in fresh and canned peaches after pre- and postharvest treatment, *J. Agric. Food Chem.*, 43: 1357–1360.

Lentza-Rizos, Ch. and Tsioumplekou, M. (2001) Residues of aldicarb in oranges: a unit-to-unit variability study, *Food Add. Contam.*, 18: 886–897.

Liapis, K.S., Miliadis, G.E., and Aplada-Sarlis, P. (1995) Dicofol residues on field sprayed apricots and in apricot juice, *Bull. Environ. Contam. Toxicol.*, 54: 579–583.

Lund, A.E. and Narahashi, T. (1981) Kinetics of sodium channel modification by the insecticide tetramethrin, in squid axon membranes, *J. Pharmacol. Exper. Therap.*, 219: 464–473.

Maynard, M.S., Ku, C.C., and Jacob, T.A. (1989) Fate of avermectin B_1a on citrus fruits. 2. Distribution and magnitude of the avermectin B_1a and ^{14}C residue on fruits from a picked fruit study, *J. Agric. Food Chem.*, 37: 184–189.

Mazzali, G., Reggiani, C., Boccelli, R., and Capri, E. (1993) Les résidus de pesticides dans les poires traitées avec la lutte intégrée, *A.N.P.P.–B.C.P.C., Second Int. Symp. on Pesticides, Applications, and Techniques*, Association Nationale de protection des plantes, Strasbourg, Sept. 22–23, 1993, pp. 437–443.

Meister, R.T. (2002) *Farm Chemicals Handbook*, Global Guide to Crop Protection Resources, Willoughby, OH.

Mestres, R. and Mestres, G. (1992) Deltamethrin: uses and environmental safety, *Rev. Environ. Contam. Toxicol.*, 124: 1–18.

Miliadis, G.E., Tsiropoulos, N.G., and Aplada-Sarlis, P.G. (1999) High-performance liquid chromatographic determination of benzoylurea insecticide residues in grapes and wine using liquid and solid-phase extraction, *J. Chromatogr. A,* 835: 113–120.

Minelli, E.V., Angioni, A., Cabras, P., Garau, V.L., Melis, M., Pirisi, F.M., Cabitza, F., and Cubeddu, M. (1996) Persistence of some pesticides in peach fruit, *Ital. J. Food Sci.,* 8: 57–62.

Morgan, D.P. (1982) *Recognition and Management of Pesticide Poisonings,* 3rd ed., Environmental Protection Agency, Washington, D.C.

Mott, L. and Snyder, K. (1987) *Pesticide Alert: A Guide to Pesticides in Fruits and Vegetables,* Sierra Club, San Franscico, CA.

Nath, A., Patyal, S.K., and Sharma, I.D. (1997) Persistence and bioefficacy of endosulfan and chlorpyrifos on apple, *Pest. Res. J.,* 9: 92–96.

Nauen, R. (1995) Behaviour modifying effects of low systemic concentrations of imidacloprid on *Myzus persicae* with special reference to an antifeeding response, *Pest. Sci.,* 44: 145–153.

Nauen, R., Ebbinghaus, U., and Tietjen, K. (1999) Ligands of the nicotinic acetylcholine receptor as insecticides, *Pest. Sci.,* 55: 608–610.

Nazer, I.K. (1986) Analysis for quinalphos residues on and in lemon fruits, *J. Agric. Entomol.,* 3: 304–309.

NIOSH. (1995) *Registry of Toxic Effects of Chemical Substances,* National Institute for Occupational Safety and Health, Cincinnati, OH.

NLM. (1995) *Hazardous Substances Data Bank,* U.S. National Library of Medicine, Bethesda, MD.

NRC. (1987) *Regulating Pesticides in Food: The Delaney Paradox,* National Academy Press, Washington, D.C..

Papadopoulou-Mourkidou, E., Kotopoulou, A., and Stylianidis, D. (1989) Field dissipation of the pyrethroid insecticide/acaricide biphenthrin on the foliage of peach trees, in the peel and pulp of peaches, and in tomatoes, *Ann. Appl. Biol.,* 115: 405–416.

Peto, R., Pike, M.C., Bernstein, L., Gold, L.S., and Ames, B.N. (1984) The TD_{50}: a proposed general convention for the numerical description of the carcinogenic potency of chemicals in chronic-exposure animal experiments, *Environ. Health Persp.,* 58: 1–8.

PHS. (1995) *Hazardous Substance Data Bank,* Public Health Service, Washington, D.C.

Powell, D.M., Maitlen, J.C., and Mondor, W.T. (1978) Spring migrant green peach aphid: control on peach and apricot with systemic insecticides and resultant residues, *J. Econ. Entomol.,* 71: 192–194.

Ray, D.E. (1991) Pesticides derived from plants and other organisms, in *Handbook of Pesticide Toxicology,* Hayes, W.J., Jr., and Laws, E.R., Jr., Eds., Academic Press, San Diego, CA, pp. 585–636.

Ripley, B.D., Cox, D.F., Wiebe, J., and Frank, R. (1978) Residues of dikar and ethylenethiourea in treated grapes and commercial grape products, *J. Agric. Food Chem.,* 26: 134–136.

Ryan, J.J., Pilon, J.C., and Leduc, R. (1982) Composite sampling in the determination of pyrethrins in fruit samples, *J. AOAC Int.,* 65: 904–908.

Sarode, S.V., Lalitha, P., and Krishnamurthy, P.N. (1981) Residues of fenthion in/on muskmelon, *J. Entomol. Res.,* 5: 179–181.

Sawyer, C., Peto, R., Bernstein, L., and Pike., M.C. (1984) Calculation of carcinogenic potency from long-term carcinogenesis experiments, *Biometrics,* 40: 27–40.

Scrano, L., Faretra, F., Cariddi, C., Antonacci, E., and Bufo, S.A. (1991) Evaluation of dicarboximide residues in cold-stored grapes exposed to field and post-harvest treatments, *Pest. Sci.,* 31: 37–44.

Sharma, S.K. and Bharat, N.K. (1994) Persistence of carbendazim on apple fruit and leaves, *Plant Dis. Res.*, 9: 204–206.

Sharma, S.K., Singh, I., Singh, B., and Singh, G. (1992) Estimation of cabofuran residues in peach (*Prunus persica* Bastch.) fruit, *J. Insect Sci.*, 5: 105.

Sharma, I.D., Nath, A., and Patyal, S.K. (1996) Estimation of *N*-dodecylaguanidine acetate (dodine) residues in apple (*Malus domestica*), *Pest. Res. J.*, 8: 191–194.

Smith, G.J. (1993) *Toxicology and Pesticide Use in Relation to Wildlife: Organophosphorus and Carbamate Compounds*, C.K. Smoley, Boca Raton, FL, pp. 5–7.

Sone S., Nagata, K., Tsuboi, S., and Shono, T. (1994) Toxic symptoms and neural effect of a new class of insecticide, imidacloprid, on the American cockroach, *Periplaneta americana* (L.), *Pest. Sci.*, 19: 69–72.

Stein, E.R. and Wolfenbarger, D.A. (1989) Methyl bromide residues in fumigated mangos, *J. Agric. Food Chem.*, 37: 1507–1509.

Sundaram, K.M.S, Boyonoski, N., Wing, R.W., and Cadogan, B.L. (1987) Simultaneous determination of fenitrothion and aminocarb in blueberry foliage and fruits: application to the analysis of residues in field samples, *J. Environ. Sci. Health*, B22: 565–578.

Suwanketnikom, R. and Sasiprapa, W. (1991) Degradation and residues of dimefuron in pineapple, *Kasetsart J. (Nat. Sci.)*, 25: 100–106.

Szeto, S.Y., Wan, M.T., Price, P., and Roland, J. (1990) Distribution and persistence of diazinion in a cranberry bog, *J. Agric. Food Chem.*, 38: 281–285.

Thakur, V.S. and Gupta, G.K. (1992) Persistence of dodine residue on apple (*Malus domestica*) fruits, *Indian J. Agric. Sci.*, 62: 566–569.

Tsiropoulos, N.G., Aplada-Sarlis, P.G., and Miliadis, G.E. (1999) Evaluation of teflubenzuron residue levels in grapes exposed to field treatments and in the must and wine produced from them, *J. Agric. Food Chem.*, 47: 4583–4586.

Tucker, S.B. and Flannigan, S.A. (1983) Cutaneous effects from occupational exposure to fenvalerate, *Arch. Toxicol.*, 54: 195–202.

USEPA. (1983–1985) *Chemical Information Fact Sheet*, Technical Sheet 766C, U.S. Environmental Protection Agency, Washington, D.C.

USEPA. (1986) Guidelines for carcinogen risk assessment, *Fed. Reg.*, 51: 33992–34003.

USEPA. (1987a) *Health Advisory Summary: Methomyl*, Office of Drinking Water, U.S. Environmental Protection Agency, Washington, D.C.

USEPA. (1987b) *Mancozeb*, Pesticide Fact Sheet 125, Office of Pesticides and Toxic Substances, U.S. Environmental Protection Agency, Washington, D.C.

USEPA. (1988) *Guidance for the Registration of Pesticide Products Containing Maneb as the Active Ingredient*, U.S. Environmental Protection Agency, Washington, D.C., pp. 4–11.

USEPA. (1989) Captan — intent to cancel registrations: conclusion of special reviews, *Fed. Reg.*, 54: 8116–8150.

USEPA. (1990a) Final rule: pesticide tolerance for iprodione, *Fed. Reg.*, 55: 2834–2835.

USEPA. (1990b) *Avermectin B1*, Pesticide Fact Sheet 89.2, Office of Pesticides and Toxic Substances, U.S. Environmental Protection Agency, Washington, D.C.

USEPA. (1995a) Imidacloprid: pesticide tolerances, *Fed. Reg.*, 60: 34943–34945.

USEPA. (1995b) *List of Chemicals Evaluated for Carcinogenic Potential*, Office of Pesticides Programs, Health Effects Division, U.S. Environmental Protection Agency, Washington, D.C.

USEPA. (1996) Proposed guidelines for carcinogen risk assessment, *Fed. Reg.*, 61: 17960–18011.

USFDA. (1986) *The FDA Surveillance Index*, National Technical Information Service, U.S. Food and Drug Administration, Springfield, VA, pp. 5–92.

Vijverberg, H.P.M., Van der Zalm, J.M., and Van der Bercken, J. (1982) Similar mode of action of pyrethroids and DDT on sodium channel gating in myelinated nerves, *Nature*, 295: 601–603.

Winter, C. (1992) Pesticide tolerances and their relevance as safety standards, *Regul. Toxicol. Pharmacol.*, 15: 137–150.

Woodham, D.W., Hatchett, J.C., and Bond, C.A. (1974) Comparison of dimethoate and dimethoxon residues in citrus leaves and grapefruit following foliar treatment with dimethoate wettable powder with and without surfactant, *J. Agric. Food Chem.*, 22: 239–242.

Yoshida, S., Kusuno, S., and Imaida, M. (1988) Distribution of pesticide residues in melon, *J. Agric. Chem. Soc. Jpn.*, 62: 35–37.

TABLE 8.1
A Summary of Pesticide Residue Levels in Different Fruit Crops

Country/ Year	Pesticide	Dose (Active Ingredient)	No. of Treatments	Interval to Last Treatment[a]	Residues (ppm, unless specified otherwise)/Comments			Refs.
Apples								
Canada 1975	Ethylene dibromide	8–24 m L^{-1}	1	13	<0.1 when held at 13°C			Dumas and Bond (1975)
				28	<0.1 when held at 4°C			
Canada 1985					**Whole Apple**	**Pulp**	**Peel**	Bélanger et al. (1985)
	Permethrin	200 g ha^{-1}	3	35	0.121	0.019	2.140	
	Cypermethrin	50 g ha^{-1}	3	35	0.193	0.100	1.940	
	Fenvalerate	70 g ha^{-1}	3	35	0.121	0.050	1.445	
	Azinphos-methyl	1100 g ha^{-1}	3	35	0.070	0.035	0.960	
India 1992	Dodine	0.98 kg ha^{-1}	1	15		0.62		Thakur and Gupta (1992)
		1.95 kg ha^{-1}	1	15		1.07		
		2.93 kg ha^{-1}	1	15		1.32		
India 1994	Carbendazim	0.05%	1	35		0.73		Sharma and Bharat (1994)
		to run-off	2	35		0.75		
			3	35		0.87		
			4	35		0.89		
			All	45	Below detectable level			
India 1996	Dodine	1.95 kg ha^{-1}	2	15	**Site I**	**Site II[b]**		Sharma et al. (1996)
		3.90 kg ha^{-1}	2	15	0.11	0.58		
					0.17	0.95		

TABLE 8.1 (cont.)
A Summary of Pesticide Residue Levels in Different Fruit Crops

Country/Year	Pesticide	Dose (Active Ingredient)	No. of Treatments	Interval to Last Treatment[a]	Residues (ppm, unless specified otherwise)/Comments	Refs.
Apples (cont.)						
India 1997	Endosulfan	0.05%	2	10		Nath et al. (1997)
		0.1%	2	10		
					Endosulfan 35 WP: Site I ND, Site II 0.386; Endosulfan 50 WP: Site I 0.182, Site II 0.399	
					Endosulfan 35 WP: Site I 0.137, Site II 0.424; Endosulfan 50 WP: Site I 0.166, Site II 0.535	
					The 50 WP is more persistent than the 35 WP.	
	Chlorpyrifos	0.02%	2	10		
		0.04%	2	10		
					Chlorpyrifos WP: Site I ND, Site II ND; Chlorpyrifos EC: Site I 0.147	
					Chlorpyrifos WP: Site I ND, Site II ND; Chlorpyrifos EC: Site I 0.632	
					The EC formulation is more persistent than the WP.	
Israel 1981	Fenvalerate	450 g ha^{-1}	1	30	0.45	Greenberg (1981)
					A 41% decrease from the residue level was recorded just after application.	
Portugal 1987	Dimethoate	50 g hl^{-1}	7	14		Ferreira et al. (1987)
			5	14		
					Dimethoate 1.50; Omethoate 0.14	
					Dimethoate 0.86; Omethoate 0.09	

	Pesticide	Treatment	No.	Interval	Whole Apple / Unprocessed Fruit	Wet Pommace / Processed Product / Fresh Fruit	Dried Pommace / Juice	Cider / Loss / Juice	Reference
United Kingdom 1976	Fenitrothion	0.05% to run-off	2	63 and 84				0.01	Hameed and Allen (1976)
	Methidathion			63 and 84				0.01	
	Phosalone			63 and 84				0.71	
	Phosmet			63 and 84				0.02	
	Tetrachlorvinphos			63 and 84				0.06	
	Triazophos			63 and 84				1.28	
	Permethrin			40				0.57	
United States 1997	Diphenyl amine	Red Delicious: 2000 ppm	1	9 months	3.18	3.30	1.90	0.039	Johnson et al. (1997)
		Granny Smith: 2200 ppm	1	—	1.01	6.03	2.95	0.083	
Apricots									
France 1992	Deltamethrin	Market basket survey	—	—	0.03	<0.01	<0.01	>66%	Mestres and Mestres (1992)
Greece 1995	Dicofol	30.8 g 100 L^{-1}	1	14		0.1	0.05		Liapis et al. (1995)
		38.5 g 100 L^{-1}	1	14		0.17	0.08		
		30.8 g 100 L^{-1}	1	32		0.05	ND		
		38.5 g 100 L^{-1}	1	32		0.09	ND		

(For United States 1997: "Red Delicious" values in the Whole Apple row = 3.18; "Granny Smith" values = 1.01.)

TABLE 8.1 (cont.)
A Summary of Pesticide Residue Levels in Different Fruit Crops

Country/Year	Pesticide	Dose (Active Ingredient)	No. of Treatments	Interval to Last Treatment[a]	Residues (ppm, unless specified otherwise)/Comments			Refs.

Apricots (cont.)

Italy 1997

					Fresh Fruit	Oven-Drying Rehydration		Cabras et al. (1997)
	Dimethoate	216.6 g ha⁻¹	1	38	0.12	0.09		
	Omethoate[c]	–	—	38	0.05	0.08		
	Fenitrothion	16 g ha⁻¹	1	38	0.03	<0.01		
	Ziram	217 g ha⁻¹	1	38	0.12	0.22		

Oven-drying caused a fruit concentration of 5.3. Omethoate and ziram residues doubled while the residues of other pesticides remained at fresh-fruit levels.

Italy 1998

					Fresh Fruit	Sunlight-Drying Rehydration	Oven-Drying Rehydration	Cabras et al. (1998a)
	Phosalone	225.8 g ha⁻¹	1	21	0.48	0.64	1.43	
	Iprodione	375 g ha⁻¹	1	21	1.09	0.29	1.25	
	Diazinon	90.25 g ha⁻¹	1	21	<0.01	<0.01	<0.01	
	Procymidone	375 g ha⁻¹	1	21	0.65	0.24	0.35	
	Bitertanol	75 g ha⁻¹	1	21	0.50	0.27	0.52	

Sun drying caused a fruit concentration factor of 5.6; however residues decreased by 50% except phosalone. Oven drying caused a fruit concentration factor of 5.6 to 6.5. Residue values were almost the same as fresh fruit, except for phosalone, which increased by threefold.

Elkins et al. (1972)

United States 1972

		Initial Level	Heat Processed	Stored 1 Year at Room Temperature	Stored 1 Year at 37.8°C
Captan	1	88.5	2.7	0.88	0
Endosulfan	1	1.79	1.60	1.40	0.27
Diazinon	1	0.45	0	0	0
Azinphos-methyl	1	1.00	0.39	0	0
Malathion	1	7.63	5.20	1.22	0
Methyl parathion	1	0.85	0.39	0	0
Zineb	1	6.7	5.36	3.89	3.48
Ziram	1	5.0	3.00	0.60	0.30
Maneb	1	9.8	5.88	4.61	4.51
Carbaryl	1	11.4	10.03	9.58	9.46

Storage at elevated temperatures resulted in substantial decreases in endosulfan residues. Thermal processing degraded captan, and storage at ambient temperature resulted in further losses. Storage at elevated temperatures for 1 year resulted in complete degradation of residues.

The organophosphate insecticides, diazinon, azinphos-methyl, malathion, and methyl parathion, were all degraded at different rates by the heat processing. Subsequent storage at ambient temperature further destroyed the remaining residues.

The carbamate pesticides appeared to be more resistant to heat degradation then the organophosphate insecticides. Ziram was the only fungicide evaluated that decreased to very low levels when stored at elevated temperatures following heat treatment. Carbaryl appears to be relatively stable in acid-type products such as apricots.

TABLE 8.1 (cont.)
A Summary of Pesticide Residue Levels in Different Fruit Crops

Country/Year	Pesticide	Dose (Active Ingredient)	No. of Treatments	Interval to Last Treatment[a]	Residues (ppm, unless specified otherwise)/Comments			Refs.
Bananas								
Germany 1993	Thiabendazole	Market basket survey	—	—	0.7 µg g^{-1} in the whole fruit and 0.1 µg g^{-1} in the edible portion. Contamination of the edible portion by the peel during peeling was found to be low. Washing the fruit prior to peeling eliminates the contamination.			Königer and Wallnöfer (1993)
Blueberries								
Canada 1987	Fenitrothion	210 g ha^{-1}	2	15	0.03			Sundaram et al. (1987)
	Aminocarb	70 g ha^{-1}	2	15	0.02			
Cherries			Unprocessed Fruit	Processed Product	Juice			
France 1992	Deltamethrin	Market basket survey	—	—	<0.01	<0.01	<0.01	Mestres and Mestres (1992)

Italy 1997	Acephate	Market basket survey	—	1 out 4 samples had 0.03-ppm residues.	Bicchi et al. (1997)
	Diazinon		—	All samples showed no residues.	
	Dimethoate		—	All samples showed no residues.	
	Fenitrothion		—	1 out of 4 samples had 0.01-ppm residues.	
	Malathion		—	1 out of 4 samples had 0.04-ppm residues	
	Pirimicarb		—	1 out of 4 samples had 0.05-ppm residues.	
	Trichlorfon		—	All samples showed no residues.	
	Bromopropylate		—	1 out of 4 samples had 0.07-ppm residues.	
	Dicofol		—	1 out of 4 samples had 0.06-ppm residues; another had 0.08-ppm residues.	
	Tetradifon		—	1 out of 4 samples had 0.06-ppm residues.	
Cranberries					
Canada 1990	Diazinon	6 kg ha^{-1}	2		Szeto et al. (1990)
			14	12 ppb	
			21	6 ppb	
			28	7 ppb	
				No detectable residues after 36 days. The tolerance is established at 250 ppb.	
Grapefruit					
United States 1974	Dimethoate Surfactant	15.6 mL 100 L^{-1} + 62.5 mL	1 14	Addition of a surfactant to the tank mix resulted in a more rapid penetration of the insecticide into the leaf than when no surfactant was used. Disappearance was about equal, but residues on leaves were less subject to wash-off by rainfall and other weathering factors. Residues in the pulp were 0.03 ppm of dimethoate and <0.05 dimethoxon, below the 2-ppm allowable tolerance. Residues in the peels were higher, with an average of 3.29 ppm (14 days after treatment). This was due to either translocation from the treated leaves or direct deposition in the fruit, or a combination of the two.	Woodham et al. (1974)

TABLE 8.1 (cont.)
A Summary of Pesticide Residue Levels in Different Fruit Crops

Country/Year	Pesticide	Dose (Active Ingredient)	No. of Treatments	Interval to Last Treatment[a]	Residues (ppm, unless specified otherwise)/Comments	Refs.
Grapefruit (cont.)						
United States 1977	Phenthoate	4.2 kg ha^{-1}	1	45	Washing 3 days after treatment removed 50% of the residues on the rind.	Iwata et al. (1977)
					Residues in rind after 45 days: 0.25 ppm not washed and 0.22 ppm washed. It was detected in the pulp. On a whole-fruit basis 0.06 ppm of residues were estimated.	
United States 1981	Methyl bromide	64 g m^{-3}	—	1 hour	26.9 The fruit was fumigated for 2 hours and aerated for 15 minutes.	King et al. (1981)
				48 hours	0.52 The rapid decrease was probably due to desorption plus a small amount of hydrolysis to yield inorganic bromide.	
Grapes						
France 1983	Phosalone	Market basket survey	—	42	0.27	Barbé (1983)
	Azinphos-methyl		—	28–42	0.02	
	Parathion		—	21	ND residues	
	Malathion		—	60	ND residues	

	Pesticide	Rate	Appl.	Days	Grapes	Must	Centrifuged Must	Centrifuged Wine	Comments	Reference
Greece 1999	Teflubenzuron	12 g 100 L⁻¹	2	7	1.00	–	–	–	Teflubenzuron residues were stable with no appreciable decrease for the experimental period (49 days). During vinification residues transferred completely into the must, but, because of their high affinity for suspended matter, they were removed by approximately 98%. The very low concentrations were detected in the produced wine.	Tsiropoulos et al. (1999)
				14	1.01	1.06	0.02	0.015		
				28	0.83	0.94	0.019	0.013		
				35	0.80	0.90	0.020	0.017		
				49	0.86	–	–	–		

	Pesticide	Rate	Appl.	Days	Grapes	Wine	Comments	Reference
Greece 1999	Teflubenzuron	0.08%	1	40	0.52	0.012	Residue levels for both IGRs decreased considerably from vine to wine.	Miliadis et al. (1999)
	Flufenoxuron	0.075%	1	50	0.20	0.010		

	Pesticide	Rate	Appl.	Days	Comments	Reference
Israel 1981	Fenvalerate	37.5 g ha⁻¹	1	20	A residue level of 0.08 ppm on the day of application was reduced to 0.025 ppm 20 days later.	Greenberg (1981)
		75.0 g ha⁻¹	1	20	0.28 (almost the same level as the quantity of residues measured just after application)	

TABLE 8.1 (cont.)
A Summary of Pesticide Residue Levels in Different Fruit Crops

Country/ Year	Pesticide	Dose (Active Ingredient)	No. of Treatments	Interval to Last Treatment[a]	Residues (ppm, unless specified otherwise)/Comments				Refs.
Grapes (cont.)									
Italy 1991	Dichlozolinate	1000 g ha⁻¹	1	80	1.5				Scrano et al. (1991)
	Iprodione	1000 g ha⁻¹	1	80	1.6				
	Procymidone	750 g ha⁻¹	1	80	1.4				
	Vinclozolin	1000 g ha⁻¹	1	80	1.0				
	Procymidone	750 g ha⁻¹ + fumigation 5 g 100 m⁻²	1	80	1.7				
	Vinclozolin	1000 g ha⁻¹ + fumigation 5 g 100 m⁻²	1	80	1.4				
					Post-harvest fumigation caused only a slight increase of residue levels when compared to field applications.				
					Fresh Fruit	Sun-Dried Fruit	Oven-Dried Fruit		
							Washing	Drying	
Italy 1998	Benalaxyl	4.8 g ha⁻¹	2	22	0.05	0.04	0.04	0.07	Cabras et al. (1998b)
	Dimethoate	130 g ha⁻¹	2	22	1.02	0.19	1.06	0.28	
	Ipridione	225 g ha⁻¹	2	22	1.74	2.79	0.75	0.81	
	Metalaxyl	2.9 g ha⁻¹	2	22	0.13	0.10	0.12	0.09	
	Phosalone	135.4 g ha⁻¹	2	22	0.97	0.69	1.08	2.73	
	Procymidone	225 g ha⁻¹	2	22	2.63	2.42	1.55	1.58	
	Vinclozolin	300 g ha⁻¹	2	22	0.30	0.08	0.30	0.19	
	Parathion	54.7 g ha⁻¹	2	22	<0.01	—	—	—	

The drying process caused a concentration factor of 4; therefore, residues should increase fourfold if no losses occurred due to dehydration. In sunlight drying, the residue level in raisins was identical to that in fresh fruits for benalaxyl, metalaxyl, and phosalone. It was higher by 1.6 times for iprodione and lower by 1/3 and 1/5 for vinclozolin and dimethoate, respectively. The oven drying was preceded by washing, which decreased residues of iprodione and procymidone by 57 and 41%, respectively. No decrease due to washing was observed for other pesticides.

Compared to the fresh berries, during oven drying pesticide residues in raisins increased by 2.7 in phosalone and gave the same values in benalaxyl, metalaxyl, and procymidone. They were lower in vinclozolin and dimethoate. The two drying processes caused different residue decreases for different pesticides. The same finding was observed only with benalaxyl and metalaxyl. Sunlight drying decreased more residues in phosalone and vinclozolin, whereas oven drying decreased more residues of iprodione and procymidone. The decrease in dimethoate was due to heat, and the decrease in benalaxyl, procymidone, and phosalone was due to co-distillation. Iprodione and metalaxyl residues decreased due to heat and co-distillation.

TABLE 8.1 (cont.)
A Summary of Pesticide Residue Levels in Different Fruit Crops

Country/Year	Pesticide	Dose (Active Ingredient)	No. of Treatments	Interval to Last Treatment[a]	Residues (ppm, unless specified otherwise)/Comments	Refs.
Kiwis						
Chile 1994	Azinphos-methyl	1.05 kg ha^{-1}	1	57	0.91	Gonzalez and Curkovic (1994)
	Phosmet	1.25 kg ha^{-1}	1	42	1.66	
	Dicofol	777 g ha^{-1}	1	20	2.21	
	Methidathion	1.36 kg ha^{-1}	1	33	1.91	
	Methidathion	975 g ha^{-1}	1	26	0.61	
	Methidathion	0.4 kg ha^{-1}	1	46	0.06	
	Chlorpyrifos	812 g ha^{-1}	1	85	0.08	
	Chlorpyrifos	1.11 kg ha^{-1}	1	20	0.28	
	Diazinon	1.73 kg ha^{-1}	1	33	0.12	
New Zealand 1982	Iprodione	37.5 g 100 L^{-1}	5	4	0: 3.4; 1 day: 3.2; 3 days: 3.4; 7 days: 2.1; 14 days: 2.1; 22 days: 1.4. 22 days after the last application, the average residue level was 1.4 ppm.	FAO (1981)

Lemons

Location/Year	Chemical	Application	No.	Days	Quinalphos — Rind	Quinalphos — Pulp	Quinalphos — Whole Fruit	2-Hydroxy-Quinoxaline — Rind	2-Hydroxy-Quinoxaline — Pulp	2-Hydroxy-Quinoxaline — Whole Fruit	Reference
Jordan 1986	Quinalphos	0.125%	1	4	4.02	0.04	0.79	ND	ND	ND	Nazer (1986)
	Quinalphos-oxygen analog		—	8	1.01	0.01	0.20	0.114	ND	0.023	
	2-Hydroxy-quinoxaline		—	16	1.00	0.007	0.20	0.076	ND	0.015	

The oxygen analog was always below detectable levels. The amount of 0.04 ppm quinalphos in the pulp after 4 days was within the tolerance level; however, the estimated residue of 0.79 ppm on the whole fruit was above the tolerance limit.

Location/Year	Chemical	Application	No.	Days	Value	Reference
United States 1977	Phenthoate	7.00 kg ha⁻¹	1	68	1	Iwata et al. (1977)
		3.49 kg ha⁻¹	1	48	0.7	
		1.75 kg ha⁻¹	1	68	0.4	

Residues found on and in the rind:

Phenthoate residues above 0.01 ppm were not detected in the pulp of lemons. Low-volume treatment resulted in higher residues on the rind.

United States 1985	Avermectin B₁a	Immersion of branches in 3-ppm solution	1	60		Iwata et al. (1985a)

Residues were <0.001 μg g^{-1} in pulp of treated lemon and 0.004 μg cm^{-2} in the rind.

TABLE 8.1 (cont.)
A Summary of Pesticide Residue Levels in Different Fruit Crops

Country/Year	Pesticide	Dose (Active Ingredient)	No. of Treatments	Interval to Last Treatment[a]	Residues (ppm, unless specified otherwise)/Comments				Refs.
					0 (1 hr)	3 days	10 days	21 days	
Lemons and Oranges									
United States 1979	Carbaryl	12.5 kg ha⁻¹	1	Oranges: 52	No measurable residue levels could be noted with chlorobenzilate, dimethoate, or trichlorfon in the pulp of oranges and lemons. Carbaryl was detected only in 1 of 6 samples with 0.05-ppm residues in the pulp.				Iwata et al. (1979)
	Chlorobenzilate	3.36 kg ha⁻¹	1	Lemons: 59					
	Dimethoate	1.4 kg ha⁻¹	1						
	Trichlorfon	4.5 kg ha⁻¹	1						
Mangos									
India 1988	Permethrin	0.02%	1	—	1.26	0.80	0.39	0.08	Awasthi (1988)
	Permethrin	0.03%	1	—	1.78	1.31	0.44	0.11	
	Fenvalerate	0.01%	1	—	0.87	0.64	0.22	0.053	
	Fenvalerate	0.02%	1	—	1.38	1.02	0.34	0.075	
	Cypermethrin	0.02%	1	—	0.83	0.57	0.19	0.035	
	Cypermethrin	0.03%	1	—	1.43	0.92	0.33	0.061	
	Deltamethrin	0.002%	1	—	0.17	0.11	ND	—	
	Deltamethrin	0.003%	1	—	0.23	0.13	ND	—	

Residues were detected in the flesh of the mangos; nonsystemic and highly lipophylic, these pyrethroids persisted in the fruit.

Location/Year	Pesticide	Dose		Observations	Reference
United States 1989	Methyl bromide	16 g m⁻³ 48 g m⁻³ 56 g m⁻³ 64 g m⁻³	— — — —	Residues in the peel and flesh were above 20 ppm at 0.17 hours after fumigation; 1 hour after fumigation, residue levels were below 15 ppm. Analyses of the peel at 0.17, 1, 2, 5, 24, and 48 hours after fumigation showed that the methyl bromide. residues followed an exponential regression, decreasing rapidly during the first hour followed by a gradual decline. Total residues were <0.01 ppm at the highest concentration 24 hours after treatment and not detectable after 48 hours.	Stein and Wolfenbarger (1989)

Melons

Location/Year	Pesticide	Dose	Observations	Reference
Japan 1988	Chlorinated hydrocarbons	—	Ten years after the banning of organochlorine pesticides in Japan, endrin, dieldrin, p,p′-DDT, p,p′-DDE, heptachlor epoxide, and β-HCH were detected in melons. Endrin, dieldrin, and heptachlor epoxide concentrations in the melons were as follows: seed ≥ rind > sarcocarp (edible region); p,p′-DDT and p,p′-DDE concentrations were rind > sarcocarp > seed. β-HCH was detected only in the rind.	Yoshida et al. (1988)

Muskmelons

Location/Year	Pesticide	Dose		Whole Fruit	Pulp	Observations	Reference
India 1981	Fenthion	0.5 kg ha⁻¹ 1 kg ha⁻¹	1 1				Sarode et al. (1981)
		Initial levels (0 hour)		0.96	0.35		
		Initial levels (0 hour)		1.4	0.60		

The residues (initial) dissipated below detectable levels on the 5th day for the lower concentration and on the 7th day for the higher concentration. Washing the fruit resulted in a 43.5 to 74.2% reduction in residues in the whole fruit and a 38.0 to 52.0% reduction in the pulp.

TABLE 8.1 (cont.)
A Summary of Pesticide Residue Levels in Different Fruit Crops

Country/ Year	Pesticide	Dose (Active Ingredient)	No. of Treatments	Interval to Last Treatment[a]	Residues (ppm, unless specified otherwise)/Comments	Refs.
Nectarines						
Italy 1995	Pirimicarb	262.5 g ha^{-1}	—	0 7 14 21	0.51 0.22 0.17 0.09	Cabras et al (1995b)
					Dilution effect caused by the fruit growth along with volatilization and photodegradation contributed to residue dissipation. Repeated use could lead to active ingredient accumulation in nectarines with the likelihood of residues being above the legal limit at harvest.	
Oranges						
Greece 2001	Aldicarb	2 g ai/tree	1	120	At this rate, no detectable residues were noted for the parent, the sulfoxide, or the sulfone; however, 88 days after harvest, 0.03 and 0.04 ppm of aldicarb sulfoxide and sulfone were recorded in samples from 3 trees out of 18.	Lentza-Rizos and Tsioumplekou (2001)

					Whole Fruit	Pulp	Peel	MRL[d]/PHI[e]	
Italy 1995	Chlorpyrifos-methyl	121.5 g ha⁻¹	2	21	0.03	ND	0.09	0.3/15 days	Cabras et al. (1995a)
	Dimethoate	171.0 g ha⁻¹	2	—	0.17	ND	0.41	1.0/20 days	
	Fenthion	174.2 g ha⁻¹	2	28	0.04	ND	0.16	0.3/28 days	
	Methidathion	102.6 g ha⁻¹	2	69	0.31	ND	0.94	0.2/20 days	
	Parathion	4.9 g ha⁻¹	2	21	0.03	ND	0.20	0.5/20 days	
	Methyl parathion	51.2 g ha⁻¹	2	28	0.08	ND	0.47	0.2/20 days	
	Quinalphos	93.8 g ha⁻¹	2	28	0.06	ND	0.20	0.1/21 days	

Methidathion showed remarkable persistence after 69 days. It was still over the MRL used in Italy. Quinalphos was borderline.

					Whole Fruit	Pulp	Peel		
United States 1977	Phenthoate	3.4 kg (x) in 5678 L	1	56			0.6		Iwata et al. (1977)
		1.7 kg in 5678 L	1				0.4		
		0.9 kg (y) in 5678 L	1				0.18		
		3.4 kg in 379 L	1				1.7		

Orange rind: Residues dissipated quickly in the first 4 weeks then at a slower pace for the remaining 4 weeks.

Residues from low-volume treatment were twice those for the dilute spray (8.4 kg ha⁻¹). The low-volume application is more economical as less water per hectare is required and more pesticide is deposited on the tree. No phenthoate was detected in the pulp in any time. Valencia oranges are 18.7% rind by weight, so at a 15-day interval residues on a whole-fruit basis would range from 0.8 ppm (x) to 0.1 ppm (y). Washing had no effect on residues on the rind.

TABLE 8.1 (cont.)
A Summary of Pesticide Residue Levels in Different Fruit Crops

Country/ Year	Pesticide	Dose (Active Ingredient)	No. of Treatments	Interval to Last Treatment[a]	Residues (ppm, unless specified otherwise)/Comments		Refs.
					Rind	**Unwashed Whole Fruit**	
Oranges							
United States 1985							Iwata et al. (1985b)
	Acephate	1.12 kg ha^{-1}	1	32	0.16	0.04	
	Amitraz	2.11 kg ha^{-1}	1	24	0.98	0.26	
	Chlorpyrifos	1.68 kg ha^{-1}	2	45	1.1	0.27	
	Formetanate hydrochloride	1.03 kg ha^{-1}	1	31	0.85	0.21	
					All residues were below U.S. tolerance limits.		
United States 1989	Avermectin B$_1$a	0.028 kg ha^{-1}	1	4 weeks	Pulp residue: 2 ppb		Maynard et al. (1989)
Oranges, Grapefruit, Tangerines, Tangors							
United States 1991	Methyl bromide	24–48 g m^{-3} for 2 hours	1	—	At any dose, residues were higher in oranges and tangerines than in grapefruit. Oranges, tangerines, and tangors sorbed 1.4–1.9 times more methyl bromide than grapefruit.		King and Benschoter (1991)

Oranges, Plums, Pears

			Unprocessed Peach	Processed Peach (Cooking)		
Canada 1982	Pyrethrins	Market basket survey	—		Plums: 97 ppb of pyrethrin I; Oranges: 116 ppb of pyrethrin II; Pears: 45 ppb of pyrethrin I. A total of 130 samples were analyzed: 1 out of 22 plum samples (4.5%) had the residues reported above; 3 out of 25 orange samples (12%) had the residues reported above; and 1 out of 22 pear samples (4.5%) had the residues reported above.	Ryan et al. (1982)

Peaches

			Unprocessed Peach	Processed Peach (Cooking)		
France 1992	Deltamethrin	Market basket survey	0.04	<0.01	—	Mestres and Mestres (1992)
Greece 1989	Biphenthrin	2 g 100 L^{-1} 4 g 100 L^{-1}	3	21	Residues in peach peel: 247 mg g^{-1} for the low concentration and 367 mg g^{-1} for the high concentration. In the pulp, the level was not detectable for either concentration.	Papadopoulou-Mourkidou et al. (1989)

TABLE 8.1 (cont.)
A Summary of Pesticide Residue Levels in Different Fruit Crops

Country/ Year	Pesticide	Dose (Active Ingredient)	No. of Treatments	Interval to Last Treatment[a]	Residues (ppm, unless specified otherwise)/Comments	Refs.
Peaches (cont.)						
Greece 1995	Iprodione	0.05%	1	14	1.30, in the pulp	Lentza-Rizos (1995)
					1.23, in the whole fruit (pulp and stone)	
					After washing, 0.61 ppm in the pulp and 0.57 ppm in the whole fruit.	
					0.10 in the pulp when peeled after storage for 15 days and 0.015 ppm in cans stored at room temperature for 8 months.	
					After dipping for 3 minutes in 500 ppm of iprodione: 5.35 ppm in the pulp (skin and flesh), 5.06 in the fruit (flesh and stone), 0.35 ppm when stored for 15 days and then peeled, and 0.08 ppm in cans stored for 8 months at room temperature.	
					For peaches not treated before harvest, 4.20 ppm in the pulp and 3.99 ppm in the whole fruit (flesh and stone).	
India 1992	Carbofuran	3 g/plant (drench)	1	61	<0.05	Sharma et al. (1992)

Location	Pesticide	Rate	Applications	Days	Residues	Notes	Reference
Italy 1995	Pirimicarb	262.5 g ha⁻¹	1	0 / 7 / 14 / 21	0.62 / 0.40 / 0.17 / 0.10	Dilution effect caused by the fruit growth along with volatilization and photodegradation contributed to residue dissipation. Repeated use could lead to active ingredient accumulation in peaches with the likelihood of residues being above the legal limit at harvest.	Cabras et al. (1995b)
Italy 1996	Carbendazim	104.25 g ha⁻¹	2	—	0 days: 0.84; 21 days: 0.16		Minelli et al. (1996)
	Dimethoate	171 g ha⁻¹	2	—	0 days: 0.97; 21 days: 0.12		
	Azinphos-methyl	84 g ha⁻¹	2	—	0 days: 1.89; 21 days: 0.25		
	Diazinon	76 g ha⁻¹	2	—	0 days: 0.60; 21 days: 0.01		
	Acephate	21.3 g ha⁻¹	1	—	0 days: 2.00; 21 days: 0.39	Diazinon had the fastest rate of decay	
Spain 1995	Carbosulfan	2 kg ha⁻¹ 0.750 kg ha⁻¹	—	2 hours / 14 days / 21 days / 30 days	6.19; 57 days later, 0.11 / 0.23 / 0.12 / 0.12	The MRL[d] established by the European Union is 1 ppm.	Barba et al. (1995)
Peaches and Apricots							
United States 1978	Oxydemeton-methyl	—	1	—		No residues could be found in apricots or peaches by foliar spray (0.37 g ai/L) but soil injection of 7 g ai 2.5 cm⁻¹ of trunk diameter produced the following residues: Peaches, 0.09 (152 days after) Apricots, 0.55 (105 days after)	Powell et al. (1978)

TABLE 8.1 (cont.)
A Summary of Pesticide Residue Levels in Different Fruit Crops

Country/ Year	Pesticide	Dose (Active Ingredient)	No. of Treatments	Interval to Last Treatment[a]	Residues (ppm, unless specified otherwise/Comments)			Refs.
					>50% of the Tolerance Level	<50% of the Tolerance Level	Over the Tolerance Level	
Pears								
Italy 1993	Captan	Market basket survey	—	—	1	9	0	Mazzali et al. (1993)
	Procymidone		—	—	1	6	0	
	Dichlofluanid		—	—	0	0	0	
	Myclobutanil		—	—	0	0	0	
	Dodine		—	—	0	1	0	
	Dithianon		—	—	0	1	0	
	Penconazole		—	—	0	0	0	
	Amitraz		—	—	4	0	0	
	Carbaryl		—	—	0	4	0	
	Pirimicarb		—	—	0	0	0	
	Azinphos-methyl		—	—	2	12	0	
	Quinalphos		—	—	3	2	0	
	Fenitrothion		—	—	0	1	0	
	Phosalone		—	—	1	1	0	

Pineapples

Thailand 1991	Dimefuron	2.5 kg ha⁻¹	1	16 months	Dimefuron and its metabolites were absorbed via the roots and/or shoots and transported to the fruit. Residues (μg g^{-1}) found in pineapples grown from crowns and tillers were:	Suwanketnikom and Sasiprapa (1991)

	Flesh	Peel	Crown
Crown	0.045	0.049	0.087
Tillers	0.064	0.058	0.0128

Plums

Italy 1998	Iprodione	350 g ha⁻¹	1	21	Although the drying process caused a fruit concentration factor of 3, the residues on the dried fruit were not higher than on the fresh fruit. Residues in fresh fruit (F) and after washing, drying, and rehydration (WDR) were:
	Phosalone	225.8 g ha⁻¹	1	—	
	Bitertanol	75 g ha⁻¹	1	—	
	Procymidone	350 g ha⁻¹	1	—	

Cabras et al. (1998d)

	Iprodione	Phosalone	Bitertanol	Procymidone
F	0.68	0.21	0.16	0.37
WDR	0.30	0.24	0.05	0.22

Phosalone showed the same residue level; the other pesticides were 0.6, 2.3, and 3.2 times lower.

TABLE 8.1 (cont.)
A Summary of Pesticide Residue Levels in Different Fruit Crops

Country/Year	Pesticide	Dose (Active Ingredient)	No. of Treatments	Interval to Last Treatment[a]	Residues (ppm, unless specified otherwise)/Comments			Refs.
					0	**14 days**	**28 days**	
Plums and Prunes								
Italy 1998	Dimethoate	750 g ha^{-1}	1	—	1.08	<0.01	<0.01	Cabras et al. (1998c)
	Vinclozolin	12.5 g ha^{-1}	1	—	2.29	0.66	0.15	
	Cyproconazole	456 g ha^{-1}	1	—	0.01	<0.01	<0.01	
						Dried	**Oven-Dried and Rehydrated Fruits**	
	Dimethoate	—	1	—		<0.01	<0.01	
	Vinclozolin	—	1	—		<0.01	<0.01	
	Cyproconazole	—	1	—		<0.01	<0.01	

Only vinclozolin residues were detected in the fresh fruit 28 days after harvest; the other two compounds were at a negligible residue level.

Strawberries

			n	0	1 days	2 days	7 days	14 days	21 days	
Australia 1985	Dimethoate	60 mg L⁻¹	4	2.81	1.98	1.57	0.64	0.30	0.18	Goodwin et al. (1985)
		90 mg L⁻¹	4	3.65	2.56	1.90	0.69	0.25	0.30	
		150 mg L⁻¹	4	6.30	5.18	3.58	0.99	0.53	0.38	

90 mg ai/L resulted in mean residues below maximum residue limit of 2 ppm 2 days after the trial spray; therefore, a 3-day waiting period would be appropriate.

			n							
Brazil 1988	Dicofol and endosulfan	Market basket survey	—							Guindani and Ungaro (1988)

Residues were noted in the range of 0.02 to 2.61 ppm for dicofol and 0.01 to 0.5 ppm for endosulfan. The Brazilian tolerance is 1 ppm for dicofol and 2 ppm for ensdosulfan. 28.3% had illegal residues of dicofol, 29.4% had illegal residues of endosulfan, and 14.1% had illegal residues of both products. Only 28.2% of the berries had residues within the tolerance limits.

			n							
Canada 1978	Disulfoton	1.68 kg ha⁻¹	1	12 months	<0.01–0.13					Chisholm and Specht (1978)
		3.36 kg ha⁻¹	1							
		6.72 kg ha⁻¹	1							
		13.44 kg ha⁻¹	1							

Sulfone and sulfoxide residues were found in berries 12 months later and traces (0.01 ppm) of the sulfone 24 months later. Residues of disulfoton metabolites remained in the soil 2 years following application.

			n	0	1 days	3 days	7 days	14 days	
Egypt 1995	Methomyl	675 g ha⁻¹	1	Unwashed	2.2	1.9	1.2	0.55	0.17	Ahmed and Ismail (1995)
			—	Washed	1.2	1.1	0.79ª	0.37	0.12	
		Market basket survey					0.18			

Thorough rinsing with tap water reduced methomyl residues on the berries by 0.05 ppm.

TABLE 8.1 (cont.)
A Summary of Pesticide Residue Levels in Different Fruit Crops

Country/Year	Pesticide	Dose (Active Ingredient)	No. of Treatments	Interval to Last Treatment[a]	Residues (ppm, unless specified otherwise)/Comments				Refs.
					0	3 days	7 days	14 days	
Strawberries (cont.)									
Spain 1991	Bromopropylate	625 g ha^{-1}	1	—	11.97	4.23	2.33	0.53	Barba et al. (1991)
		937 g ha^{-1}	1	—	13.76	7.46	2.62	0.63	
					After 14 days, residue levels were within the MRL^{d} of 0.7 ppm recommended by the FAO.				
United States 1977	Carbofuran	292 mL ha^{-1} and 584 mL ha^{-1}	1		The combined residues of carbofuran and its metabolites never exceeded the tolerance level of 0.5 ppm, nor did the carbamate fraction exceed 0.2 ppm 6 days after application.				Archer et al. (1977)

292.1 mL ha^{-1}

	Carbofuran	3-OH	3-Oxo	Total	Phenol 3-7-Diol
1	0.420	<0.01	0.103	0.523	0.073
3	0.110	<0.01	0.015	0.125	0.010
5	<0.050	<0.01	<0.010	0.060	0.012
7	<0.050	<0.01	<0.010	<0.050	0.025

	Carbofuran	3-OH	3-Oxo	Total	Phenol 3-7-Diol
	\multicolumn{5}{c}{584.2 mL ha^{-1}}				Archer et al. (1977)
1	0.740	0.012	0.014	0.766	0.094
3	0.183	<0.010	<0.010	0.183	0.010
5	0.075	<0.010	0.054	0.129	0.011
7	0.056	<0.010	<0.010	0.056	<0.010

[a] In days, unless specified differently.
[b] Applied in site II later than in site I; site II received 170 mm less rain.
[c] Omethoate is a metabolite of dimethoate.
[d] Maximum residual level.
[e] Pre-harvest interval.

9 Behavior of Polyhalogenated and Polycyclic Aromatic Hydrocarbons in Food-Producing Animals

Ron (L.A.P.) Hoogenboom

CONTENTS

Abstract Food products of animal origin may contribute significantly to the exposure of consumers to environmental contaminants. This is particularly true for the more lipophilic and persistent compounds such as many chlorinated and brominated hydrocarbons. For regulatory purposes, it is essential to have information on the relation between levels in feed and edible products such as milk, eggs, and meat. For this reason, many studies have been performed on the carryover of polychlorinated biphenyls (PCBs) and dioxins in milk and to a lesser extent eggs. Similar is the case for non-lactating cows. Much less information is available on the fate of these compounds in fast-growing animals such as broilers and pigs. Older studies have shown the carryover of polybrominated biphenyls, following the FireMaster incident in 1973. However, no information is available on the fate of other polybrominated flame retardants, although recent data show that animal-derived products do contribute to the overall exposure to these compounds. Very remarkable is the almost complete absence of data on the carryover of polyaromatic hydrocarbons and in particular their active metabolites in food-producing animals, despite the frequent occurrence of these compounds in dried feed ingredients and the environment of the animals. This chapter describes the current knowledge on the fate of polyhalogenated and polycyclic aromatic hydrocarbons in food-producing animals, including data from the major feed incidents with these compounds.

Abbreviations   AHH, arylhydrocarbon hydroxylase; BCF, bioconcentration factor; BTF, biotransfer factor; bw, body weight; COR, carryover rate; DDT, 1,1,1-trichloro-2,2-bis(4-chlorophenyl)ethane; EROD, ethoxyresorufin-O-deethylase; GC–ECD, gas chromatography–electron capture detection; HBCD, hexabromocyclododecane; HCB, hexachlorobenzene; HpCDD, heptachlorodibenzo-p-dioxin; HpCDF, heptachlorodibenzofuran; HxCDD, hexachlorodibenzo-p-dioxin; HxCDF, hexachlorodibenzofuran; MWI, municipal waste incinerator; OCDD, octachlorodibenzo-p-dioxin; OCDF, octachlorodibenzofuran; p,p'-DDE, 1,1-dichloro-2,2-bis(4-chlorophenyl)ethylene; PAHs, polycyclic aromatic hydrocarbons; PBBs, polybrominated biphenyls; PBDEs, polybrominated diphenylethers; PCBs, polychlorinated biphenyls; PCDD, polychlorinated dibenzo-p-dioxins; PCDF, polychlorinated dibenzofurans; PCP, pentachlorophenol; PeCDD, pentachlorodibenzo-p-dioxin; PeCDF, pentachlorodibenzofuran; SCF, Scientific Committee on Food; TCDD, 2,3,7,8-tetrachlorodibenzo-p-dioxin; TCDF, 2,3,7,8-tetrachlorodibenzofuran; TEQ, toxic equivalent; 2,4,5-T, 2,4,5-trichlorophenoxyacetic acid; WHO, World Health Organization; ww, wet weight

Key Words   *carryover, contaminants, flame retardants, food incidents, food-producing animals, polychlorinated aromatic hydrocarbons, polycyclic aromatic hydrocarbons, polychlorinated biphenyls*

INTRODUCTION

Feed and feed ingredients can be contaminated with environmental contaminants, possibly resulting in a health risk for both the food-producing animal and the human consumer. Furthermore, such contaminants may also be present in the environment of the animals, both inside and outside. Several major incidents, such as the chicken edema disease (1957–1969), the Michigan FireMaster (1973), and the Belgium PCB (1999) incidents have revealed the impact of contaminations on animal health, the economy, and possibly human health. Strict policies, including limits for feed and food, have been developed to deal with these problems. Increased monitoring may reveal novel sources, as in the case of contaminated kaolinic and ball clay, cholin chloride mixed with contaminated wood, and recently bakery waste dried on open fires from waste wood. In each case, the first question is the effect on the levels in food products and the health risk for the consumer; therefore, it is essential to obtain information on the sources leading to the introduction of such compounds into the food chain and on the behavior of these compounds in food-producing animals.

In most cases, xenobiotic compounds may be effectively metabolized by the animal and thus absent in edible products. In some cases, however, metabolism may not be equal to complete detoxification, and metabolites may still present a potential risk. This has been shown, for example, in the case of the mycotoxin aflatoxin B_1, which in lactating cows is metabolized to aflatoxin M_1, resulting in small amounts of this carcinogenic metabolite being present in milk. In the case of the nitrofuran drug furazolidone, metabolism resulted in the formation of so-called protein-bound residues characterized by a long half-life and which are still suspected carcinogenic compounds (Hoogenboom et al., 2002b). For many other contaminants, such as polycyclic aromatic hydrocarbons, metabolic pathways in food-producing animals and possible residues of toxic metabolites in edible products have not been examined.

Another group of contaminants, such as certain dioxins and PCBs, is poorly metabolized, and due to their lipophilic nature these contaminants will accumulate in tissue fat or be transferred to the fat fraction of milk and eggs. The same is true for organochlorine pesticides such as hexachlorobenzene (HCB), 1,1,1-trichloro-2,2-bis(4-chlorophenyl)ethane (DDT), and dieldrin in egg yolk, the levels of which can considerably exceed levels in feed (Kan, 1978). Although levels of most of these pesticides have decreased dramatically, some problems may still remain such as, for example, toxaphene (Schwind and Kaltenecker, 2000; Kan, 2002). This chapter summarizes the existing knowledge on the fate of polyhalogenated and polycyclic aromatic hydrocarbons and focuses on some of the incidents with feed and animal-derived products.

DIOXINS AND POLYCHLORINATED BIPHENYLS

Incidents with polychlorinated biphenyls (PCBs) and dioxins have shown that these compounds pose a major threat to edible products derived from food-producing animals. Dioxins are produced as by-products in the synthesis of certain chemicals, such as pentachlorophenol and 2,4,5-trichlorophenoxyacetic acid (2,4,5-T), and during incineration of waste (see Figure 9.1). These compounds bind to the so-called Ah-receptor present in mammalian cells, thus resulting in the transcription of a large number of genes. In laboratory animals, exposure results in tumors in the liver and, at even lower levels, affects the immune and reproductive systems, as well as resulting in impaired learning. Based on these studies, the World Health Organization (WHO) and Scientific Committee on Food (SCF) have set very low exposure limits of, respectively, 1 to 4 pg TEQ (toxic equivalent) per kg bw per day (WHO, 2000)

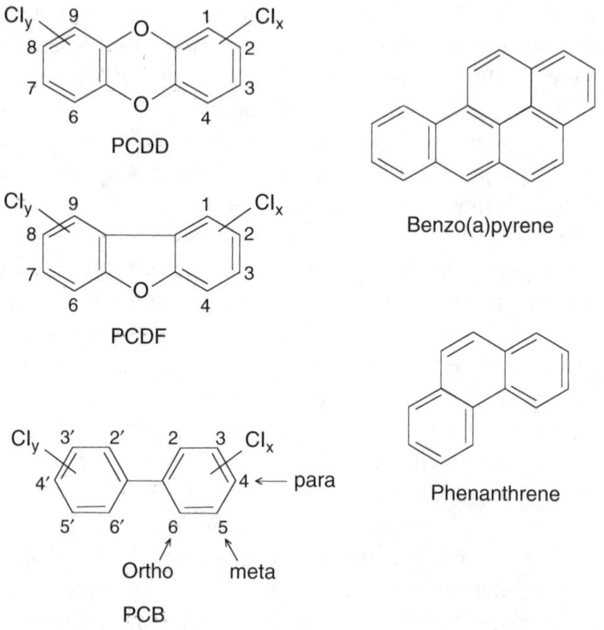

FIGURE 9.1 Structures of polychlorinated dibenzo-*p*-dioxins (PCDDs) and dibenzofurans (PCDFs), polychlorinated biphenyls (PCBs), and two polycyclic aromatic hydrocarbons: benzo(*a*)pyrene and phenanthrene.

and 14 pg TEQ per kg bw per week (SCF, 2001). These limits include the 17 toxic dioxins as well as 12 so-called planar PCBs, which have properties similar to those of dioxins.

Several studies have subsequently shown that, at present, the exposure of some of the populations in Western countries exceeds these limits; therefore, the EU has developed a strategy for further reducing the exposure that includes the establishment of residue limits for food products: 1 ng TEQ per kg fat for pork, 2 ng TEQ per kg fat for poultry, and 3 ng TEQ per kg fat for beef, milk, and eggs (EC, 2001). In addition, limits have been set for feed (0.75 ng TEQ per kg) and feed ingredients (0.75–6 ng per kg TEQ) (EC, 2002). The so-called TEQ principle is based on the fact that the concentrations of the different congeners are multiplied by a toxic equivalency factor (TEF) that expresses their relative toxicity to the most toxic congener 2,3,7,8-tetrachlorodibenzo-*p*-dioxin (TCDD) (Berg et al., 1998). At this stage, planar dioxins (such as PCBs) are included in the exposure limits but not yet in the EU food and feed limits. Based on more detailed information on current levels of these PCBs, the EU limits will be adapted in the near future.

Polychlorinated biphenyls are a group of 209 different congeners that have been produced as technical mixtures (such as Aroclor 1254) and have been used in large amounts as, for example, heat-transfer fluids, hydraulic lubricants, and dielectric fluids for capacitors and transformers. Twelve of these congeners have a planar structure and have similar properties as dioxins. Other PCBs have been shown to affect brain development (Schmidt, 1999) and appear to be responsible for the tumor promotion effects of these mixtures (Plas et al., 2001). In addition, metabolites of non-dioxin-like PCBs interfere with the homeostasis of vitamin A and thyroid hormones (Safe, 1994). In practice, the consumer will be exposed to a mixture of both dioxins, dioxin-like PCBs, and other PCBs, and the toxicology of these mixtures is even more complex. As a result, no exposure limits for non-dioxin-like PCBs have been established thus far, contrary to limits for PCBs in food. In order to avoid the difficulty of analyzing all 209 congeners, it is often customary to analyze only seven so-called indicator PCBs that represent the various technical mixtures. These include PCBs 28, 53, 101, 138, 153, and 180, but also PCB 118, which is a dioxin-like mono-ortho-PCB. It is important to realize that the total amount of PCBs in a technical mixture may be three- to fourfold higher. As is described in this chapter, this relative contribution may change in animal-derived products due to selective absorption, metabolism, carryover, and accumulation of the different congeners.

The high toxicity of dioxins and PCBs is partly due to their lipophilic nature and resistance to metabolic degradation, resulting in accumulation in the body. Eventually, this may result in body burdens that are higher than critical levels, thus resulting in the adverse effects described earlier. One of the few mechanisms leading to a significant reduction in body burden levels is excretion of these compounds in the milk. The same is true for food-producing animals, where dioxins are transferred into milk and eggs.

TRANSFER OF POLYCHLORINATED BIPHENYLS IN LACTATING COWS

Two of the greatest incidents with contaminants in food were the Yusho and Yu-Cheng incidents with PCB-contaminated rice oils in Japan (1968) and Taiwan (1979). The contamination of the oil, used directly for human consumption, was caused by leakage of PCB oil used as heat-transfer fluid in heating equipment. In 1970, shortly after the first rice oil incident, PCBs were detected for the first time in milk in the eastern part of the United States. The source was shown to be feed silos coated with the Aroclor 1254-containing product Cumar (Willett and Hess, 1975). Levels in silage near the coated wall varied between 10 and 60 mg/kg, with occasional levels over 7 g/kg. A survey showed that about 7% of the milk samples had detectable levels of PCBs, but only few exceeded the limit of 2.5 mg/kg fat. This discovery triggered studies on the relationship between PCBs in feed and milk in order to allow management of the risks evolving from this type of contamination. Fries et al. (1973) treated 9 cows with 200 mg Aroclor 1254 for 60 days followed by a withdrawal period on clean feed for another 60 days. Individual PCBs could not be identified at that time. PCB levels in milk increased rapidly, and a steady state was reached after 40 days, with average PCB levels in milk of 61 mg/kg fat. Concentrations in body fat (determined in fat biopsy samples) obtained after 30 and 60 days of exposure were, respectively, 20 and 42 mg/kg. During the elimination period, levels in milk fat declined 50% within 15 days but then slowed down. Levels in body fat decreased much more slowly, with average levels of 36 and 30 mg/kg at 90 and 120 days, respectively. During this period, several other studies were carried out with Aroclor 1254, with reported dose levels varying between 3.5 and 1000 mg/day. Willett et al. (1990) evaluated these studies, starting by standardization of the PCB levels determined by gas chromatography and electron capture detection (GC–ECD). When focusing on cows exposed for 60 days or longer, the following relations were obtained between daily dose (in mg) and, respectively, milk and body fat levels (in mg/kg):

$$[PCB]_{\text{milk fat}} = 0.28 \times (\text{daily dose})^{0.82}$$
$$[PCB]_{\text{body fat}} = 0.16 \times (\text{daily dose})^{0.85}$$

McLachlan et al. (1990, 1993) investigated the transfer of dioxins, PCBs, and organochlorine pesticides at normal background levels from feed to milk of one lactating cow. Contaminants were analyzed in milk, urine, and feces. Daily exposure to contaminants came primarily from the feed and varied between 30 and 7600 ng for PCBs. It was shown that, in general, the transfer to milk increased with higher chlorination of the PCBs, particularly when a congener is substituted at the 4 and 4′ positions. Under these steady-state conditions, the carryover rates from feed to milk varied between 12% for the labile congeners (such as PCB 28) to more than 78% for the most persistent congeners, including indicator PCBs 118, 138, 153, and 180. In this study, the carryover rate (COR) was defined as the ratio of the amount excreted in milk and the total amount excreted in milk and feces. The pesticides hexachlorobenzene (HCB) and p,p′-DDE (1,1-dichloro-2,2-bis(4-chlorophenyl)eth-ylene) showed similarly high CORs.

Similar carryover rates were obtained by Thomas et al. (1999a,b), who performed a 3-month carryover study with five lactating cows. Animals were exposed at back-ground levels (54 µg total PCB per day; 53 congeners analyzed), using "naturally incorporated" feed stuffs (Figure 9.2). The seven indicator PCBs contributed 10%

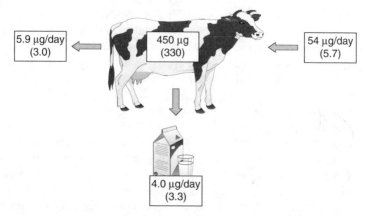

FIGURE 9.2 Mass-balance of PCB intake and efflux in lactating cows as determined by Thomas et al. (1999a,b). Figures present the sum of 53 congeners and the sum of the 7 indicator PCBs between brackets. Level in the cow presents the total amount of PCBs in the animal (body burden), primarily present in the body fat.

to this intake. In this study, total daily PCB excretion in milk tended to decrease with increasing lactation period, partly due to decreasing milk gift and partly due to decreasing levels. No difference was found in PCB levels between morning and afternoon milkings. Average PCB levels in milk were 3.9 µg/kg fat for the indicator PCBs (i.e., 118, 138, 153, and 180), which contributed 79%. Due to the loss of body fat during the lactation period, the input–output balance (i.e., the relative ratio between the intake through the feed and output through the milk) reached levels of 134, 116, 124, and 112% for the more stable PCBs 118, 138, 153, and 180, respectively. PCB levels and congener patterns in the body fat of these animals were very similar within the different tissues and organs and reflected those in the milk. Levels in liver on a fat base were threefold higher, indicating specific binding of certain PCBs, as is also the case for higher chlorinated dioxins (see below). Total body burden in these animals was estimated to be 450 µg, with indicator PCBs contributing 73%. The 95 kg of body fat contained 97.7% of this body burden; the muscle tissues, 1.8% (total body weight, 631 kg).

Transfer of Dioxins in Lactating Cows

Many studies have been performed to investigate the transfer of dioxins into milk. Firestone et al. (1979) and Jensen and Hummel (1982) exposed lactating cows to, respectively, pentachlorophenol (PCP) and 2,4,5-trichlorophenoxyacetic acid (2,4,5-T) contaminated with dioxins. The PCP contained primarily the higher chlorinated 1,2,3,6,7,8-hexachlorodibenzo-p-dioxin (HxCDD), heptachlorodibenzo-p-dioxin (HpCDD), and octachlorodibenzo-p-dioxin (OCDD) congeners; the 2,4,5-T, only TCDD. Both studies were carried out with relatively high dioxin levels (20 and a range of 0.09–9 µg TEQ per day, respectively); therefore, they might not be representative of general practice. Interestingly, the half-life of 41 days for TCDD, calculated after terminating the 11-week exposure of cows with 2,4,5-T, was similar as determined at lower levels in later studies. The same is true for the half-lives (76, 88, and 274 days, respectively) obtained after the 70-day exposure period for the hexa-, hepta-, and octa-CDD (Firestone et al., 1979).

Jones et al. (1987, 1989) studied the fate of radiolabeled TCDD in lactating cows given a high single dose of grain spiked with either 30 µg or 45 mg (0.05 and 75 µg/kg body weight). Seven days after treatment with the high dose, most of the radiolabel was excreted in the feces, with lesser amounts in milk and urine. Fat and liver tissue contained the highest levels of radiolabel at 116 and 76 µg/kg (ww) tissue, respectively (levels not corrected for fat content). In the 2 low-dosed animals, killed after 14 days, levels in fat and liver differed more, being 104 and 8 ng/kg, respectively. Blood and milk levels showed a very similar pattern, with a peak at 1 to 2 days of 6.5 and 70 ng/kg, respectively, for cow 1, and 4.5 and 86 ng/kg, respectively, for cow 2. Also, 16 and 11%, respectively, of the radiolabel was excreted in the milk of these two cows. The depletion showed the typical two-phase distribution (i.e., a rapid first elimination and a much slower second elimination). The activity of ethoxyresorufin-O-deethylase (EROD) and arylhydrocarbon hydroxylase (AHH) in the liver, as measured 7 and 14 days after slaughter, showed a strong and moderate increase in the high- and low-dosed animals. Induction of the cytochrome

P-450 might be involved in the relative high retention of TCDD in the liver, particularly in the case of the high-dosed cow. This may also influence the extrapolation of data from a high-dose exposure to more realistic levels that may have no effect on liver enzymes. In the same study, when 2 lactating cows received a dose of 0.05 µg/kg radiolabeled TCDD spiked to soil (Jones et al., 1989), 12 and 14% of the dose was excreted into the milk during the study period of 14 days. Although peak levels in blood and milk appeared to be lower, these data do not suggest a big difference in the uptake of TCDD added to either grain or soil.

Later studies were performed under more realistic conditions with long-term exposures. Under steady-state and at background exposure levels, McLachlan et al. (1990) found carryover rates of 25 to 35% for the most toxic congeners: 2,3,7,8-TCDD, 1,2,3,7,8-pentachlorodibenzo-*p*-dioxin (PeCDD), and 2,3,4,7,8-pentachlorodibenzofuran (PeCDF); 15% for the hexachlorinated congeners; and less than 5% for the hepta- and octachlorinated congeners (Table 9.1). Cows were exposed to 7.5 ng TEQ per day and excreted 1.6 ng TEQ per day (21%) into milk and 4.2 ng TEQ per day (56%) in the feces. The remaining 23% was not accounted for, in particular due to the loss of 2,3,7,8-tetrachlorodibenzofuran (TCDF), PeCDF, and HpCDD, which are most likely metabolized. Lower chlorinated congeners were better absorbed than higher chlorinated congeners, an observation confirmed by other studies. Similar congener-specific effects were observed by Fürst et al. (1993), who investigated the relationship between levels in soil and milk and levels in grass and milk at a number of sites. Their data clearly show that grass but not soil levels are important for milk levels. Fries (1987) and Derks et al. (1994) came to the same conclusions, the latter based on the decrease of dioxin levels in milk and grass but not soil near waste incinerators.

One of the first incidents with dioxins in The Netherlands was the presence of these compounds in milk from cows grazing in the vicinity of a municipal waste incinerator (MWI) (Olie et al., 1977; Liem et al., 1991). Levels exceeded 6 ng TEQ per kg, the Dutch limit at that time. The area was closed for dairy cows, the MWIs were adapted, and the cows were transferred to a rural area. Several studies were carried out to investigate the carryover to milk, particularly the depletion kinetics. Olling et al. (1991) exposed 4 cows to a high single dose of 8 congeners each at 3.7 or 37 ng/kg body weight dissolved in oil. Half-lives in milk fat varied from 27 to 34 days for the heptachlorinated congeners, and 40 to 49 days for the tetra-, penta-, and hexachlorinated dibenzo-*p*-dioxins (PCDD/Fs). TCDF showed a half-life of 1 day and was not detected in the body fat, again demonstrating that this compound is actively metabolized. Levels in milk and body fat were of the same order of magnitude, with the exception of the liver, which showed relatively high levels. The latter may be explained by the binding of the higher chlorinated congeners to specific proteins.

In a follow-up study, Slob et al. (1995) treated lactating cows with a single dose of contaminated fly ash (14 µg TEQ) and obtained very low carryover rates of 0.35 and 0.53% for the total TEQ level. This study also included a field study with cows on a farm in the vicinity of a waste incinerator. Levels in grass were around 10 ng TEQ per kg, and levels in milk were around 10 ng TEQ per kg fat. Carryover rates were calculated to vary between 15% for TCDD and less than 1% for the hepta-

and octachlorinated congeners TCDF and 1,2,3,7,8-PeCDF (Table 9.1). The carry-over rate for the total TEQ was only 7.5%, which is threefold lower than the rate reported by McLachlan et al. (1990). This study was the only one that included carryover of the dioxin-like non-ortho PCBs 77, 126, and 169, which had carryover rates of 1.2, 35, and 31%, respectively. These data show that the most important dioxin-like PCB 126 has a high carryover rate.

Another carryover study with 4 cows was carried out to investigate the depletion kinetics of the different dioxin congeners (Tuinstra et al., 1992). Cows were fed with contaminated grass and an additional amount of dioxins spiked to briquettes, which resulted in dioxin levels in milk of around 50 ng TEQ per kg fat. Cows were subsequently fed clean grass. As in previous studies, it was shown that the elimination half-lives for the 3 most important dioxin congeners in these cows varied between 63 and 76 days. Schuler et al. (1997a) performed a field study near a modern waste incinerator and calculated transfer rates from both air to grass and grass to milk. Total TEQ in grass was around 0.6 ng TEQ per kg dry weight, and the daily intake of dioxins was about 10 ng TEQ, leading to concentrations in milk of 1 to 3 ng TEQ per kg fat. Carryover rates were similar to those described by other authors: about 10 to 20% for total TEQ (Table 9.1).

McLachlan and Richter (1998) repeated their earlier study, this time with 4 lactating cows. After 12 weeks of exposure at background levels, cows were fed with grass obtained from a field that had received repeated applications with sewage sludge for 24 days. In particular, the intake of hexa-, hepta-, and octachlorinated PCDDs and hepta- and octachlorinated polychlorinated dibenzofurans (PCDFs) increased dramatically. Despite the low TEF values of these congeners, total TEQ increased from about 1.5 to 12 ng TEQ per day. As before, carryover rates to milk decreased with increasing chlorination, from about 40% for TCDD and PeCDD to 0.5% for OCDD during the first phase (Table 9.1). In phase 2, carryover rates for those congeners for which the intake clearly increased were a factor of 2 lower. This can be explained by the fact that the grass was fed for only 17 days prior to sampling. As a result, most of the compounds are likely to be accumulated in the body fat and liver and steady state is not yet obtained. In this study, the levels in the different tissues were very similar when based on fat. Low levels in feces and absence in milk again indicate that TCDF and 1,2,3,7,8-PeCDF are metabolized in cows. In general, the fraction excreted in the feces increased with higher chlorination grade, indicating a lower absorption of these more lipophilic compounds. The authors conclude that the sewage sludge has no effect on the absorption and carryover to milk. Fries et al. (1999) studied the fate of the higher chlorinated dioxins by feeding dairy cows with PCP-contaminated wood. Four Holstein cows received a daily dose of 70 ng TEQ for 58 days. Steady state was obtained at the first sampling point at 30 days with milk levels of 6 ng TEQ per kg fat. Carryover rates for individual congeners are in the range reported by other authors (Table 9.1). About 9% of the total ingested TEQ level was excreted into the milk. This rather low figure can be explained by the high chlorination of the congeners, with HpCDD contributing almost 50% to the total TEQ intake.

An unusual incident with lactating cows was discovered in 1998 in Southwest Germany, where a gradual increase in milk levels was traced back to the use of

TABLE 9.1
Carryover Rates as Determined in Lactating Cows

						Reference				
	Firestone et al. (1979)[a]	McLachlan et al. (1990)[a]	Olling et al. (1991)[b]	Slob et al. (1995)[a]	Schuler et al. (1997a)	McLachlan (1998)[a]		Fries (1999)[a]	Malisch (2000)[a]
Variables									
Daily dose (ng TEQ per kg bw per day)	36.4	0.012	11.1	0.20	0.014	0.002	0.018	0.11	0.02
Source	Pentachloro-phenol	Natural	Standards	Municipal waste incinerator	Municipal waste incinerator	Natural	Sludge	Pentachloro-phenol	Citrus pulp
Number of cows	3	1	4	Many	41	4	4	4	Many
Duration exposure (days)	70	35	1	30	395	84	56	24	180
Milk fat/day (kg)	0.4	1.4	—	1.0	0.9	0.9	1.0	0.9	1.2
Carryover Rates (%)									
2,3,7,8-TCDD	—	35	30	15	30	38	51	35	58
1,2,3,7,8-PeCDD	—	33	28	10	20	39	27	39	49
1,2,3,4,7,8-HxCDD	—	17	—	5.6	8	33	21	15	51

1,2,3,6,7,8-HxCDD	13	14	27	6.4	—	33	13	18	77
1,2,3,7,8,9-HxCDD	—	18	—	3.1	—	16	10	13	35
1,2,3,4,6,7,8-HpCDD	1.3	3	1.6	0.6	2	3.4	2.0	3.3	18
1,2,3,4,6,7,8,9-OCDD	0.2	4	—	0.1	0.8	0.7	0.3	0.4	3.7
2,3,7,8-TCDF	—	—	—	—	2	ND	ND	<0.1	2.8
1,2,3,7,8-PeCDF	—	—	—	—	4	ND	ND	<0.1	3.8
2,3,4,7,8-PeCDF	—	25	36	12	50	40	65	17	58
1,2,3,4,7,8-HxCDF	—	—	18	4.3	7	24	23	14	33
1,2,3,6,7,8-HxCDF	—	16	—	3.6	—	19	27	15	30
2,3,4,6,7,8-HxCDF	—	14	—	4.2	—	19	20	9	19
1,2,3,7,8,9-HxCDF	—	—	—	—	—	—	—	<0.1	ND
1,2,3,4,6,7,8-HpCDF	—	3	1.7	0.4	1	3.4	1.9	3.5	3.1
1,2,3,4,7,8,9-HpCDF	—	8	—	0.5	—	ND	3.6	4.3	4.2
1,2,3,4,6,7,8,9-OCDF	—	1	—	—	1	—	0.3	0.3	0.4
PCB77	—	—	—	1.2	—	—	—	—	—
PCB126	—	—	—	35	—	—	—	—	—
PCB169	—	—	—	31	—	—	—	—	—

a Carryover rates are estimated from the intake through the feed and excretion in milk at steady state.
b Carryover rates are estimated from the total intake and excretion in milk during depletion.

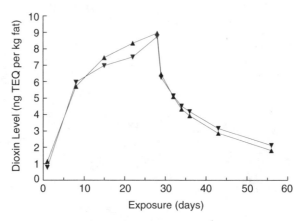

FIGURE 9.3 Dioxin levels in milk from two cows fed 5.4 kg of citrus pulp per day for 4 weeks at a level of 10 ng TEQ per kg. Subsequently, cows received clean feed for another 4 weeks. (Adapted from Traag et al., 1999.)

contaminated citrus pulp from Brazil (Malisch, 2000). The contamination was actually caused by the use of contaminated lime, derived from a polyvinyl chloride (PVC) production plant. Levels up to 7.9 and 4.3 ng international toxic equivalents (I-TEQ) per kg fat were measured in milk and veal fat, respectively. In The Netherlands, levels in pooled milk samples during this period increased to a maximum of 5 ng TEQ per kg fat as compared to maximum levels of 2 and 1 pg TEQ per kg by the end of 1999 and 2001, respectively (Baumann et al., 2002). Using one batch of contaminated citrus pulp, a carryover study was carried out with lactating cows. Figure 9.3 shows the levels in milk from 2 cows that were fed the contaminated citrus pulp daily for a period of 4 weeks (Traag et al., 1999). The pulp was contaminated with 10 ng TEQ dioxins per kg, a level that is about 15 times the current limit of 0.75 ng TEQ per kg. It is evident that this exposure rapidly led to increased dioxin levels in milk but also to an initial rapid decrease after termination of the exposure. The depletion showed the typical two-phase disposition profile, and the half-life of elimination was calculated to be 20 days. This half-life was shorter than the half-life calculated by Malisch (2000) for cows on a farm that had received contaminated pulp for 6 months; in this case, the half-life was 8 to 10 weeks for the total TEQ level and the levels of the two most important congeners, 2,3,7,8-TCDD and 1,2,3,7,8-PeCDD. A possible explanation is a much more extensive distribution and higher storage in lower perfused fat tissues at prolonged exposure. Carryover rates were also estimated and are shown in Table 9.1. The rate for the total WHO TEQ was estimated to be 44%.

FATE OF DIOXINS IN BEEF ANIMALS

The first study on the fate of dioxins in beef cattle was carried out by Jensen et al. (1981), who treated calves with feed mixed with 2,4,5-T contaminated with 0.06 mg/kg TCDD. Seven animals of about 200 kg received a daily dose of 0.15 ng TCDD per day for 28 days, amounting to a total dose of 4.2 µg. At that time, 3 animals were slaughtered; the others were followed for depletion kinetics and slaughtered after 50 weeks. Levels of TCDD in fat, liver, and muscle just after the exposure period were 84, 9, and 2 ng/kg tissue, respectively. Correction for the fat content in muscle (2%) showed that the levels on a fat base were similar in fat and muscle tissue, leading to the conclusion that fat is the most suitable tissue for monitoring TCDD exposure. Using a 3 to 4% fat content in liver (Feil et al., 2000), TCDD levels in liver fat would be 200 to 300 ng/kg, indicating selective retention in liver. During the elimination period, the half-life for TCDD was calculated to be 16.5 weeks, based on levels in fat biopsy samples. It should be noted that, during this 50-week withdrawal period, animal weights increased from 210 to 313 kg. This implies that at least part of the decrease in the levels is due to a dilution by the increase of body weight and, more important, body fat. It is unclear whether the high dose of 2.5 g 2,4,5-T per day had any influence on the kinetic behavior of TCDD.

In order to determine bioconcentration factors (BCFs) in beef animals, Feil et al. (2000) fed 4 growing calves with feed enriched with a number of selected dioxins and dioxin-like PCBs for 120 days. Animals received a daily dose of 225 ng TEQ (83–750 ng/congener). During this period, the weight of the animals increased from 250 to 350 kg, and the percentage of body fat increased from 4 to 10%. In addition, 4 control animals were included, and analysis of the tissues of these animals showed that a second contamination source was present. This source was shown to be wood posts treated with PCP. As a result, both the control and dosed animals showed high levels (100 to 1500 ng/kg fat) of hexa-, hepta-, and octachlorinated dioxins, which are typical contaminants in PCP. Both the hepta- and octachlorinated congeners accumulated in the liver. The tetra- and pentachlorinated dioxins and furans were only observed in the dosed animals and reached levels in back and perirenal fat of up to 300 (TCDD), 100 (PeCDD), 5 (TCDF), and 100 (2,3,4,7,8-PeCDF) ng/kg. Fat-based levels of TCDD in ribeye were twice as high. TEQ levels reached maximum levels of 260 and 20 ng TEQ per kg fat in back fat of dosed and control animals. Based on these data, about 30 to 50% of the TCDD, PeCDD, and PeCDF was retained. As in other animals, TCDF was only retained at a level of 1%. A recent follow-up study on PCP-contaminated wood in animal facilities showed that this source may still be responsible for a large portion of the increased beef residues in U.S. cattle (Fries et al., 2002a). A close relationship was observed between dioxin and PCP levels in wood, showing that the latter may serve as a good indicator for contamination.

Thorpe et al. (2001) treated 10 Holstein–Friesian heifers with 5 lower chlorinated dioxin congeners for 4 weeks at a dose of 150 ng/congener/day or 405 ng TEQ per day. This regimen was followed by withdrawal periods of 1, 14, and 27 weeks. Initial levels in fat varied from 48 for TCDD to 22 ng/kg for 1,2,3,6,7,8-HxCDD but decreased three- to fourfold during the next 26 weeks. During this period, animal weights increased from 340 to 490 kg, again showing that part of the decrease in the levels can be attributed to the increase in body fat. Half-lives calculated in fat tissue were calculated to be 93 days for 2,3,7,8-TCDD, 126 days for 1,2,3,7,8-PeCDD, 148 days for 1,2,3,6,7,8-HxCDD, 106 days for 2,3,4,7,8-PeCDF, and 124 days for 1,2,3,4,7,8-hexachlorodibenzofuran (HxCDF). Levels in muscle fat were initially 6 times higher than in body fat but decreased to about 2 times at weeks 14

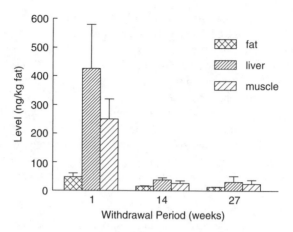

FIGURE 9.4 Levels of TCDD in subcutaneous fat, liver, and muscle tissue from cows treated for 4 weeks followed by withdrawal periods of 1, 14, and 27 weeks. Similar results were obtained for the other four congeners. (Adapted from Thorpe et al., 2001.)

and 27 (Figure 9.4). This finding is in line with the observation of Feil et al. (2000). Based on these results, the authors concluded that levels in fat samples taken shortly after exposure may seriously underestimate the levels in other tissues, including meat. A possible explanation is the fact that perfusion (and, therefore, distribution to the fat) is much slower.

In a parallel study of their experiment with lactating cows, Richter and McLachlan (2001) fed 4 non-lactating cows with grass contaminated at background levels (0.2 ng TEQ per kg) for 11.5 weeks, followed by 4 weeks on grass contaminated with sludge (1.6 ng TEQ per kg). Two cows each were slaughtered at the end of phase 1 and 2. Average exposures during phases 1 and 2 were, respectively, 1.4 and 12.5 ng TEQ per day, the increase primarily coming from higher chlorinated PCDDs. Based on the intake and excretion in feces, apparent lower absorption with higher chlorination rate was again observed. Very remarkable was the fact that even at the still relatively low levels of exposure during phase 2, the higher chlorinated congeners accumulated in the liver. Based on organ weights, it was calculated that, at the end of this phase, approximately 4, 6, 12, 50, and 73% of the total increase in the body burdens of, respectively, 1,2,3,7,8-PeCDD, 1,2,3,6,7,8-HxCDD, 1,2,3,7,8,9-HxCDD, HpCDD, and OCDD were present in the liver. The authors hypothesized that initially all the dioxins are retained in liver and are subsequently distributed to other tissues. The higher blood/liver partition coefficient for the lower chlorinated compounds subsequently results in a more rapid distribution of these congeners to the other tissues.

Dioxins and PCBs in Chickens

One of the first reported incidents with dioxins in chickens was the chicken edema syndrome, which was reported in 1957 (Sanger et al., 1958; Schmittle et al., 1958). Millions of chicken became ill or died after eating a feed with toxic fatty acids,

These were produced from fat scrapings of cowhides, which were later shown to have been treated with polychlorophenols (reviewed by Firestone, 1973). It took until 1966 to determine that dioxins were the causal agent. It was shown that the toxic fat contained dioxin levels as high as 260 µg TEQ per kg (Higginbotham et al., 1968; Hayward et al., 1999). In 1969, another outbreak of chicken edema disease occurred in North Carolina. The cause was traced back to the accidental contamination of vegetable oil with wastewater from a pesticide plant (Firestone, 1973).

In a nationwide survey in 1996 by the U.S. Environmental Protection Agency, elevated dioxin levels were found in 2 out of 80 chicken samples (Ferrario et al., 1997; Ferrario and Byrne, 2000). Levels in these 2 samples were about 37 ng TEQ per kg, mainly derived from TCDD (50 to 60%). The contamination was traced back to the use of contaminated ball clay as an anti-caking agent in the feed. Further studies on different batches of ball clay revealed average levels around 1 µg TEQ per kg product, which had fortunately been used at a rate of less than 1% in feed for chickens, catfish, and cows (Ferrario et al., 2000). After termination of this use, the Food and Drug Administration investigated dioxin levels in catfish and eggs, focusing on the presence of TCDD only as a screening method. In 24 egg samples, all derived from hens exposed to ball clay, TCDD levels varied between 0.6 and 2.5 ng TEQ per kg wet weight. Based on the 60% contribution of TCDD to the total TEQ and 10% fat in the egg, this indicates levels of about 10 to 30 ng TEQ per kg fat. Interestingly, the highest levels in this survey were obtained from a producer who used feed without ball clay but who had fortified the feed with fat from contaminated chickens. A similar problem, due to rendering of contaminated fat, occurred during a large food incident that occurred in January 1999.

In April 1999, RIKILT (The Netherlands) became involved in the Belgian dioxin crisis after detecting dioxin levels of 0.78 µg TEQ per kg in chicken feed, 0.96 µg TEQ per kg in chicken fat, and 0.71 µg TEQ per kg in egg fat (Hoogenboom et al., 1999). Guided by the congener pattern (primarily PCDFs), PCBs were analyzed and shown to be the source, with indicator PCB levels of 31.7, 36.9, and 35.1 mg/kg product in feed, chicken fat, and egg fat, respectively (Hoogenboom et al., 1999). Based on these data, it became apparent that the 80,000 kg of fat used for the production of chicken and pig feed in January had been contaminated by at least 200 kg of PCB oil contaminated with high levels of in particular dibenzofurans (PCDFs) (Bernard et al., 1999; Larebeke et al., 2001). The difference in the quantity of 50 kg described in the chapter by De Bont et al. (2005) can be explained by the use of indicator PCBs, which represent only 30 to 40% of an Aroclor 1254/1260 technical mixture. Feed and food samples were eventually sent to RIKILT because of problems with the hatching success of eggs, the viability of the young chickens, and symptoms in adult chickens resembling the chicken edema syndrome, pointing in the direction of dioxins. Because the incident was discovered 3 months after it had occurred, the contamination could spread across the food chain and required the analysis of many food items for dioxins. Unfortunately, the analysis of dioxins is very difficult and expensive and only a limited capacity was available. At the end of June, it was therefore decided to accept PCB analysis as an indicator for dioxins. Based on a ratio of 50,000 between the sum of the so-called indicator PCBs (PCBs 28, 53, 101, 118. 138, 153, and 180) and dioxins (expressed in TEQs), PCB limits

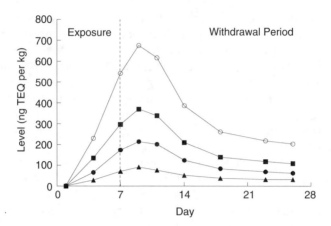

FIGURE 9.5 Levels of dioxins (closed circles), non-ortho-PCBs (closed triangles), and mono-ortho-PCBs (closed cubes), as well as total TEQ levels (open circles) in chicken eggs. Chickens were exposed for 7 days and subsequently fed clean feed.

of 200 ng/g fat for animal and egg fat and 100 ng/g fat for milk fat were established in Belgium. It was assumed that the ratio would be constant over time; that is, kinetics for the indicator PCBs and dioxins in animals were assumed to be identical. Although some studies had been performed in chickens on either dioxins or PCBs, no studies were available to support this assumption.

TRANSFER OF DIOXINS AND PCBS FROM FEED TO EGGS

In order to study the similarity in kinetics of dioxins and PCBs, carryover studies were performed with broilers, laying hens, and pigs fed with Belgian feed (Traag et al., 2001; Hoogenboom et al., 2002a). The studies focused on the depletion of dioxins and PCBs following a short exposure period of 1 week. The mixture of two original chicken feeds, containing 1 and 4% contaminated fat, was diluted tenfold for this study. Levels of dioxins, non-ortho-PCBs, and mono-ortho-PCBs were, respectively, 61, 23, and 116 ng TEQ per kg. In addition, the feed contained 3.2 mg/kg of indicator PCBs, resulting in a ratio between the indicator PCBs and dioxins of 52,000. Figure 9.5 shows the levels of dioxins and non-ortho- and mono-ortho-PCBs in egg fat. The levels showed a maximum at day 10 (i.e., 3 days after termination of the exposure). This can be explained by the production process of an egg in the ovarium of the hen, which requires about 10 days. Maximum levels of dioxins and total TEQ levels (dioxins and PCBs) were 214 and 675 ng TEQ per kg fat, respectively. Based on the 10- to 15-fold dilution of the original feed, this suggests that, during the first weeks of the incident, total TEQ levels as high as 10 µg TEQ per kg or 60 µg TEQ per egg might have occurred. Such levels were never measured because the first eggs and chickens were sampled several weeks after the feed had been replaced by clean feed.

Indicator PCB levels followed a pattern similar to that for dioxins with a maximum level of 17 mg/kg egg fat at day 10. Lower chlorinated PCBs 28, 52, and 101 were less present in the fat and more rapidly excreted during the depletion period than PCBs 118, 138, 153, and 180.

Dioxins in Eggs from Free-Range Chickens

In 2001, a new monitoring program was started in The Netherlands to investigate products of animal origin, such as meat and eggs. Both in 2001 and 2002, over 300 samples were screened in the CALUX bioassay (Hoogenboom, 2002) and suspected samples were investigated by gas chromatography/mass spectrometry (GC/MS). In addition, samples collected in each quarter of the year were pooled per type of sample and analyzed by GC/MS in order to investigate the average background level of dioxins and co-planar PCBs in these products. In 2001, 57 egg samples were screened; 2 of these eggs (3.5%) showed a positive response and were shown to contain dioxin levels of 5.0 and 7.7 ng TEQ per kg fat and total TEQ levels (including PCBs) of 5.5 and 11.3 ng TEQ per kg. The latter sample was traced back to a small farm with free-ranging chickens which sold its eggs locally. For comparison, dioxin levels determined in 4 pool samples prepared from the 57 egg samples varied between 0.5 and 0.7 ng TEQ per kg, and total TEQ levels varied between 0.8 and 1.5 ng TEQ per kg. Because this observation indicated that many more farms with free-range chickens might produce eggs with dioxin levels over the residue limit, 17 farms were selected and visited. Eight of these farms were considered free-range and allowed but did not force their chickens to go outside. As a result, these chickens foraged outside for only a limited part of the day. Nine other farms were so-called organic farms, forcing their chickens to forage outside the stable for at least 8 hours per day. Screening of the 17 egg samples revealed 6 positive samples, all coming from the organic farms. The 6 positive samples were analyzed by GC/MS, and 1 sample had a dioxin level above the Dutch limit at that time of 5 ng TEQ per kg, and 2 other samples had a level at or above the new EU limit of 3 ng TEQ per kg. Total TEQ levels varied between 2.9 and 10.5 ng TEQ per kg, showing that dioxin-like PCBs may contribute significantly to the residue levels.

An attempt was made to find the source of the contamination at the first farm. Feed samples were negative in the CALUX assay (i.e., lower than 0.4 ng TEQ per kg). Furthermore, similar feed was used in farms without free-ranging chickens and as such seems unlikely to contribute more than 1 ng TEQ per kg fat. Water samples did not contain significant levels; therefore, it seemed likely that the source of the contamination was outside the stable and possibly related to the ingestion of contaminated soil. Samples of soil and straw collected outside and inside the stable contained dioxin levels of 1.1 and 1.6 ng TEQ per kg, respectively, and total TEQ levels of 1.3 and 3.0 ng TEQ per kg, respectively, which are not abnormal levels in Western countries. However, assuming a complete transfer of dioxins to the egg and a fat content of 6 g per egg, a total of at least 60 pg total TEQ should be ingested per day or at least 46 g of the soil contaminated at 1.3 ng TEQ per kg; therefore, it cannot be excluded that worms or insects, able to accumulate dioxins, may play a role in the contamination.

Schuler et al. (1997b) performed a field survey on chickens from 5 farms. Soil samples taken from a depth of 0 to 10 cm were analyzed and shown to contain 11,

13, 1.8, 1.3, and 1.4 ng I-TEQ per kg dry weight. Corresponding levels in single eggs were 3.1 and 6.1, 19 and 12, 4.6 and 2.3, 6.1, and 3.5 ng I-TEQ per kg fat, respectively. The relatively low levels in eggs from the first farm were hypothesized to be due to the high density of chickens on this particular farm as compared to the other farms, resulting in the disappearance of soil organisms.

Harnly et al. (2000) described a more controlled study on a contaminated area close to a pentachlorophenol wood treatment facility in Oroville, California. Soil concentrations of around 6 ng I-TEQ per kg (range, 1.5–46) resulted in egg levels of 20 to 50 ng I-TEQ per kg fat (range, 0.8–140). The fraction of eggs exceeding 10 ng I-TEQ per kg was around 70 to 90%. Modeling of the data indicated that, for confined chickens, a soil level of 2.7 ng TEQ per kg was required to result in an egg level of 10 ng I-TEQ per kg fat; however, a soil level of only 0.4 ng TEQ per kg was required for chickens that had a larger area to forage. Again, this suggests a role for worms and insects, as their presence is more likely at lower densities.

Wågman et al. (2001) showed that worms fed contaminated food are able to accumulate, in particular, the more chlorinated PCBs, mainly due to a slower elimination of these congeners. Matscheko et al. (2002) studied levels in soil and worms and observed that the accumulation of certain PCBs from soil to worms is higher than that of 2,3,7,8-substituted dioxins. In general, the ratios between worm lipids and soil organic matter were on the order of 1 to 20 for PCBs and 0.1 to 1 for dioxins, with higher accumulation of the tetra- and penta-chlorinated PCDD/Fs. Regarding the lipid content of worms (1–2%) and percentage of organic matter in soil (2–6%), levels of PCBs in worms on a wet weight basis in general exceeded those in soil. For dioxins, this seems to be less so.

In general, these studies confirm that very low soil levels already result in high levels in eggs, which appear to be a very sensitive product. In fact, preliminary data obtained at RIKILT show that the new EU limit for feed is actually too high to guarantee egg levels below the new EU limit for eggs (Traag et al., 2003).

DIOXINS AND PCBS IN BROILERS

As described earlier, a carryover study was performed on broilers with the Belgian feed (Traag et al., 2001; Hoogenboom et al., 2004). Broilers were fed for 1 week with the diluted feed described above, followed by periods on clean feed for 1 or 3 weeks. Table 9.2 shows the levels of dioxins, dioxin-like non- and mono-ortho-PCBs, and indicator PCBs. The major decrease in tissue levels appears to be due to the growth of the animals. Based on normal growth curves, body weight will increase from 800 at week 0 to 1500 and 2500 g at weeks 1 and 3, respectively. Fat levels will increase from 13 to 14 and 16%, resulting in body fat levels of about 100, 200, and 400 g, respectively. As can be seen from Table 9.2, dioxin and PCB levels showed a similar two- and fourfold reduction, thus suggesting very little metabolism and excretion. No congener-specific accumulation and depletion were observed, with the exception of levels of PCB 77 which were relatively low at week 0 and decreased more than sixfold during the depletion phase.

Vos et al. (2003) performed a carryover study with the 7 indicator PCBs at levels as low as 3 and 12 µg/kg feed, which are below the Belgium limit of 200 µg/kg fat.

TABLE 9.2

Levels of Dioxins, Non-Ortho-PCBs, Mono-PCBs, and Indicator PCBs in Fat of Broilers Fed with Contaminated Feed for 1 Week Followed by Clean Feed for 1 or 3 Weeks[a]

Week	Dioxins (ng TEQ per kg)	Non-Ortho-PCBs (ng TEQ per kg)	Mono-Ortho-PCBs (ng TEQ per kg)	Total	Indicator PCBs (μg/kg)
0	102	84	216	402	6234
1	55	41	121	217	3165
3	26	22	61	109	1522

[a] Fat samples from 5 broilers per sampling point were pooled.

Broiler chickens were exposed during their 6-week lifetime. Fat levels in feed were also varied (4, 6, or 8%). During the last 29 to 42 days, the intake and output through feces were monitored, resulting in bioavailability rates of 68 and 82% for the 3 and 12 μg/kg feeds, respectively. Levels in abdominal fat, thighs, and breast were 26, 20, and 63 μg/kg, respectively, at the lower PCB level, and 117, 41, and 107 μg/kg, respectively, at the high level. The percentage of fat in the feed did not influence the bioavailability and levels in the tissues. These data suggest that levels in abdominal fat may not be representative for other tissues; in particular, the percentage of fat in the breast is very low which may easily lead to variations in the figures. No congener specific data were presented.

Dioxins in Pigs

Table 9.3 shows the levels of dioxins and dioxin-like and indicator PCBs in back fat of 3-month-old pigs fed tenfold-diluted Belgian feed for 1 week, followed by clean feed for up to 12 weeks (Hoogenboom et al., 2004). By age 3 months, pigs will normally grow from an initial 20 kg (11% fat) to 110 kg (28%) during the experimental period, resulting in an increase in body fat content of 2.2 to 30 kg. The 14-fold increase in body fat reflects a decrease in PCB levels of about 13-fold. Dioxin levels, however, seem to decrease somewhat more rapidly (20-fold). As in the case of cows, both TCDF and 1,2,3,7,8-PeCDF were barely detectable in the fat, and levels decreased very rapidly during the elimination phase. The same was true for PCBs 28 and 77. Relative levels of other dioxin-like and indicator PCBs initially reflected feed levels, but the lower chlorinated congeners (e.g., PCBs 101, 118, 126) were eliminated more quickly than the higher chlorinated PCBs (e.g., 138, 153 and 180).

POLYCYCLIC AROMATIC HYDROCARBONS

Incomplete combustion may result in the production of polycyclic aromatic hydrocarbons (PAHs). Many different PAHs have been identified, and a number of these compounds have been shown to be potent carcinogens, both in animals and humans.

TABLE 9.3

Levels of Dioxins, Non-Ortho-PCBs, Mono-PCBs, and 7 Indicator PCBs in Fat of Pigs Fed with Contaminated Feed for 1 Week Followed by Clean Feed for 15 Weeks

Week	Dioxins (ng TEQ per kg)	Non-Ortho-PCBs (ng TEQ per kg)	Mono-Ortho-PCBs (ng TEQ per kg)	Total	Indicator PCBs (µg/kg)
0	26.1	15.3	81.9	123.3	3614
1	21.8	10.3	63.0	95.1	2566
2	15.0	6.4	48.1	69.5	1787
4	7.4	3.0	29.4	39.8	1244
8	3.3	1.3	17.7	22.3	866
12	1.3	0.6	10.3	11.9	603

Note: Biopsy samples were obtained from 5 pigs and pooled prior to analysis. Levels of the 7 indicator PCBs were determined in fat from individual pigs ($n = 5$ per sampling point).

The most notorious congener is benzo(a)pyrene. In a recent report, the Scientific Committee on Food of the EU has recommended a reduction in exposure to these compounds as much as possible. High levels of PAHs may be present in feed or feed ingredients, in particular when dried, as well as in the environment of the animals. In general, however, the relative contribution of food of animal origin to the oral intake of PAHs by consumers appears to be low. This is most likely due to the fact that PAHs can be extensively metabolized; however, data on the possible transfer from feed to food are scarce (IPCS, 1998).

Laurent et al. (2001) fed two growing pigs with 1 L of milk spiked with radiolabeled benzo(a)pyrene (233 µg/L) or phenanthrene (49 µg/L). The amount of radiolabel was analyzed in blood samples taken from the vena porta and the brachiocephalic artery. As shown in Figure 9.6, both compounds were rapidly absorbed, and within 24 hours most of the radiolabel was eliminated from the blood. Despite the fact that the dose of phenanthrene was 5 times less, much higher plasma levels were reached with this compound, indicating a higher absorption or lower distribution in tissues. The authors did not investigate whether the radiolabel was present as the parent compound or its metabolites. In addition, no studies were performed on the presence of radiolabel in edible tissues.

Grova et al. (2002a) studied the fate of ^{14}C-labeled phenanthrene, pyrene, benzo-(a)pyrene, and TCDD in lactating goats, at single oral doses of 219, 233, 316, and 479 µg, respectively. Levels of the radiolabel in blood, measured 7 hours after dosing, were highest for pyrene and phenanthrene, with five- to tenfold lower levels for TCDD and benzo(a)pyrene. Levels decreased subsequently for all 4 compounds. Levels in milk were highest for TCDD at 22 hours (9 ng/mL), with a gradual decrease. Fivefold lower levels of radiolabel were present in the case of pyrene and phenanthrene, with peaks at 22 and 7 hours, respectively. Almost no benzo(a)pyrene-related radioactivity was detected in milk. Total amounts of radiolabel excreted in

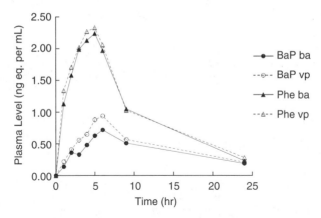

FIGURE 9.6 Levels of radiolabeled compounds in blood taken from the portal vein (vp) or branchiocephalic artery (ba) of two pigs fed with milk containing benzo(a)pyrene (BaP) or phenanthrene (Phe). (Adapted from Laurent et al., 2001.)

milk within the first 103 hours were 1.5, 1.9, 0.2, and 7.8% for phenanthrene, pyrene, benzo(a)pyrene, and TCDD, respectively. In the same period, amounts excreted into urine were 40.4, 11.4, 6.3, and 0.7% and in feces 21.7, 25.5, 88.2, and 20.3%, respectively.

These data show that the more toxic congener benzo(a)pyrene is poorly absorbed from the gastrointestinal tract and transferred to milk, either unchanged or as metabolites. The relatively low levels in blood for benzo(a)pyrene seem to exclude the possibility that most of this compound is metabolized and excreted in the bile. The less lipophilic PAHs are effectively absorbed and to a small extent excreted in the milk. These data could explain the rather low levels of PAHs and absence of benzo(a)pyrene in milk from cows grazing in the vicinity of possible sources (Grova et al., 2002b).

Ciganek et al. (2002) used 1-hydroxypyrene in urine as a marker of exposure for cows and pigs on 5 Czech farms. Average urinary excretions of this metabolite of pyrene were found to be 0.46 and 189 µg/day for pigs and cows, respectively. These excretions were estimated to represent about 3.2 and 11.9% of the total daily exposure. Assuming that all pyrene is excreted in urine as this metabolite, the figure of 11.9% is remarkably close to that obtained by Grova et al. (2002a) for goats. Ciganek et al. (2002) also estimated total exposure of pigs and cows to total and carcinogenic PAHs through feed, water, and air. For pigs, the daily intake was 0.26 mg total PAHs (2.6 µg/kg bw per day), with about a 4% contribution of carcinogenic PAHs. Primarily due to the intake of forages, the figures for cows were much higher: 14 mg/day (35 µg/kg bw per day) and 16%, respectively.

BROMINATED FLAME RETARDANTS

The appearance of brominated flame retardants in the environment and the food chain has caused increasing concern. Several different classes of compounds are or have been used (Figure 9.7), such as polybrominated biphenyls (PBBs), polybrominated

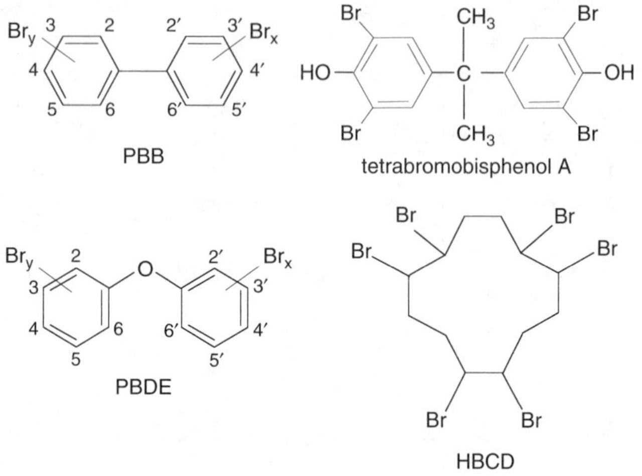

FIGURE 9.7 Structures of polybrominated flame retardants.

diphenylethers (PBDEs), and hexabromocyclododecane (HBCD). Several of these compounds have been shown to be very persistent in the environment and to accumulate in fatty tissues.

One of the most tragic accidents involving food-producing animals was the Michigan incident that occurred in the fall of 1973 (Carter, 1976). The feed additive NutriMaster (magnesium oxide) was accidentally substituted with FireMaster FF-1, a flame retardant based on polybrominated biphenyls (PBBs). Total PBB intakes as high as 250 g per cow in about 16 days were estimated, initially resulting in symptoms such as body-weight loss, decreased milk production, and a very typical effect on hoof growth. Fries (1985) estimated that up to 250 kg of FireMaster was fed to the livestock, of which 125 kg was eliminated through the feces and 94 kg ended up in human food before regulation. The main constituents of FireMaster are PBB 153 (2,2′,4,4′,5,5′-hexabromobiphenyl; 47%) and PBB 180 (2,2′,3,4,4′,5,5′-heptabromobiphenyl; 24%). As in the case of the Belgian PCB incident, most of the contaminated food was consumed before the problem was discovered. And, very similar to that crisis, the cause was only discovered due to the action of individual persons who kept looking for the agent causing the death and disease of the animals. After elucidating the cause, 9 months after the actual incident, Fries et al. (1978) were able to obtain 32 cows that had been exposed to 200 to 400 g PBB over 14 days. Six cows were slaughtered directly, and 12 others died or had to be killed within 3 months. The latter group contained the highest body fat levels (0.2–4 g/kg). Milk fat levels in these cows were 0.1 to 0.7 g/kg. Fourteen cows were kept on clean feed for 6 to 9 months and at the end showed body fat and milk fat levels of 20 to 150 and 16 to 51 µg/kg, respectively. The half-life in milk fat averaged 60 days (range, 36–301 days) (Cook et al., 1978). During this depletion phase, a good correlation between body and milk fat was observed, with the latter being 42% of the former. A small part of the PBBs was excreted through the feces (10 mg/day), as compared to 65 mg/day via the milk. This finding indicates active elimination of this type of compound through the feces. Based on the half-life, it can be estimated that the initial PBB levels in milk were 2 to 3 g/kg.

Even before this incident, Fries and Marrow (1975) performed a carryover study with 4 lactating cows exposed for 60 days to 10 mg/day of the related product FireMaster BP-6, which contained the same major congeners although with a higher hexa- to hepta- ratio. Cows produced on average 0.6 kg milk fat per day. Maximum levels of the hexa-PBB were 3 µg/g fat and were reached after 20 days. This steady-state condition was reached earlier than in the case of PCBs and DDE, the major metabolite of DDT. After termination of the exposure, a two-phase elimination was obtained with a very rapid first phase and a second phase with a half-life of 58 days. Again, the decline of 71% during the first 15 days was greater than in the case of PCBs (48%) and DDE (39%). As in the case of PCBs, the hepta- congener was not transferred as well to milk.

Similar findings were observed for the carryover of these PBB congeners to eggs (Fries et al., 1976). The study was carried out because chicken feed became contaminated by cross-contamination in mixing plants and perhaps also through the rendering of animal material. Ten laying hens were exposed for 63 days with a diet containing 20 mg/kg of FireMaster BP-6, followed by a period of 59 days on clean feed. The hepta- congener was excreted in feces to a higher extent than the hexa- congener (15 vs. 9% of intake, respectively). It was estimated that about 50 and 45% of the hepta- and hexa- congeners were excreted in the eggs during the first 63 days. Levels of the hexa- and hepta- congeners in eggs reached a plateau of about 10 and 2 mg/kg egg within 21 days and showed the typical biphasic decrease when the exposure stopped. Levels in body fat of both the hexa- and hepta- congener were 40 and 3 mg/kg at day 63 and decreased very slowly during the next 59 days. These data indicate that the PBBs in the body fat are poorly mobilized and transferred to the eggs.

Recent studies have shown the presence of PBDEs in U.S. chicken meat (2–40 ng/g fat) (Huwe et al., 2002) and in various food products in Sweden, including meat, eggs, and dairy products (Lind et al., 2002). In the latter study, the estimated intake of HBCD (162 ng/day) was about fourfold higher than that of PBDEs, with a relative contribution from meat, dairy products, and eggs of 8, 14, and 7%, respectively. No data are available on the carryover of PBDEs and HBCDs in food-producing animals, either from feed or the environment.

GENERAL DISCUSSION

This chapter has summarized the major incidents involving polyhalogenated hydrocarbons and the carryover studies that were often initiated due to a lack of required information at the time of the incidents. It is important to realize that a dramatic improvement of analytical methods was achieved during the period of more than 3 decades in which the studies described above were carried out. First, packed gas chromatography columns were replaced by capillary columns, thus achieving a much better separation of the different congeners in these complex mixtures. Second, the use of electron capture detection (ECD) was replaced by much more specific mass spectrometry detection. Many of the older studies on PCBs and PBBs were carried out with packed columns and ECD, which did not permit the study of specific congeners. Most of the selectivity was obtained by the use of specific clean-up procedures such as the use of acid silica, and most of the conclusions drawn from these studies are still valid. The dramatic improvements in analytical techniques allowed a scaling down of the doses used toward the more realistic doses obtained in practice.

The studies described in this chapter show that the carryover of contaminants from feed to edible products can be influenced by many different factors, beginning with absorption of the compounds being dependent on not only the physical properties (e.g., lipophilicity) but also the source of the contaminant. Compounds bound to air particles and deposited as such on feed may be differently absorbed than compounds present in fat ingredients in the feed. In the case of dioxins, PCBs, and PBBs, as well as PAHs, it appears that the higher chlorinated and more lipophilic congeners are more poorly absorbed than the lower chlorinated congeners. At the same time, the toxic 2,3,7,8-substituted dioxin congeners seem to be less well absorbed than the less toxic congeners (McLachlan et al., 1990). It should be pointed out that this may also indicate a more efficient excretion of the toxic congeners into the bile. This process is normally not taken into account when determining the bioavailability of compounds; however, studies with PBBs in lactating cows indicate that these compounds are actively excreted into the bile and subsequently the feces (Cook et al., 1978). A very interesting observation is the possible formation of octa- and possibly HpCDD in the gastrointestinal tract or feces of cows (Fries et al., 2002b), although the significance with respect to the consumer might be low.

Although many polyhalogenated contaminants are very persistent, metabolism is a second important factor in the carryover. Many PCBs and a number of the toxic dioxins appear to be metabolized in food-producing animals, thus explaining their poor recoveries in mass-balance studies. PAHs are very actively metabolized, in fact leading to the formation of reactive intermediates that are responsible for the adverse effects. Whether such metabolites are present in edible products has not been examined.

Last, but not least, is storage or excretion into edible products. Both the carryover into milk and eggs and the accumulation in body fat or other tissues are dependent on the physical properties of the compounds. In the case of dioxins, the carryover of the lower chlorinated and less lipophilic congeners is higher than that of the higher chlorinated congeners, whereas the non-toxic analogs are not excreted in milk at all. The higher chlorinated compounds tend to accumulate in the liver. Especially at prolonged exposure, distribution plays an important role. In both laying hens and dairy cows an equilibrium exists between the body fat and the fat in eggs and milk. This equilibrium will eventually result in a steady-state situation where a balance is obtained between the input through the feed and the output into the milk or eggs. For some compounds, this equilibrium is reached much earlier than for other compounds. In the case of growing animals such as calves, pigs, and broilers, the fat compartment will continuously increase, and such steady-state conditions will not be obtained. The data obtained by Thorpe et al. (2001) indicate that especially during the first days of exposure the levels in body fat may underestimate the levels in the fat in the meat. This may be explained by a poorer perfusion of the fat tissues in comparison to the muscle tissues.

Following termination of the exposure, the body burden plays an important role, being the sole source for transfer of contaminants to the milk or egg. In general, the depletion of persistent dioxins, PCBs, and PBBs is characterized by two phases: a rapid initial (distribution) phase and a much slower second (elimination) phase. The first phase is probably based on the uptake, distribution, and excretion of contaminants present in the gastrointestinal tract and blood. The second part represents the mobilization of contaminants from body fat and liver. It is important to realize that levels in both milk and eggs normally decrease by more than 50% during this first phase; however, in eggs, the start of the elimination phase is delayed due to the fact that the production of an egg requires about 10 days. In growing animals, dilution by increasing fat volumes is very important.

A number of groups have modeled the carryover of persistent contaminants, particularly in the lactating cow. Novel approaches are based on physiologically based pharmacokinetic modeling (PB-PK modeling) and ideally take into account the size of the different tissues and organs and factors such as blood flow and milk production (Derks et al., 1994). Several parameters have been introduced to describe the behavior. The bioconcentration factor (BCF) is used as the ratio of the concentrations in feed and milk, possibly based on a wet weight or lipid basis. This factor is influenced by the amount of feed consumed and as such by factors such as water content and energetic value; therefore, the biotransfer factor (BTF), defined as the ratio of the concentration in the milk and the total ingested quantity of contaminant, seems to be more appropriate, where the concentration in milk is ideally expressed on a fat base. The more useful parameter is the carryover rate (COR), defined as the percentage of the total amount ingested that, for example, is excreted into the milk. In most cases, this is based on the daily intake and excretion when steady-state conditions are reached, but, in the absence of such conditions, total intake and (extrapolated) excretion during the study period are also used (Table 9.1). Sometimes, the carryover rate is used as a synonym of bioavailability, being the fraction of the contaminant absorbed in the gastrointestinal tract. This does not recognize the possibility that part of the compound is excreted in the bile and feces or metabolized after mobilization from the body fat. Carryover rates can be used to determine the impact of a certain feed contamination on, for example, levels in milk; however, as long as no equilibrium exists between intake and output, such as during the first days or weeks of exposure, this will lead to an overestimation of the actual milk levels due to the fact that during this period part of the contaminants will be stored in the liver and body fat.

Current regulations for environmental contaminants tend to be based on the sum of a number of congeners, after applying the toxic equivalency principle. For toxicological reasons, this is a very good approach as it takes into account the additive nature of mixtures of compounds; however, when trying to model the behavior of contaminants in animals, it is necessary to base such modeling on individual congeners with regard to the differences in behavior described in this chapter. A feed contamination of lower chlorinated dioxins (e.g., as in 2,4,5-T) will give much higher TEQ levels in milk than a feed contamination with a similar TEQ level but derived from higher chlorinated compounds (as in PCP). The same is true for PCB mixtures, although the variations in congener patterns found in practice might be much lower;

however, a rendered fat derived from exposed animals might contain the more stable congeners and as such give a much higher carryover.

CONCLUSIONS

This chapter shows that contamination of feed and the environment with contaminants imposes a major threat to the quality of food of animal origin. Increasing knowledge on the toxic effects of these compounds often results in a further reduction of exposure limits and in most cases a reduction of maximum residue levels in food and feed. In order to allow proper tuning of limits in food and feed, it is important to understand the fate of contaminants in food-producing animals. Such information can best be obtained from controlled animal studies, ideally performed with incurred feed and accompanied by modeling of the different parameters. Important factors are the length of the exposure, the levels used in the study as compared to the actual levels observed in practice, the congener pattern of the contamination, and whether or not the absorption can be influenced by the matrix. Such information is also essential when evaluating the consequences of a feed incident for the general public. At present, most data refer to the carryover of dioxins from feed to milk in dairy cows, with clear information on the maximum transfer of the different dioxin and PCB congeners, as expressed in the carryover rates, as well as half-lives after termination of exposure. Much less information is available on pigs, broilers, and laying hens, although in particular the contamination of eggs from free-range chickens presents a problem. Data on the carryover of flame retardants such as PBDEs and HBCD, as well as the PAHs, are scarce, although these compounds can be present in feed and the environment of food-producing animals; however, recent studies indicate that the carryover of carcinogenic polyaromatic hydrocarbons to milk is low.

REFERENCES

Baumann, R.A., Den Boer, A.C., Groenemeijer, G.S., Den Hartog, R.S., Hijman, W.C., Liem, A.K.D., Marsman, J.A., and Hoogerbrugge, R. (2002) Dioxinen en dioxineachtige PCBs in Nederlandse consumptiemelk: trendonderzoek 1997–2001, *RIVM rapport* 639102024/2002, Bilthoven, The Netherlands.

Berg, M. van den, Birnbaum, L.S., Bosveld, A.T.C., Brunström, B., Cook, Ph., Feeley, M., Giesy, J.P., Hanberg, A., Hasegawa, R., Kennedy, S.W., Kubiak, T., Larsen, J.C., Leeuwen, F.X.R. van, Liem, A.K.D., Nolt, C., Peterson, R.E., Poellinger, L., Safe, S., Schrenk, D., Tillitt, D., Tysklind, M., Younes, M., Wärn, F., and Zacharewski, T. (1998) Toxic equivalency factors (TEFs) for PCBs, PCDDs, PCDFs for humans and wildlife, *Environ. Health Persp.*, 106: 775–792.

Bernard, A., Hermans, C., Broeckaert, F., Poorter, G. de, Cock, A. de, and Hoins, G. (1999) Food contamination by PCBs and dioxins; an isolated episode in Belgium is unlikely to have affected public health, *Nature*, 401: 231–232.

Carter, L.J. (1976) Michigan's PBB incident: chemical mix-up leads to disaster, *Science*, 192: 240–243.

Cigenek, M., Ulrich, R., Neca, J., and Raszyk, J. (2002) Exposure of pig fatteners and dairy cows to polycyclic aromatic hydrocarbons, *Veterinari Medicina*, 47: 137–142.

Cook, R.M. Prewitt, L.R., and Fries, G.F. (1978) Effects of activated carbon, phenobarbital, and vitamins A, D, and E on polybrominated biphenyl excretion in cows, *J. Dairy Sci.*, 61, 414–419.

De Bont, R., Elskens, M., Baeyens, W., Hens, L., and Larebeke, N. van (2005) A survey of 3 PCB and dioxin contamination episodes: from contamination of food items to body burdens, in *Reviews in Food and Nutrition Toxicity*, Preedy, V.R. and Watson, R.R., Eds., CRC Press, Boca Raton, FL.

Derks, H.J.G.M., Berende, P.L.M., Olling, M., Everts, H., Liem, A.K.D., and Jong, A.P.J.M. de (1994) Pharmacokinetic modeling of polychlorinated dibenzo-*p*-dioxins (PCDDs) and furans (PCDFs) in cows, *Chemosphere*, 28: 711–715.

EC (2001) Council regulation (EC) No. 2375/2001 of November 29, 2001, amending Commission Regulation (EC) No. 466/2001 setting maximum levels for certain contaminants in foodstuffs, *Off. J. Eur. Commun.*, L321: 1–5.

EC (2002) Council directive 2001/102/EC of November 27, 2001, amending Directive a999/29/EC on the undesirable substances and products in animal nutrition, *Off. J. Eur. Commun.*, L6: 45–49.

Feil, V.J., Huwe, J.K., Zaylskie, R.G., Davison, K.L., Anderson, V.L., Marchello, M., and Tiernan, T.O. (2000) Chlorinated dibenzo-*p*-dioxin and dibenzofuran concentrations in beef animals from a feeding study, *J. Agric. Food Chem.*, 48: 6163–6173.

Ferrario, J.P. and Byrne, C.J. (2000) The concentration and distribution of 2,3,7,8–dibenzo-*p*-dioxins/-furans in chickens, *Chemosphere*, 40: 221–224.

Ferrario, J., Byrne, C., Lorber, M., Saunders, P., Leese, W., Dupuy, A., Winters, D., Cleverly, D., Schaum, J., Pinsky, P., Deyrup, C., Ellis, R., and Walcott, J. (1997) A statistical survey of dioxin-like compounds in United States poultry fat, *Organohalogen Comp.*, 32: 245–251.

Ferrario, J.P., Byrne, C.J., and Cleverly, D.H. (2000) 2,3,7,8-Dibenzo-*p*-dioxins in mined clay products from the United States: evidence for possible natural origin, *Environ. Sci. Technol.*, 34: 4524–4532.

Firestone, D. (1973) Etiology of chick edema disease, *Environ. Health Persp.*, 5: 59–66.

Firestone, D., Clower, M., Borsetti, A.P., Teske, R.H., and Long, P.E. (1979) Polychlorodibenzo-*p*-dioxin and pentachlorophenol residues in milk and blood of cows fed technical pentachlorophenol, *J. Agric. Food Chem.*, 27: 1171–1177.

Fries, G.F. (1985) The PBB episode in Michigan: an overall appraisal, *CRC Crit. Rev. Toxicol.*, 16: 105–156.

Fries, G.F. (1987) Assessment of potential residues in foods derived from animals exposed to TCDD-contaminated soil, *Chemosphere*, 16: 2123–2128.

Fries, G.F. and Marrow, G.S. (1975) Excretion of polybrominated biphenyls into the milk of cows, *J. Dairy Sci.*, 58, 947–951.

Fries, G.F., Marrow, G.S., and Gordon, C.H. (1973) Long-term studies of residue retention and excretion by cows fed a polychlorinated biphenyl (Arochlor 1254), *J. Agric. Food Chem.*, 21: 117–121.

Fries, G.F., Cecil, H.C., Bitman, J., and Lillie, R.J. (1976) Retention and excretion of polybrominated biphenyls by hens, *Bull. Environ. Contam. Toxicol.*, 15: 278–282.

Fries, G.F., Cook, R.M., and Prewitt, L.R. (1978) Distribution of polybrominated biphenyl residues in the tissues of environmentally contaminated dairy cows, *J. Dairy Sci.*, 61, 420–425.

Fries, G.F., Paustenbach, D.J., Mather, D.B., and Luksemburg, W.J. (1999) A congener specific evaluation of transfer of chlorinated dibenzo-*p*-dioxins and dibenzofurans to milk of cows following ingestion of pentachlorophenol-treated wood, *Environ. Sci. Technol.*, 33: 1165–1170.

Fries, G.F., Veil, V.J., Zaylskie, R.G., Bialek, K.M., and Rice, C.P. (2002a) Treated wood in livestock facilities: relationships among residues of pentachlorophenol, dioxins, and furans in wood and beef, *Environ. Pollut.*, 116: 301–307.

Fries, G.F., Paustenbach, D.J., and Luksemburg, W.J. (2002b) Complete mass balance of dietary polychlorinated dibenzo-*p*-dioxins and dibenzofurans in dairy cattle and characterization of the apparent synthesis of hepta- and octachlorodioxins, *J. Agric. Food Chem.*, 50: 4226–4231.

Fürst, P., Krause, G.H.M., Hein, D., Delschen, T., and Wilmers, K. (1993) PCDD/PCDF in cow's milk in relation to their levels in grass and soil, *Chemosphere*, 27: 1349–1357.

Grova, N., Feidt, C., Laurent, C., and Rychen, G. (2002a) [^{14}C] milk, urine and faeces excretion kinetics in lactating goats after an oral administration of [^{14}C] polycyclic aromatic hydrocarbons, *Int. Dairy Sci.*, 12: 1025–1031.

Grova, N., Feidt, C., Crépineau, C., Laurent, C., Lafargue, P.E., Hachimi, A., and Rychen, G. (2002b) Detection of polycyclic aromatic hydrocarbon levels in milk collected near potential contamination sources, *J. Agric. Food Chem.*, 50: 4640–4642.

Harnly, M.E., Petreas, M.X., Flattery, J., and Goldman, L.R. (2000) Polychlorinated dibenzo-*p*-dioxin and polychlorinated dibenzofuran contamination in soil and home-produced chicken eggs near pentachlorophenol sources, *Environ. Sci. Technol.*, 34: 1143–1149.

Hayward, D.G., Nortrup, D., Gardner, A., and Clower, M. (1999) Elevated TCDD in chicken eggs and farm-raised catfish fed a diet with ball clay from a Southern United States mine, *Environ. Res. A*, 81: 248–256.

Higginbotham, G.R., Huang, A., Firestone, D., Verrett, J., Ress, J., and Campbell, A.D. (1968) Chemical and toxicological evaluations of isolated and synthetic chloro derivatives of dibenzo-*p*-dioxin, *Nature*, 220: 702–703.

Hoogenboom, L.A.P. (2002) The combined use of the CALUX bioassay and the HRGC/HRMS method for the detection of novel dioxin sources and new dioxin-like compounds, *Environ. Sci. Pollut. Res.*, 9: 9–11.

Hoogenboom, L.A.P., Traag, W.A., and Mengelers, M.J.B. (1999) The Belgian Dioxin Crisis: Involvement of RIKILT, poster presented at Dioxin '99, Venice, Italy.

Hoogenboom, L.A.P., Traag, W.A., Kan, C.A., Bovee, T.F.H., Weg, G. van der, Onstenk, C., and Portier, L. (2002a) Residues of dioxins and PCBs in eggs following short-term exposure of laying hens to feed from the Belgian crisis, *Organohalogen Comp.*, 57: 241–244.

Hoogenboom, L.A.P., Bruchem, G.D. van, Sonne, K., Enninga, I.C., Rhijn, J.A. van, Heskamp, H., Huveneers-Oorsprong, M.B.M., Hoeven, J.C.M. van der, and Kuiper, H.A. (2002b) Absorption of a mutagenic metabolite released from protein-bound residues of furazolidone, *Environ. Toxicol. Pharmacol.*, 11: 273–287.

Hoogenboom, L.A.P., Kan, C.A., Bovee, T.F.H., Weg, G., van der, Onstenk, C., and Traag, W.A. (2004) Residues of dioxins and indicator PCBs in fat of growing pigs and broilers fed contaminated feed, *Chemosphere*, in press.

Huwe, J.K., Lorentzsen, M., Thuresson, K., and Bergman, A. (2002) Analysis of mono- to deca-brominated diphenyl ethers in chickens at the part per billion level, *Chemosphere*, 46(5): 635–640.

IPCS. (1998) *Selected Non-Heterocyclic Polycyclic Aromatic Hydrocarbons*, Environmental Health Criteria 202, International Programme on Chemical Safety, WHO, Geneva.

Jensen, D.J. and Hummel, R.A. (1982) Secretion of TCDD in milk and cream following the feeding of TCDD to lactating dairy cows, *Bull. Environ. Contam. Toxicol.*, 29: 440–446.

Jensen, D.J., Hummel, R.A., Mahle, N.H., Kocher, C.W., and Higgins H.S. (1981) A residue study on beef cattle consuming 2,3,7,8-tetrachlorodibenzo-*p*-dioxin, *J. Agric. Food Chem.*, 29: 265–268.

Jones, D., Safe, S., Morcom, E., Holcomb, M., Coppock, C., and Ivie, W. (1987) Bioavailability of tritiated 2,3,7,8-tetrachlorodibenzo-*p*-dioxin (TCDD) administered to Holstein dairy cows, *Chemosphere*, 16: 1743–1748.

Jones, D., Safe, S., Morcom, E., Holcomb, M., Coppock, C., and Ivie, W. (1989) Bioavailability of grain and soil-borne tritiated 2,3,7,8-tetrachlorodibenzo-*p*-dioxin (TCDD) administered to lactating Holstein cows, *Chemosphere*, 18: 1257–1263.

Kan, C.A. (1978) Accumulation of organochlorine pesticides in poultry: a review, *J. Agric. Food Chem.*, 26: 1051–1055.

Kan, C.A. (2002) Prevention and control of contaminants of industrial processes and pesticides in the poultry production chain, *Worlds Poultry Sci. J.*, 58: 159–167.

Larebeke, N. van, Hens, L., Schepens, P., Covaci, A., Bayens, J., Everaert, K., Bernheim, J.L., Vlietinck, R., and Poorter, G. de (2001) The Belgian PCB and dioxin incident of January–June 1999: exposure data and potential impact on health, *Environ. Health Persp.*, 109: 265–273.

Laurent, C., Feidt, C., Lichtfouse, E., Grova, N., Laurent, F., and Rychen, G. (2001) Milk–blood transfer of ^{14}C-tagged polycyclic aromatic hydrocarbons (PAHs) in pigs, *J. Agric. Food Chem.*, 49: 2493–2496.

Liem, A.K.D., Hoogerbrugge, R., Kootstra, P.R., Van der Velde, E.G., and De Jong, A.P.J.M. (1991) Occurrence of dioxins in cow's milk in the vicinity of municipal waste incinerators and a metal reclamation plant in The Netherlands, *Chemosphere*, 23: 1975–1984.

Lind, Y., Aune, M., Atuma, S., Becker, W., Bjerselius, R., Glynn, R., and Darnerud, P.O. (2002) Food intake of the polybrominated flame retardants PBDEs and HBCD in Sweden, *Organohalogen Comp.*, 58: 181–184.

Malisch, R. (2000) Increase of the PCDD/F-contamination of milk, butter and meat samples by use of contaminated citrus pulp, *Chemosphere*, 40: 1041–1053.

Matscheko, N., Tylskind, M., Wit, C. de, Bergek, S., Andersson, R., and Sellström, U. (2002) Application of sewage sludge to arable land-soil concentrations of polybrominated diphenyl ethers and polychlorinated dibenzo-*p*-dioxins, dibenzofurans, and biphenyls and their accumulation in earthworms, *Environ. Toxicol. Chem.*, 21: 2515–2525.

McLachlan, M.S. (1993) Mass balance of polychlorinated biphenyls and other organochlorine compounds in a lactating cow, *J. Agric. Food Chem.*, 41: 474–480.

McLachlan, M.S. and Richter, W. (1998) Uptake and transfer of PCDD/Fs by cattle fed naturally contaminated feedstuffs and feed contaminated as a result of sewage sludge application. 1. Lactating cows, *J. Agric. Food Chem.*, 46: 1166–1172.

McLachlan, M.S., Thoma, H., Reissinger, M., and Hutzinger, O. (1990) PCDD/F in an agricultural food chain; part 1: PCDD/F mass balance of a lactating cow, *Chemosphere*, 20: 1013–1020.

Olie, K., Vermeulen, P.L., and Hutzinger, O. (1977) Chlorodibenzo-*p*-dioxins and chlorodibenzofurans are trace components of fly ash and flue gas of some municipal incinerators in The Netherlands, *Chemosphere*, 8: 455–459.

Olling, M., Derks, H.J.G.M., Berende, P.L.M., Liem, A.D.K., and Jong, A.P.J.M. de (1991) Toxicokinetics of eight ^{13}C-labelled polychlorinated dibenzo-*p*-dioxins and -furans in lactating cows, *Chemosphere*, 23: 1377–1385.

Plas, S.A. van der, Sundberg, H., Berg, H. van den, Scheu, G., Wester, P., Jensen, S., Bergman, A., de Boer, J., Koeman, J.H., and Brouwer, A. (2001) Contribution of planar (0–1 *ortho*) and non-planar (2–4 *ortho*) fractions of Arochlor 1260 to the induction of altered hepatic foci in female Spague–Dawley rats, *Toxicol. Appl. Pharmacol.*, 169: 255–268.

Richter, W. and McLachlan, M.S. (2001) Uptake and transfer of PCDD/Fs by cattle fed naturally contaminated feedstuffs and feed contaminated as a result of sewage sludge application. 2. Non-lactating cows, *J. Agric. Food Chem.*, 49: 5857–5865.

Safe, S.H. (1994) Polychlorinated biphenyls (PCBs): environmental impact, biochemical and toxic responses, and implications for risk assessment, *CRC Crit. Rev. Toxicol.*, 24: 87–149.

Sanger, V.L., Scott, L., Hamdy, A., Gale, C., and Pounden W.D. (1958) Alimentary toxemia in chickens, *J. Am. Vet. Med. Assoc.*, 133: 172–176.

SCF (2001) *Opinion of the Scientific Committee on Food on the Risk Assessment of Dioxins and Dioxin-Like PCBs in Food*, Scientific Committee on Food report CS/CNTM/ DIOXIN/20 final, http://europa.eu.int/comm/food/fs/sc/scf/out90_en.pdf.

Schmidt, C.W. (1999) Poisoning young minds, *Environ. Health Persp.*, 107: 302–307.

Schmittle, S.C., Edwards, H.M., and Morris, D. (1958) A disorder of chickens probably due to a toxic feed: preliminary report, *J. Am. Vet. Med. Assoc.*, 132: 216–219.

Schuler, F., Schmid, P., and Schlatter, Ch. (1997a) Transfer of airborne polychlorinated dibenzo-*p*-dioxins and dibenzofurans into dairy milk, *J. Agric. Food Chem.*, 45: 4162–4167.

Schuler, F., Schmid, P., and Schlatter, Ch. (1997b) The transfer of polychlorinated dibenzo-*p*-dioxins and dibenzofurans from soil into eggs of foraging chicken, *Chemosphere*, 34: 711–718.

Schwind, K.J. and Kaltenecker, M. (2000) Toxaphen in fleisch und eiern, ein mögliches importiertes rückstandsproblem, *Fleischwirtschaft*, 80: 71–74.

Slob, W., Olling, M., Derks, H.J.G.M., and Jong, A.P.J.M. de (1995) Congener-specific bioavailability of PCDD/Fs and coplanar PCBs in cows: laboratory and field measurements, *Chemosphere*, 31: 3827–3838.

Thomas, G.O., Sweetman, A.J., and Jones, K.C. (1999a) Input–output balance of polychlorinated biphenyls in a long-term study of lactating dairy cows, *Environ. Sci. Technol.*, 33: 104–112.

Thomas, G.O., Sweetman, A.J., and Jones, K.C. (1999b) Metabolism and body-burden of PCBs in lactating dairy cows, *Chemosphere*, 39: 1533–1544.

Thorpe, S., Kelly, M., Startin, J., Harrison, N., and Rose, M. (2001) Concentration changes for 5 PCDD/F congeners after administration in beef cattle, *Chemosphere*, 43: 869–879.

Traag, W.A., Mengelers, M.J.B., Kan, C.A., and Malisch, R. (1999) Studies on the uptake and carry-over of polychlorinated debenzodioxins and dibenzofurans from contaminated citrus pulp pellets to cow's milk, *Organohalogen Comp.*, 42: 201–204.

Traag, W.A., Kan, C.A., Bovee, T.F.H., Weg, G. van der, Onstenk, C., Portier, L., and Hoogenboom, L.A.P. (2001) Dioxin and PCB levels in fat of pigs and broilers fed with feed from the Belgian crisis, *Organohalogen Comp.*, 51: 291–294.

Traag, W.A., Portier, L., Bovee, T.F.H., Weg, G. van der, Onstenk, C., Elghouch, N., Coors, R., Kraats, C. van de, and Hoogenboom, L.A.P. (2002) Residues of dioxins and coplanar PCBs in eggs of free range chickens, *Organohalogen Comp.*, 57: 245–248.

Traag, W.A., Kan, C.A., Zeilmaker, M., and Hoogenboom, L.A.P. (2003) Carry-over of dioxins and PCBs at low levels from feed to eggs, *Organohalogen Comp.*, 61: 381–384.

Tuinstra, L.G.M.Th., Roos, A.H., Berende, P.L.M., van Rhijn, J.A., Traag, W.A., and Mengelers, J.B. (1992) Excretion of polychlorinated dibenzo-*p*-dioxins and -furans in milk of cows fed on dioxins in the dry period, *J. Agric. Food Chem.*, 40: 1772–1776.

Vos, S. de, Maervoet, J., Schepens, P., and Schrijver, R. de (2003) Polychlorinated biphenyls in broiler diets: their digestibility and incorporation in body tissues, *Chemosphere*, 51: 7–11.

Wågman, N., Strandberg, B., and Tylskind, M. (2001) Dietary uptake and elimination of selected polychlorinated biphenyl congeners and hexachlorobenzene in earthworms, *Environ. Toxicol. Chem.*, 20: 1778–1784.

WHO (2000) Consultation on assessment of the health risk of dioxins — re-evaluation of the tolerable daily intake (TDI): executive summary, *Food Add. Contam.*, 17: 223–240.

Willett, L.B. and Hess, J.F. (1975) Polychlorinated biphenyl residues in silos in the United States, *Residue Rev.*, 55: 135–147.

Willett, L.B., Liu, T.-T.Y., and Fries, G.F. (1990) Reevaluation of polychlorinated biphenyl concentrations in milk and body fat of lactating cows, *J. Dairy Sci.*, 73: 2136–2142.

10 A Survey of Three PCB and Dioxin Contamination Episodes: From Contamination of Food Items to Body Burdens

Rinne De Bont, Marc Elskens, Willy Baeyens, Luc Hens, and Nik van Larebeke

CONTENTS

0-8493-2757-1/05/$0.00+$1.50

Abstract Belgian citizens face a high background exposure to dioxins and poly-chlorinated biphenyls (PCBs). During the past 3 years, three episodes of animal feed contamination have added to this exposure. This chapter calculates the body burdens (body burden defined as the concentration of a persistent substance accumulated in a relevant tissue or body fluid) resulting from these exposures and compares the results with measured body burden data in the Belgian population. Geometric mean PCB (sum of seven indicator congeners) background concentrations in Belgian food items range between 16.6 ng/g fat for milk and 72.1 ng/g fat for poultry. Corresponding geometric mean dioxin concentrations range between 0.8 pg TEQ per g fat for pork and 2.4 pg TEQ per g fat for poultry. On top of this, Belgium has faced three animal feed contamination episodes: a major one in 1999, one in 2000, and one in 2002. During the 1999 crisis, a substantial part of the human food chain was contaminated, with PCB concentrations in poultry up to 56,856 ng/g fat and dioxin concentrations up to 2613.4 pg TEQ per g. In 1999, and to a lesser extent in 2001, occasional incidents of isolated contamination also increased concentrations in food items, the contribution of which to body burdens should not be neglected.

Based on background exposure levels, the body burdens of Belgian female adolescents and women (ages 50 to 65) have been calculated. Calculated PCB body burdens are 75.5 µg/kg body weight for female adolescents and 147.0 µg/kg body weight for adult women, and dioxin body burdens are 3.7 ng TEQ per kg body weight for female adolescents and 7.1 ng TEQ per kg body weight for women. Measured dioxin body burdens are substantially higher and amount to 8.8 ng TEQ per kg body weight for female adolescents and 14.7 ng TEQ per kg body weight for female adults. The difference between calculated and observed values might stem from higher background levels in the past, from episodes of widespread contamination, and from exposure through other routes. Calculated PCB body burdens are 20% higher than the measured ones (57.1 µg/kg body weight for female adolescents and 121.6 µg/kg body weight for women). This difference might be explained by assumptions regarding the half-life of PCBs which overestimate the actual half-life. It was estimated that the 1999 crisis resulted in an increase of PCB body burdens by 28% and of dioxin body burdens by 4.3%. As to PCB body burdens, measurements before and after the crisis are concordant with this estimate.

INTRODUCTION

Dioxins are a group of synthetic organic chemicals that contain 210 structurally related individual chlorinated dibenzo-p-dioxins (CDDs) and chlorinated dibenzo-furans (CDFs). Of these, 17 congeners are toxicologically significant; these congeners are substituted with chlorine at the 2, 3, 7, and 8 positions on the molecule, and 2,3,7,8-tetrachlorodibenzo-p-dioxin (TCDD) is the prototype of this group of aromatic hydrocarbons. Dioxins have never been intentionally produced, except in small quantities for research. Although natural sources such as forest fires may produce dioxins, these sources are small compared to anthropogenic sources, including incineration and combustion processes, chlorine bleaching in pulp and paper mills, and chlorinated organic chemicals. Dioxins have long half-life times which explains their wide distribution in the environment. Because dioxins have a very low solubility in water and low volatility, most are contained in soil and sediments. This environmental compartment serves as a reservoir from which dioxins may be released over a long period of time.

In contrast to dioxins, PCBs did have commercial uses. Because of their stability and persistence they were used as dielectric, heat-exchange, and hydraulic fluids in capacitors and transformers. Their production ceased decades ago, but they are still among the priority global contaminants. The 209 PCB congeners differ by number and position of chlorine atoms. Dietary intake is the most important source of exposure to dioxins and dioxin-like PCBs for the general population. Meat, dairy products, fish, and other seafood products contribute more than 90% of the daily intake of the general population. Non-food sources and pathways such as air, soil, paper, smoking, and drinking water are of minor importance for human dioxin exposure. The chemical and physical stability of dioxins and PCBs explains their bioaccumulation and biomagnification in plant and animal tissues. Because they are lipophylic chemicals, dioxins and PCBs mainly accumulate in fatty tissues. In humans, the bioavailability of dioxins and dioxin-like PCBs from food containing fat or oil is known to be higher than 75%. Distribution in the body is dose and congener dependent. Dioxins and PCBs are not easily disposed of without release into the environment and the contamination of human and animal food supplies. The three animal feed and/or food incidents caused by PCBs and dioxins that have recently occurred in Belgium are described below.

THE BELGIAN PCB/DIOXIN INCIDENT OF JANUARY–JUNE 1999

Melted animal fat and household waste fat are used in the production of animal-food products. In January 1999, 60 to 80 tons of this recycled fat were contaminated with approximately 50 kg of PCBs and 1 g of dioxins originating from oil from discarded transformers. The entire amount was delivered to 10 animal-feed producers, which resulted in the contamination of 500 tons of animal feed. More than 1500 Belgian animal farms used this contaminated animal feed. The 500 tons of contaminated feed represented a limited percentage of the total amount of feed produced and used in Belgium, which is estimated to exceed 28,000 tons/week (van Larebeke et al., 2001). The first clinical signs of contamination were observed in early February 1999 on several poultry farms. The symptoms included a decrease in egg production and hatching and an epidemic of chicken edema disease. By March, toxicological analysis showed the presence of exceptionally high levels of dioxins in the animal feed, chickens, and eggs. In late May, the crisis became public. At that moment, the authorities mobilized all available laboratories for analytical work. As a result, between the end of May and the end of December 1999, over 50,000 food analyses were performed. The exposure of the population was estimated to be 4 months (February to May) (van Larebeke et al., 2001). In February 2000, the Belgian Ministry of Public Health established a Federal Agency for the Safety of the Food Chain (FAVV). This agency introduced CONSUM, a monitoring system that traces PCBs and dioxins in the food chain. Every year, 15,000 samples are analyzed. In the animal feed sector, this involves a systematic monitoring of ingredients (animal fat, fishmeal) and a representative screening of the finished product.

PCB/DIOXIN INCIDENT OF MAY–JULY 2000

In May 2000, routine CONSUM tests showed 12,587 ng PCBs per g fat in bovine feed of the animal feed company Bauduin-Cambier (Feluy, Belgium). Distribution of these products was blocked, and 201 farms underwent veterinary inspection because they used fodder delivered by this company. The feed these companies purchased from Bauduin-Cambier was analyzed, and maximum PCB levels of 213,146 ng/g fat were detected. None of the already slaughtered pigs and cows appeared to be contaminated. The contaminated feed was mainly consumed by breeding calves. Milk from different companies was analyzed. One out of 102 samples was weakly positive (208 ng/g fat) but had a different PCB profile, indicating that the contamination originated from another source.

PCB INCIDENT OF JANUARY 2002

A routine CONSUM check in January 2002 revealed that the animal-feed producer Hanekop had produced contaminated chicken feed that contained 1600 ng PCB per g fat or eight times the 200 ng/kg standard. The distribution of 19 chicken farms was blocked, and 5 of these farms were prohibited from releasing their products on the market for a longer period. Three of these companies already had their chickens slaughtered for consumption; nevertheless, the sale of the entire production of one of these companies and of a part of the production of the other two could be prevented. Only chickens for meat consumption and no laying hens were affected. Consequently, there was no contamination of eggs and their derivatives. By the end of January 2002, two samples of pig feed produced by Hanekop were shown to contain high PCB concentrations (821 and 1569 ng/g fat). The distribution of the products of 7 companies that received pig feed from Hanekop was prohibited. Analysis of the animals of these companies failed to show concentrations exceeding the standard of 200 ng/g fat. The cause of this contamination episode remains unclear.

BODY BURDEN

During these last two incidents it is unclear as to what extent the Belgian population was exposed to PCBs in food products, because no data are available on the number and nature of these contaminated food products, nor on the amount released for consumption. As a consequence of the three incidents and because background dioxin and PCB levels in Belgian food products are high, it can be assumed that Belgians are exposed to high levels of these toxicants. The toxicity of dioxins and PCBs is related to the amount accumulated in the body during one's lifetime — the so-called body burden (BB), where body burden is defined as the concentration of a persistent substance accumulated in a relevant tissue or body fluid. This BB is used to assess the toxic effects of dioxins, as it is a much better estimate of chronic exposure than the daily intake. The question arises as to what extent high background dioxin and PCB levels in combination with recurrent incidents result in high BBs in Belgium. Moreover, it is important to find out whether the incidents increased the BBs in a measurable way. The objectives of the study reported here are thus fourfold: (1) to overview the background and crisis-related levels of contamination in human food items and animal feed in Belgium; (2) to calculate the body burdens of PCBs and dioxins in Belgian women based on measurements of background dioxin and PCB concentrations in food and on available food consumption data, sufficiently representative for the Belgian population; (3) to compare these calculated body burdens to measured concentrations of PCBs and dioxins in Belgian female adolescents and adults; and (4) to evaluate the impact of the three Belgian PCB and dioxin incidents.

MATERIALS AND METHODS

Exposure: Dioxin and PCB Levels in Animal Feed, Animals, and Food Products

The PCB/Dioxin Incident of 1999

During the initial period (January to end of May) of the 1999 PCB/dioxin contamination episode, only a few measurements were performed, as the incident was dealt with in a "confidential" manner. Large-scale sampling and laboratory testing were performed after the crisis went public on May 27. We used two datasets: one with samples that were processed before September 1999 and one consisting of samples that were processed between September and December 1999. In this study, samples were categorized into two sets of data: incident-related samples (samples assumed to be affected by the feed incident) and non-incident-related samples (samples that are assumed not to be affected by the feed incident and are thus considered as background or, in the case of high levels, as linked to occasional incidents of isolated contamination).

Polychlorinated biphenyl measurements include seven marker congeners (PCBs 28, 52, 101, 118, 138, 153, and 180) and are expressed as the sum of these congeners in nanograms per gram of fat. For polychlorinated dibenzo-p-dioxins (PCDDs)/polychlorinated dibenzofurans (PCDFs), congeners with chlorine substitution of at least the 2, 3, 7, and 8 positions were measured, and the total dioxin content of the sample was expressed in picogram TEQ per gram of fat using the WHO toxic equivalency factor (TEF) values (Van den Berg et al., 1998). Dioxins were measured using mass spectrometry. PCBs were quantified using gas chromatographic techniques followed by electron capture or mass spectrometry. A pool of 23 laboratories performed the PCB measurements; 18 accredited laboratories performed dioxin measurements.

In the dataset, results below a defined detection limit were arbitrarily replaced by half the detection limit. To determine the mean PCB and dioxin concentrations, laboratories handling too high detection limits (>80 ng PCB per g fat in more than 5% of the samples) were excluded from the study. This was done to avoid an overestimation of the mean PCB and dioxin concentrations due to incorporation of results reflecting high detection limits. The numbers of samples analyzed are shown in Tables 10.2, 10.3, 10.5, and 10.6. Maximum concentrations and the percentage of samples with PCB concentrations exceeding 200 and 1000 ng PCB per g fat and with dioxin concentrations exceeding 2 and 5 pg TEQ per g fat were calculated. To get a general picture of these percentages, we did not exclude any laboratory. The numbers of samples are shown in Tables 10.2, 10.3, 10.5, and 10.6.

Background Concentrations 2001

The year 2001 had no documented PCB or dioxin incidents, and the PCB data provided by CONSUM can therefore be considered as background values. During this period, no dioxin concentrations were measured.

The PCB/Dioxin Episodes of 2000 and 2002

Data on contamination during these episodes were provided by CONSUM. They mainly concern animal feed samples. For the crisis in 2000 (Bauduin-Cambier), results of 342 PCB measurements and 10 dioxin measurements are available. For the crisis in 2002 (Hanekop), 407 PCB and 4 dioxin measurements are included. The PCB and dioxin values of these samples are compared to background values of 1999 and 2001 and to values of contaminated samples measured during the 1999 crisis.

Occasional Incidents of Isolated Contamination

Some samples, not related to any incident, showed high levels of contamination. It can be assumed that these events are related to occasional incidents of isolated contamination. To assess the extent to which these gave rise to high PCB and dioxin concentrations, we calculated maximum concentrations and the percentage of samples with PCB concentrations exceeding 200 and 1000 ng PCB per g fat and with dioxin concentrations exceeding 2 and 5 pg TEQ per g fat.

Assessment of the Nature of the Contamination

The nature of the contamination during the 1999 crisis was assessed by van Larebeke et al. (2001) and Bernard et al. (2002). To characterize the origin of the PCB contamination of the 2000 and 2002 crises, the PCB congener distributions found in animal feed (with a total PCB concentration >500 ng/g fat) were compared with the profiles of seven Aroclor mixtures (A1016, A1242, A1248a, A1248g, A1254a, A1254g, and A1260) (Frame et al., 1996). Congener profiles of 29 samples of the 2000 incident and 10 samples of the 2002 incident were analyzed. Several non-crisis-related samples analyzed in 1999 showed high levels of contamination. To determine whether or not this contamination had the same origin as the contamination caused by the crisis, the crisis-related PCB profile for animal feed was compared with the PCB profile appearing in four highly contaminated animal feed samples unrelated to the crisis.

Body Burden

Estimation of the Intake of PCBs and Dioxins by Age Category

Food consumption by age category

In this study, data are presented on the PCB and dioxin body burdens of female adolescents (age 17) and adult women (ages 50–65, with a mean age of 58). Measured body burden data in blood fat are available only for these groups. Calculations of body burdens based on daily intakes were performed for the female adolescents and adult women. First, the Belgian population was categorized into eight main age groups: 0–6 months, 6–12 months, 1–4 years, 4–7 years, 7–10 years, 10–13 years, 14–18 years, and adults. Recent representative food consumption data concerning these age groups are not available. Instead, calculations are based on the following data: a food consumption study of 341 adolescent boys and girls ages 14 to 18 years performed in the spring of 1997 in the region of the city of Ghent (Dioxin Body Burden Working Group, 2001); a one-day food record involving 1340 senior citizens ages 65 to 92 years from Belgium (Dioxin Body Burden Working Group, 2001); and the results of a Dutch food consumption investigation (Voed-ingscentrum, 1998). Data from The Netherlands show that total daily fat consumption is similar in adults and in adolescents (Voedingscentrum, 1998). A preliminary analysis of food consumption habits in the 1340 elderly Belgians ages 65 to 92 years further suggests that fat intake substantially decreases after 65 years of age, whereas the origin of the fat is quite similar in adults and in adolescents. Therefore, in this chapter, the total daily fat intake for adults is considered to be the same as the intake by adolescents, but the distribution over different food items was replaced by the mean distribution for adolescents and the elderly. For children, the food items consumed by adolescents are taken into account, but the total daily fat intake is adopted accordingly to the Dutch findings (Voedingscentrum, 1998). This approach allowed calculating intake values for adults on the basis of data for milk, eggs, pork, beef, chicken, sheep, horse, fish, and vegetables. Children under the age of 1 year consume a different diet, as babies from 0 to 6 months old are considered to be solely breastfed, and babies from 6 to 12 months old are supposed to drink cow's milk and eat meat, vegetables, and fruit. These data are based on information on nutrient and energy intake for the European Community (EC, 1993) and the Dutch NEVO table (Stichting Nederlands Voedingsstoffenbestand, 1993). Intake data are expressed as the amount of PCBs and dioxins per gram of fat consumed for each type of food product (milk, eggs, pork, beef, chicken, sheep, horse, and fish), except for vegetables, for which PCBs and dioxins per gram of product are used.

Background contamination in food

The baseline body burden was calculated using background values of PCB and dioxin contamination levels of non-crisis-related samples taken during the dioxin accident of 1999 and processed after August. The data were provided by the Federal Agency for the Safety of the Food Chain. Missing data were substituted by data published in the literature, as indicated in Tables 10.9 to 10.12.

Background contamination for PCDD and PCDF

The available data, measured by CONSUM, concern concentrations in beef, poultry, and pork. The source for the additional background data for PCDD and PCDF in milk, vegetables, egg, sheep, and horse is the report by the Dioxin Body Burden Working Group (2001). Background data for these substances in fish were obtained from three different sources: Leonards et al. (2000), Jacobs et al. (2002), and Baeyens et al. (2002). The dioxin concentrations in human milk are those of the World Health Organization (WHO, 1996). Belgian samples in this international study originated from women living in Brussels, the rural area south of Brussels, and Liège, capital of the eastern Belgian province. In these samples, an average value of 34.4 pg TEQ per g milk fat was found.

Background contamination for PCBs

Background concentrations of PCBs in chicken, beef, pork, milk, and eggs were available. Concentrations in sheep and horse fat were taken from the 2001 data. Background data in fish were obtained from the RIVO Report C034/00 (Leonards et al., 2000) and from Baeyens et al. (2002). Concentrations in vegetables were taken from three different sources: Chewe et al. (1997), Lovett et al. (1997), and Schepens et al. (2001). Concentrations in mother's milk were taken from the RIVM Milieu-compendium (2000).

Intake of PCBs and dioxins per kg of body weight

The intake of PCBs and dioxins per kg of body weight was calculated. Mean body weights for the different age groups, from 1 year to adulthood, were based on data of the Dutch food consumption investigation (Voedingscentrum, 1998). The median body weights for children under 1 year relate to general data provided in the *Handbook of Pediatry* (Silver et al., 1983).

Calculated Body Burdens

Equation 10.1 provides a representation of the PCB and dioxin model used in this study to calculate the body burdens:

$$\xrightarrow[\text{Intake}]{I} X \xrightarrow[\text{Decay}]{k} \tag{10.1}$$

where X is the concentration of PCBs or dioxins per kg of body weight, I is the intake rate, and k represents the rate constant for decay. Assuming a first-order process, k is calculated from the half-life time according to:

$$\ln(X/X_o) = -k \cdot t$$

or

$$t = 1/k \cdot \ln(X_o/X)$$

or

$$t[1/2] = 1/k \cdot \ln\left[\left(2 \cdot X_o\right)/X_o\right] = 0.693/k$$

and finally:

$$k = 0.693/t_{1/2} \qquad\qquad (10.2)$$

The rate equation describing the system is:

$$dX/dt = I - k[X] \qquad\qquad (10.3)$$

where I and k are assumed to be functions of age. Concentration vs. time curves for PCBs and dioxins were generated by numerical integration according to Elskens et al. (1988).

Uncertainty exists about the half-lives of PCBs and dioxins. Shirai and Kissel (1996) mention in their review article that very short PCB half-lives (<1 year) are unlikely because the exposures required to sustain the observed body burdens are too large to be easily explained. Very long half-lives (>10 years) may be artifacts of confounding due to ongoing exposures and are also suspect. For dioxins, WHO uses a half-life of 7.5 years on average (WHO-ECEH IPCS, 1998). We assumed PCB and dioxin half-lives to be the same, as published data do not indicate that they differ substantially. Half-lives of PCBs and dioxins in children are shorter (Needham et al., 1997/1998; Wolff and Schecter, 1991); therefore, dioxin half-lives of 4 months for newborns and 5 years for 18 year olds were used (Kreuzer et al., 1997). We assumed the half-life to increase linearly with age from 4 months at birth to 5 years in 18 year olds. From 18 to 50 years old, we used a half-life of 7.5 years and from the age of 50 we considered a half-life of 10 years (Kreuzer et al., 1997). Table 10.1 shows the half-life values used in this chapter.

TABLE 10.1
Half-Life Values for PCBs and Dioxins by Age Category

Age Category (years)	Half-Life Values for PCBs and Dioxins (years)
0–0.5	0.4
0.5–1	0.5
1–4	1.0
4–7	1.8
7–10	2.6
10–13	3.4
14–18	4.4
18–50	7.5
50–60	10.0

Measured Body Burdens

The calculated body burdens of the female adolescents and adult women were compared with the body burdens of the same age and gender groups measured in a Belgian environmental health study (Vlietinck et al., 2000). Blood fat concentrations of the seven marker PCBs were measured for 47 pooled samples originating from the group of 200 adult women ages 50 to 65 (mean age, 58 years). For the 120 17-year-old female adolescents, PCBs 28, 52, 101, 138, 153, and 180 were measured. PCBs 28, 52, and 101 appeared to be below the detection limit. PCB 118 was not measured, thus for the adolescents the total PCB concentration had to be adjusted. This was done using the following formula:

$$\text{PCB total}_{\text{adolescents}} = \text{PCB total}_{\text{adults}}/(\text{PCB}138 + \text{PCB}153 + \text{PCB}180)_{\text{adults}}$$
$$\times (\text{PCB}138 + \text{PCB}153 + \text{PCB}180)_{\text{adolescents}}$$

where "total" is defined as (PCB28 + PCB52 + PCB101 + PCB138 + PCB153 + PCB180).

RESULTS

Exposure: Dioxin and PCB Levels in Animal Feed, Animals, and Food Products

Background Exposure Levels

Background values in 1999

Table 10.2 provides mean concentrations of PCBs and dioxins in a series of food samples not affected by the PCB-dioxin crisis and processed between the end of May and August 1999. The data show that the mean dioxin concentrations in beef, poultry, eggs, and pork are comparable and range between 1.4 and 5.7 pg TEQ per g fat. Although the highest mean concentration of dioxins was found in pork fat, only 13.5% of the pork samples showed dioxin levels >2 pg TEQ per g fat, while in 75% of the beef samples, 85.7% of the poultry samples, and 50% of the eggs dioxin concentrations exceeded this value. The highest mean PCB concentrations were found in poultry and pork fat (84.4 and 56.1 ng PCB per g fat, respectively) followed by eggs (46.6 ng PCB per g fat) and beef (41.0 ng PCB per g fat). Table 10.3 provides mean concentrations of PCBs and dioxins in a series of food samples not affected by the PCB/dioxin crisis and processed between September and December 1999. Mean dioxin concentrations range between 1.5 and 2.9 pg TEQ per g fat and are comparable to those found in the period before September. Compared to the period before September, a slight decrease in mean PCB concentration values was observed in all the food samples, except for animal fat of unspecified origin, animal feed, and "other food products."

TABLE 10.2

Non-Crisis-Related Dioxin and PCB Concentrations in Belgian Food and in Animal Feed Constituents Processed May–August 1999

		PCBs							Dioxins				
		Concentration (ng/g fat)		Maximum Level	Percent of Samples (ng/g fat)				Concentration (pg TEQ per g fat)		Maximum Level	Percent of Samples (pg/g fat)	
Food Item	N[c]	AM ± SD	GM	(ng/g fat)	≥200	≥1000	N[c]	AM ± SD	GM	N[d]	(pg/g fat)	≥2	≥5
Beef	337	41.0 ± 44.5	32.8	2511.0	1.6	0.4	3	3.2 ± 2.8	2.3	8	8.2	75	37.5
Poultry	200	84.4 ± 48.2	72.1	469.0	2.4	None	2	2.4 ± 0.6	2.4	7	4.8	85.7	None
Eggs	220	46.6 ± 67.6	36.5	1529.0	2.5	0.3	3	1.4 ± 0.7	1.3	4	3.1	50	None
Pork	2821	56.1 ± 139.8	42.0	5651.0	1.4	0.2	14	5.7 ± 16.9	0.8	37	64.0	13.5	5.4
Animal fat of unspecified origin[a]	29	25.6 ± 8.5	24.0	100.0	None	None	—	—	—	—	—	—	—
Animal feed	22	25.2 ± 15.1	22.3	100.0	None	None	—	—	—	—	—	—	—
Other food products[b]	2	15.0 ± 0.0	15.0	136.0	None	None	—						

[a] Animal fat not specified as being taken from cattle, pigs, or poultry.

[b] Processed food not specified as being bovine meat, pork, or chicken.

[c] Number of non-crisis-related samples analyzed during May–August 1999 used to calculate the mean values.

[d] Number of non-crisis-related samples analyzed during May–August 1999 used to calculate the maxima and the percentages of samples >200 ng PCB per g fat, >1000 ng PCB per g fat, >2 pg TEQ per g fat, and >5 pg TEQ per g fat.

Note: AM ± SD, arithmetic mean plus/minus standard deviation; GM, geometric mean; N, number.

TABLE 10.3
Non-Crisis-Related Dioxin and PCB Concentrations in Belgian Food and in Animal Feed Constituents Processed September–December 1999

		PCBs								Dioxins						
		Concentration (ng/g fat)			Maximum Level (ng/g fat)	Percent of Samples (ng/g fat)				Concentration (pg TEQ per g fat)			Maximum Level (pg/g fat)	Percent of Samples (pg/g fat)	
Food Item	N	AM ± SD	GM	N		≥200	≥1000	N	AM ± SD	GM	N		≥2	≥5
Beef	1753	35.8 ± 66.8	29.1	3050	1895.0	0.7	0.07	9	2.9 ± 2.5	1.9	17	8.3	66.7	5.6
Cattle milk	5	18.2 ± 9.4	16.6	5	34.0	None	None	—	—	—	—	—	—	—
Poultry	1773	66.3 ± 403.8	33.4	3556	3074.0	0.3	0.06	6	2.6 ± 1.3	2.4	8	13.7	87.5	25.0
Eggs	59	41.0 ± 64.2	31.5	163	508.0	0.6	None	—	—	—	—	—	—	—
Pork	5518	40.0 ± 84.2	32.2	9947	4785.0	0.8	0.06	40	1.5 ± 4.7	0.5	50	29.6	4.0	4.0
Animal fat of unspecified origin	336	31.5 ± 17.0	28.1	467	178.0	None	None	—	—	—	—	—	—	—
Fat of unspecified origin[a]	9	30.6 ± 6.3	29.7	41	100.0	None	None	—	—	—	—	—	—	—
Animal feed	399	31.0 ± 10.5	29.1	877	261.0	0.1	None	—	—	—	—	—	—	—
Other food products	27	28.7 ± 6.6	27.8	36	100.0	None	None	—	—	—	—	—	—	—

[a] Diverse fatty materials that are sometimes incorporated in animal feed, including samples of animal fat that were not labeled as being "animal fat."

Note: AM ± SD, arithmetic mean plus/minus standard deviation; GM, geometric mean; N, number.

Background Values in 2001

Table 10.4 provides mean concentrations of PCBs in a series of food items sampled from January to December of the year 2001. No dioxin concentrations were measured during this period. The highest mean PCB concentration is found in horse fat (91.6 ng PCB per g fat); 20% of the horse fat samples show concentrations above 200 ng PCB per g fat. This might be explained by the long life span of horses before consumption. The lowest mean concentration was found in sheep (21.8 ng PCB per g fat), but only 5 samples were available. Cow's milk also shows a low value (29.5 ng PCB per g fat), but in samples of other food items mean PCB concentrations of about 35.0 ng PCB per g fat were measured. These values are slightly lower than the non-crisis-related samples measured in 1999.

Episodes of Widespread Contamination

The PCB/dioxin episode of 1999

Table 10.5 shows the mean concentrations of PCBs and dioxins in a series of food samples affected by the PCB/dioxin crisis and processed between the end of May and August 1999. The data show that the highest mean dioxin concentrations were

---

TABLE 10.4

Non-Crisis-Related PCB Concentrations in Belgian Food and in Animal Feed Constituents Processed January–December 2001

		PCBs				
		Concentration (ng/g fat)		Maximum Level	Percent of Samples (ng/g fat)	
Food Item	N	AM ± SD	GM	(ng/g fat)	≥200	≥1000
Beef	312	34.2 ± 6.2	33.3	71.0	None	None
Cow's milk	190	29.5 ± 11.3	25.1	35.0	None	None
Poultry	302	35.0 ± 0.5	35.0	35.0	None	None
Eggs	345	32.8 ± 8.1	30.8	80.0	None	None
Pork	295	35.2 ± 3.5	35.0	81.0	None	None
Fat of unspecified origin	45	35.0 ± 0.0	35.0	35.0	None	None
Animal feed	8692	35.3 ± 10.1	34.8	586.0	0.05	None
Animal feed products	308	39.3 ± 23.3	36.9	304.0	0.3	None
Other food products	9	35.0 ± 0.0	35.0	35.0	None	None
Sheep	5	21.8 ± 12.2	19.2	35.0	None	None
Ostrich	4	32.7 ± 4.5	32.5	35.0	None	None
Horse	5	91.6 ± 162.6	31.7	382.0	20	None
Rabbit	5	35.0 ± 0.0	35.0	35.0	None	None
Baby food	15	35.0 ± 0.0	35.0	35.0	None	None

Note: AM ± SD, arithmetic mean plus/minus standard deviation; GM, geometric mean; N, number.

TABLE 10.5
Crisis-Related Dioxin and PCB Concentrations in Belgian Food and in Animal Feed Constituents Processed May–August 1999

	PCBs								Dioxins					
	Concentration (ng/g fat)				Maximum Level (ng/g fat)	Percent of Samples (ng/g fat)			Concentration (pg TEQ per g fat)			Maximum Level (pg/g fat)	Percent of Samples (pg/g fat)	
Food Item	N	AM ± SD	GM	N		≥200	≥1000	N	AM ± SD	GM	N		≥2	≥5
Beef	224	61.0 ± 103.6	37.8	373	2170.0	7.2	1.1	8	5.6 ± 2.1	5.3	71	19.5	94.1	47.1
Cow's milk	356	39.7 ± 43.7	28.7	721	336.0	0.6	None	11	2.8 ± 1.1	2.6	72	27.8	47.2	2.8
Poultry	328	421.3 ± 2084.8	59.6	1403	56,856.0	10.8	3.0	2	14.9 ± 1.3	14.9	39	2613.4	64.7	38.2
Eggs	45	135.5 ± 270.9	56.1	290	46,000.0	17.9	5.5	4	2.4 ± 1.4	2.2	41	713.1	68.3	36.6
Pork	3081	383.8 ± 1063.3	100.9	4998	39,700.0	30.6	11.4	118	2.1 ± 2.9	1.2	184	62.8	32.1	10.3
Animal fat of unspecified origin	329	48.0 ± 36.1	37.2	768	4092.0	0.9	0.5	—	—	—	—	—	—	—
Fat of unspecified origin	240	98.7 ± 168.0	59.4	423	3080.0	7.6	1.7	2	9.4 ± 12.6	3.1	11	45.1	90.9	90.9
Animal feed	181	994.5 ± 9447.9	38.8	615	336,000.0	12.2	3.6	10	144.6 ± 91.1	114.7	13	6144.0	100	100
Other food products	402	36.8 ± 1716.2	32.4	1096	464.0	0.5	None	—	—	—	—	—	—	—
Waste[a]	248	16,672.9	101.6	274	245,992.0	5.5	4.0	5	519.8 ± 1041.4	73.9	5	2379.4	100	100
Butter	46	41.6 ± 22.0	37.4	47	157.5	None	None	—	—	—	—	—	—	—
Animal feed products	92	80.3 ± 101.3	52.0	615	1262.0	2.9	0.4	—	—	—	—	—	—	—

[a] Waste oils that are sometimes incorporated in animal feed.

Note: AM ± SD, arithmetic mean plus/minus standard deviation; GM, geometric mean; N, number.

found in animal feed and in waste oils that are sometimes incorporated in animal feed (144.6 pg TEQ per g fat and 519.8 pg TEQ per g fat, respectively), followed by poultry fat (14.9 pg TEQ per g fat). Beef, cow's milk, eggs, and pork were also contaminated but to a lower extent. It should be realized that contamination levels in the period February to May might have been higher. The percentage of most of the samples with a dioxin concentration exceeding 2 and 5 pg TEQ per g fat is higher than for the non-crisis-related samples taken in the same period. Only poultry showed a lower percentage (>2 pg TEQ per g fat in the crisis-related samples. The mean PCB concentrations were the highest for animal feed and waste oils (994.5 and 1716.2 ng PCB per g fat), followed by poultry (421.3 ng PCB per g fat), pork (383.8 ng PCB per g fat), and eggs (135.5 ng PCB per g fat). The lowest value was found in cattle milk (39.7 ng PCB per g fat). Only 0.6% of the milk samples exceeded 200 ng PCB per g fat, and none of the samples showed values above 1000 ng PCB per g fat. Values >1000 ng PCB per g fat were found in 11.4% of the pork samples, 5.5% of the eggs, 3.6% of the animal feed samples, and 3.0% of the poultry samples.

Table 10.6 provides crisis-related dioxin and PCB concentrations in Belgian food and in animal feed constituents processed during the period September to December 1999. Dioxin measurements were available only for samples of beef, milk, pork, and animal fat of unspecified origin. The mean concentrations range between 0.4 pg TEQ per g fat for milk and 1.9 pg TEQ per g fat for beef, and they prove to be lower than the concentrations in the period before September. The PCB concentration in animal feed has dropped. This was to be expected because of the measures taken to destroy the contaminated animal feed that caused the incident. The concentrations, however, did not reach background concentrations (Table 10.2). Mean PCB concentrations in poultry, eggs, pork, animal fat of unspecified origin, and waste oil samples decreased as compared to the period before September. Mean concentrations in beef and milk increased. The percentages of the samples exceeding 200 and 1000 ng PCB per g fat decreased except for beef, milk, poultry, fat of unspecified origin, and other food products.

The PCB/dioxin episodes of 2000 and 2002
During the 2000 incident, a mean dioxin concentration of 28.3 pg TEQ per g fat was found in animal feed (Table 10.7). This is 5 times lower than the mean concentration during the 1999 crisis (144.6 pg TEQ per g fat). The mean PCB concentration, in contrast, was more than 3 times higher (3353.9 ng/g fat vs. 994.5 ng/g fat). Table 10.8 shows that, during the crisis in 2002, a mean dioxin concentration of 1.2 pg TEQ per g fat was found in animal feed. This is more than 100 times lower than the mean concentration in incident-related samples observed during the 1999 crisis. The mean PCB concentration in animal feed was more than 5 times lower than during the 1999 crisis (129.3 ng/g fat vs. 994.5 ng/g fat) but more than 3 times higher than the mean background value during the year 2001 (129.3 ng/g fat vs. 35.2 ng/g fat). The highest PCB concentration measured was 3718.0 ng/g fat, or almost 20 times the 200 ng/g fat norm. Increased PCB concentrations were found in chicken feed and to a lesser extent in pork feed. PCB concentrations in chicken fat (300 ng/g fat) seemed higher than background concentrations measured during the year 2001 (35.0 ng/g fat) and were comparable to those found during the crisis

TABLE 10.6
Crisis-Related Dioxin and PCB Concentrations in Belgian Food and in Animal Feed Constituents Processed September–December 1999

		PCBs							Dioxins					
		Concentration (ng/g fat)			Maximum Level	Percent of Samples (ng/g fat)			Concentration (pg TEQ per g fat)			Maximum Level	Percent of Samples (pg/g fat)	
Food Item	N	AM ± SD	GM	N	(ng/g fat)	≥200	≥1000	N	AM ± SD	GM	N	(pg/g fat)	≥2	≥5
Beef	169	188.5 ± 382.5	66.5	286	2731.0	19.2	2.8	2	1.9 ± 1.9	1.4	4	4.5	75.0	None
Cow's milk	65	436.1 ± 1395.0	42.5	143	7843.0	11.9	7.7	6	0.4 ± 0.6	—	47	5.0	61.7	None
Poultry	238	288.9 ± 1132.8	57.3	455	10665.0	10.9	3.6	—	—	—	—	—	—	—
Eggs	121	45.3 ± 141.0	30.7	162	38890.0	3.7	3.7	—	—	—	—	—	—	—
Pork	1936	118.8 ± 433.3	48.8	2850	8861.0	10.4	2.4	15	0.6 ± 0.8	0.3	28	2.9	3.6	None
Animal fat of unspecified origin	932	41.6 ± 48.2	36.0	1452	4218.0	0.8	0.1	1	1.7	1.7	1	1.7	None	None
Fat of unspecified origin	175	826.0 ± 1059.5	193.0	242	4208.0	36.8	24.0	—	—	—	—	—	—	—
Animal feed	124	163.5 ± 985.6	38.3	332	10,665.0	2.4	0.9	—	—	—	—	—	—	—
Other food products	470	43.1 ± 91.7	33.1	897	1875.0	1.1	0.111	—	—	—	—	—	—	—
Waste	35	73.7 ± 65.3	51.7	41	175.0	None	None	—	—	—	—	—	—	—

Note: AM ± SD, arithmetic mean plus/minus standard deviation; GM, geometric mean; N, number.

TABLE 10.7
Crisis-Related Dioxins and PCBs in Milk and in Animal Feed Constituents May–July 2000 (Bauduin–Cambier)

Food Item	PCBs						Dioxins					
	N	Concentration (ng/g fat)		Maximum Level (ng/g fat)	Percent of Samples (ng/g fat)		N	Concentration (pg TEQ per g fat)		Maximum Level (pg/g fat)	Percent of Samples (pg/g fat)	
		AM ± SD	GM		≥200	≥1000		AM ± SD	GM		≥2	≥5
Milk	3	155.0 ± 91.8	128.5	208.0	66.7	None	1	2.2	—	—	100	None
Other food products	37	794.6 ± 1399.6	168.9	6812.0	43.2	27.0	—	—	—	—	—	—
Fat of unspecified origin	2	34.7 ± 35.7	23.8	60.0	None	None	—	—	—	—	—	—
Animal feed	205	3353.9 ± 22,907.0	69.9	213,146.0	14.2	9.3	7	28.3 ± 54.8	6.6	151.7	71.4	71.4
Animal feed products	95	4911.6 ± 37,551.0	49.3	351,278.0	6.3	3.2	2	0.6 ± 0.2	0.6	0.8	None	None

Note: AM ± SD, arithmetic mean plus/minus standard deviation; GM, geometric mean; N, number.

TABLE 10.8
Crisis-Related Dioxins and PCBs January–February 2002 (Hanekop)

Food Item	PCBs						Dioxins				
		Concentration (ng/g fat)		Maximum Level (ng/g fat)	Percent of Samples (ng/g fat)			Concentration (pg TEQ per g fat)		Maximum Level (pg/g fat)	Percent of Samples (pg/g fat)
	N	AM ± SD	GM		≥200	≥1000	N	AM ± SD	GM		≥2	≥5
Pork	111	52.8 ± 52.3	42.3	341.0	2.7	None	—	—	—	—	—	—
Chicken	6	300.0 ± 298.5	139.7	678.0	50	None	—	—	—	—	—	—
Other food product	3	83.7 ± 84.3	60.5	181.0	None	None	—	—	—	—	—	—
Animal feed	222	129.3 ± 465.6	44.8	3718.0	6.8	2.7	4	1.2 ± 0.7	1.0	2.1	25	None
Animal feed product	65	36.9 ± 15.0	35.8	156.0	None	None	—	—	—	—	—	—

Note: AM ± SD, arithmetic mean plus/minus standard deviation; GM, geometric mean; N, number.

of 1999 (421.3 ng/g fat before September and 288.9 ng/g fat after September). Mean values in pork samples were comparable to background values during 1999 and 2001 (52.8 ng/g fat vs. 56.1 ng/g fat before September 1999, 40.0 ng/g fat after September 1999, and 35.2 ng/g fat during 2001).

Assessment of the Nature of the Contamination

van Larebeke et al. (2001) and Bernard et al. (2002) assessed the nature of the contamination during the 1999 crisis. van Larebeke et al. (2001) showed that the congener profile of animal feed samples heavily contaminated by the crisis exhibits a clear predominance of PCDF over PCDD congeners, a finding compatible with PCB contamination by a substance (such as transformer oil) containing PCBs rather than by dioxins originating from thermal processes such as waste incineration. To further identify the nature of the PCB oil, both studies analyzed different commercial PCB formulations under the same conditions as the contaminated feed samples. Good agreement was found between the contamination pattern for animal feed and the profiles of a 50/50 mixture of Aroclors 1254 and 1260 (van Larebeke et al., 2001) and a 25/75 mixture of these Aroclors (Bernard et al., 2002). They also revealed that for most samples with concentrations of PCBs >5000 ng/g fat, about 50,000 times more PCBs than dioxins were found, coinciding with the ratio found in transformer oil.

To evaluate the origin of the PCB contamination of the 2000 and 2002 crises, the PCB congener distributions found in animal feed were compared with 7 Aroclor mixtures (A1016, A1242, A1248a, A1248g, A1254a, A1254g, and A1260). The mean congener distribution of the 2000 crisis resembles that of A1242. The mean results for the 7 marker PCBs in 29 contaminated animal feed samples are given in Figure 10.1, which also includes the profile for Aroclor 1242. Figure 10.2 compares the mean crisis-related PCB profile of the 2002 crisis in 10 animal feed samples with the PCB profile of Aroclor 1260. The figure shows that these profiles are most comparable.

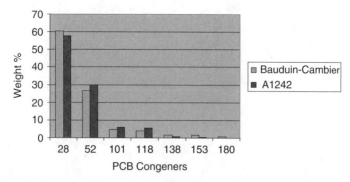

FIGURE 10.1 Weight percent distribution of 7 PCB marker congeners in 10 contaminated animal feed samples (during 2002 crisis) and in Aroclor 1260. Standard deviations of animal feed samples: 0.3, 0.7, 1.2, 0.9, 4.2, 1.6 and 1.6 for PCBs 28, 52, 101, 118, 138, 153 and 180, respectively.

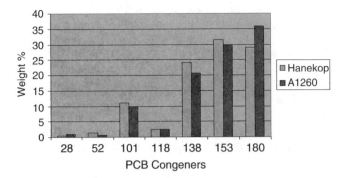

FIGURE 10.2 Weight percent distribution of 7 PCB marker congeners in 10 contaminated animal feed samples (during the 2002 crisis) and in Aroclor 1260. Standard deviations of animal feed samples: 0.3, 0.7, 1.2, 0.9, 4.2, 1.6, 1.6 for PCBs 28, 52, 101, 118, 138, 153, 180, respectively.

The PCB congener distribution in several animal feed samples from 1999 with very high PCB concentrations differs from the typical crisis-related PCB profile. van Larebeke et al. (2001) compared the crisis-related PCB profile for animal feed with the PCB profile appearing in four animal feed samples unrelated to the crisis. They showed that these five profiles differ, indicating that smaller unidentified contamination events occurred with different types of PCB mixtures, some of which resulted in high levels of contamination. The mean PCB profile for pork, reflecting the result of metabolic conversion, was compared with the crisis-related profile found in animal feed (Figure 10.3). The comparison shows that the higher PCBs (118, 138, 153, and 180) are the most persistent ones. The lower chlorinated PCBs are more easily metabolized or excreted.

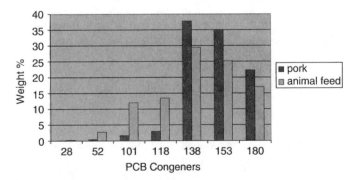

FIGURE 10.3 Crisis-related PCB profile of pork ($N = 288$) compared to the crisis-related PCB profile of animal feed. Standard deviations for pork samples: 0.5, 1.5, 3.6, 4.0, 5.7, 5.6, 4.5 for PCBs 28, 52, 101, 118, 138, 152, 180, respectively. Standard deviations for animal feed samples: 0.2, 4.1, 10.4, 3.2, 4.7, 3.8, 1.7 for PCBs 28, 52, 101, 118, 138, 152, 180, respectively.

Occasional Incidents of Isolated Contamination

During 1999 and 2001, some non-crisis-related samples showed high concentrations of PCBs and dioxins in food items. In the period before September 1999, 37% of the beef samples and 5.4% of the pork samples showed dioxin concentrations above 5 pg TEQ per g fat. After September, 5.6% of the beef samples, 25.0% of the poultry samples, and 4.0% of the pork samples exceeded this value. The maximum levels measured were 8.3 pg TEQ per g fat for beef, 13.3 pg TEQ per g fat for poultry, 3.1 pg TEQ for eggs, and 64.0 pg TEQ for pork. Non-crisis-related samples before September 1999 showed PCB levels above 200 ng PCB g/fat in no more than 2.5% of the beef, poultry, egg, and pork samples. Very high values (>1000 ng/g fat) were found in 0.4% of the beef samples, 0.3% of the eggs, and 0.2% of the pork samples. In the period after September, fewer samples showed PCB levels above 200 ng PCB per g fat than in the previous period (0.1–0.8% vs. 1.4–2.5%). Very high values (>1000 ng PCB per g fat) were reached in a most limited percentage of the samples (0.06–0.07%). In 2001, PCB concentrations did not exceed 200 ng PCB per g fat, except for horse (20%), animal feed products (0.3%), and animal feed (0.05%). Maximum PCB levels measured during 1999 were 2511.0 ng/g fat for beef, 35.0 ng/g fat for milk, 3074 ng/g fat for poultry, 1529.0 ng/g fat for eggs, 5651.0 ng/g fat for pork, and 261 ng/g fat for animal feed. Maximum levels during 2001 were substantially lower. These high concentrations are likely to be due to occasional incidents of isolated contamination.

BODY BURDEN

For lipophylic, bioaccumulating pollutants with long half-lives, biological and adverse effects are related to their availability in the body. The body burden is an indicator for this biological availability of toxins. Body burdens have been calculated that are expected to result from a diet contaminated with PCBs and dioxins at background levels prevailing in Belgium, and these body burdens were compared to body burden values measured in female adolescents and in adult women ages 50 to 65. Also, data on the increase in PCB body burden resulting from the 1999 crisis are discussed here.

Calculations of Intake of PCBs and Dioxins per kg Body Weight for Different Age Categories

Polychlorinated biphenyl and dioxin intakes were calculated using the following data:

- Consumption data of various food products (beef, pork, poultry, eggs, milk, vegetables, fish, horse, and sheep) expressed in grams fat per day or grams product per day
- Average body weight per age category
- PCB and dioxin concentrations in the different food products

TABLE 10.9
PCB and Dioxin Intakes for Babies (0–0.5 Years)

Mother's Milk Intake (mL/kg/day)	Fat Amount (g fat/100 mL)	PCB Concentration (ng/g fat)	PCB Intake (ng/kg/day)	Dioxin Concentration (pg TEQ per g fat)	Dioxin Intake (pg TEQ per kg per day)
150	4[a]	299.6[b]	1797.5	34.4[c]	206.4

[a] See Stichting Nederlands Voedingsstoffenbestand (1993).
[b] See RIVM (2000).
[c] See WHO (1996).

Note: Average body weight is 5.4 kg (Silver et al., 1983).

Source: Adapted from Silver, H.K. et al., Eds., *Handbook of Pediatry*, 14th ed., Lange Medical Publications, Los Altos, CA, 1983.

The results of these calculations are shown in Tables 10.9 to 10.12. For every table the sources of the data are provided.

Table 10.9 shows the PCB and dioxin intake for babies from 0 to 0.5 years. Breastfeeding was supposed to be their only source of intake. PCB intake was 1797.5 ng/kg/day, more than 50 times higher than the average intake by an adult. The dioxin intake was over 130 times higher than the average intake by an adult. This indicates that during 6 months of breastfeeding, Belgian babies already take in a substantial amount of their lifetime PCB and dioxin dose. The biomonitoring study on 17-year-old adolescents showed a positive correlation between PCB body burden and breastfeeding (Vlietinck et al., 2000). It is assumed that when a baby is 6 months old the breast milk is replaced by cow's milk, meat, fruit, and vegetables. The corresponding PCB and dioxin intakes are shown in Table 10.10. The PCB and dioxin concentrations in cow's milk are significantly lower than those in mother's milk. Meat is only served in small quantities (20 g/day), and fruits and vegetables contain limited amounts of PCBs and dioxins. The resulting PCB and dioxin intake is thus substantially lower than the intake during the first months of breastfeeding (more than 15 times lower for PCBs and more than 60 times lower for dioxins). Tables 10.11 and 10.12 provide PCB and dioxin intake data for children, adolescents, and adults. The main contributors to the PCB and dioxin intake are pork, milk, and vegetables. The results show a decrease in intake per kg body weight per day with age as a result of the increasing body weight.

Calculated Body Burdens

Figures 10.4 and 10.5 show the calculated PCB and dioxin body burdens as a function of age. Breastfeeding causes very high PCB and dioxin body burdens in babies younger than 0.5 years (218.63 µg/kg body weight and 25.1 ng TEQ per kg body weight, respectively). The body burden declines to a minimum of 55.85 µg/kg body

TABLE 10.10

PCB And Dioxin Intake for Babies (0.5–1 Years) with Non-Crisis-Related Meat Values September–December 1999

Food Product	Intake	Fat Amount	PCB Concentration	PCB Intake (ng/kg/day)	Dioxin Concentration (pg TEQ per g fat)	Dioxin Intake (pg TEQ per kg per day)
Cattle milk	500 mL per day	3.5 g per 100 mL[a]	29.5 ng per g fat[b]	60.1	1.4[e]	2.8
Meat	20 g per day	5.5 g per 100 g[a]	47.4 ng per g fat[c]	6.1	2.3[f]	0.3
Vegetables and fruit	500 g per day	—	0.9 ng per g product[d]	40.3	0.0003[g]	0.02
Total	—	—	—	106.5	—	3.12

[a] See Stichting Nederlands Voedingsstoffenbestand (1993).

[b] Data from 2001.

[c] Data from 1999 (September–December).

[d] Pooled data from Chewe et al. (1997), Lovett et al. (1997), and Schepens et al. (2001).

[e] See Dioxin Body Burden Working Group (2001).

[f] Data from 1999 (September–December).

[g] See Lovett et al. (1997).

Note: The average body weight is 8.6 kg (Silva et al., 1983).

Source: Adapted from Silver, H.K. et al., Eds., *Handbook of Pediatry*, 14th ed., Lange Medical Publications, Los Altos, CA, 1983.

weight for PCBs at age 4.5 years and to 3.3 ng TEQ per kg body weight for dioxins at age 7.5 years. From this point on, the body burden increases to 150.45 µg/kg body weight for PCBs and 7.24 ng TEQ per kg body weight for dioxins.

Measured Body Burdens

The calculated body burdens for 17-year-old female adolescents and 58-year old adult women were compared to the body burdens for these age and gender groups measured in blood during a Belgian environmental health study (Vlietinck et al., 2000). As shown in Table 10.13, measurements in blood fat resulted, for adolescents, in a PCB concentration of 237.0 ng/g fat, whereas the dioxin concentration was 36.6 pg TEQ per g fat. Adults showed a mean PCB concentration of 412 ng/g fat and a mean dioxin concentration of 49.7 pg TEQ per g fat. To compare these data with the calculated body burdens, the values have to be expressed in ng/kg of body weight and pg TEQ per kg of body weight. The percentage body fat of female adolescents in Belgium is estimated to be 24.1% (Vlietinck et al., 2000). The percentage body

TABLE 10.11

PCB and Dioxin Intake for Girls (1–13 Years) Based on Background Values of the Year 1999 (September–December) and Data from the Literature

Food Product	1–4 Years of Age		4–7 Years of Age		7–10 Years of Age		10–13 Years of Age	
	PCB Intake (ng/kg/day)	Dioxin Intake (pg TEQ per kg per day)	PCB Intake (ng/kg/day)	Dioxin Intake (pg TEQ per kg per day)	PCB Intake (ng/kg/day)	Dioxin Intake (pg TEQ per kg per day)	PCB Intake (ng/kg/day)	Dioxin Intake (pg TEQ per kg per day)
Chicken	3.809	0.149	3.238	0.127	2.872	0.113	2.270	0.089
Pork	16.918	0.634	14.380	0.539	12.754	0.478	10.080	0.378
Beef	6.370	0.516	5.414	0.439	4.802	0.389	3.795	0.307
Egg	4.043	0.226	3.436	0.192	3.048	0.170	2.409	0.135
Milk	13.870	1.059	11.790	0.900	10.457	0.799	8.264	0.631
Fish	9.483	0.659	8.052	0.559	7.142	0.496	5.651	0.393
Vegetable	22.119	0.149	16.917	0.127	12.560	0.112	10.005	0.089
Sheep	0.549	0.017	0.467	0.034	0.414	0.013	0.327	0.010
Horse	0.781	0.062	0.664	0.362	0.589	0.046	0.465	0.037
Total	77.942	3.471	64.358	3.278	54.637	2.616	43.267	2.068

Note: Average body weights: 1–4 years, 13.6 kg; 4–7 years, 20 kg; 7–10 years, 28.7 kg; 10–13 years, 41.5 kg.

Sources: Fat intake per food product (g fat per day) for chicken, pork, beef, eggs, milk, fish, sheep, and horse — total fat intake (Voedingscentrum, 1998); distribution (Dioxin Body Burden Working Group, 2001) (adolescents). Intake for vegetables (g product per day) (Voedingscentrum, 1998). Average weight (Voedingscentrum, 1998). PCB (ng/g fat) for chicken, pork, beef, eggs, and milk — data of non-crisis-related samples from 1999 (September–December). PCB (ng/g fat) for fish (Baeyens et al., 2002; Leonards et al., 2000; Jacobs et al., 2002). PCB (ng/g product) for vegetables (Chewe et al., 1997; Lovett et al., 1997; Schepens et al., 2001). PCB (ng/g fat) for horse and sheep — data of samples taken in 2001. Dioxin concentrations for chicken, pork, and beef — data of non-crisis-related samples from 1999 (September–December). Dioxin concentrations for fish (Leonards et al., 2000). Dioxin concentrations for vegetables, sheep, and horse (Dioxin Body Burden Working Group, 2001).

TABLE 10.12

PCB and Dioxin Intake for Adolescents (14–18 Years) and Adults (Up to 65 Years) Calculated with Non-Crisis-Related Values of the Year 1999 (September–December) and Data from the Literature

| Food Product | Adolescents | | Adults | |
	PCB Intake (ng/kg/day)	Dioxin Intake (pg TEQ per kg per day)	PCB Intake (ng/kg/day)	Dioxin Intake (pg TEQ per kg per day)
Chicken	1.790	0.070	2.104	0.082
Pork	7.951	0.298	7.070	0.265
Beef	2.994	0.243	2.296	0.186
Egg	1.900	0.106	1.375	0.077
Milk	6.519	0.498	5.791	0.442
Fish	4.456	0.310	6.553	0.455
Vegetables	7.964	0.070	7.533	0.059
Sheep	0.258	0.008	0.150	0.005
Horse	0.367	0.029	0.165	0.013
Total	34.200	1.631	33.038	1.584

Note: Average body weight for adolescents is 57.4 kg and for adults 66.9 kg.

Sources: Fat intake per food product (g fat per day) for chicken, pork, beef, eggs, milk, fish, sheep, and horse: adolescents (Dioxin Body Burden Working Group, 2001); adults — total fat intake (Dioxin Body Burden Working Group, 2001) (adolescents); distribution (Dioxin Body Burden Working Group, 2001) (average of adolescents and elderly). Intake for vegetables (g product per day) (Voedingscentrum, 1998). Average weight (Voedingscentrum, 1998). PCB (ng/g fat) for chicken, pork, beef, eggs, and milk — data of non-crisis-related samples from 1999 (September–December). PCB (ng/g fat) for fish (Baeyens et al., 2002; Leonards et al., 2000; Jacobs et al., 2002). PCB (ng/g product) for vegetables (Chewe et al., 1997; Lovett et al., 1997; Schepens et al., 2001). PCB (ng/g fat) for horse and sheep — data of samples taken in the year 2001. Dioxin concentrations for chicken, pork, and beef — data of non-crisis-related samples from 1999 (September–December). Dioxin concentrations for fish (Leonards et al., 2000). Dioxin concentrations for vegetables, sheep, and horse (Dioxin Body Burden Working Group, 2001).

fat in adult women is estimated to be 29.5% (NIH/WHO BMI Guidelines as reported by Gallagher et al., 2000). On the basis of these data, the body burdens per kg body weight were calculated (Table 10.14). The results show that the calculated PCB body burdens are comparable to and more or less 20% higher than the measured values. This indicates that the calculated values are reliable. Why the measured dioxin body burdens are about twice the calculated ones could, at least partially, be explained by contamination episodes and non-food-related routes of contamination (e.g., air) that might have contributed to actual body burdens.

Impact of the 1999 Crisis on PCB Body Burdens

Background contamination of food products in Belgium has been high and has resulted in substantial PCB and dioxin body burdens. Episodes of intense contamination can

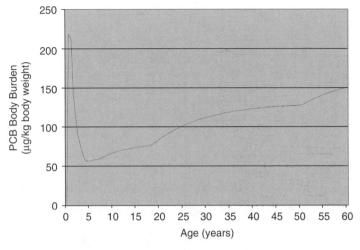

FIGURE 10.4 Calculated PCB body burden over age (μg/g fat).

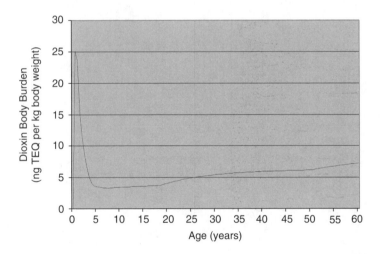

FIGURE 10.5 Calculated dioxin body burden over age (ng TEQ per g fat).

increase these body burdens. Table 10.15 shows the results of the measurements of three marker PCBs in blood fat for three groups of Belgian women (van Larebeke et al., 2002). One group was monitored before the 1999 crisis; the two other groups were studied after the crisis. The data suggest that the crisis caused a measurable increase in PCB body burden. Although these figures need to be interpreted with caution (e.g., because the three groups are not directly comparable), any increase is worrisome as body burdens of PCBs and dioxins found in Belgium reach levels that are associated with adverse effects both in animals and in humans (Koopman-Esseboom et al., 1994; Van Poucke and Willems, 1998).

TABLE 10.13

Concentrations of the Seven Marker PCBs (ng/g fat) and Dioxins (pg TEQ per g fat) in Blood of Female Adolescents (17 Years Old) and Female Adults (Average Age, 58 Years Old)

	PCB 2 (ng/g fat)	PCB 52 (ng/g fat)	PCB 101 (ng/g fat)	PCB 118 (ng/g fat)	PCB 138 (ng/g fat)	PCB 153 (ng/g fat)	PCB 180 (ng/g fat)	PCB Total (ng/g fat)	Dioxin (pg TEQ per g fat)
Female adolescents	Not measurable	Not measurable	Not measurable	Not measured	59.4	100.8	55.1	237.0	36.6
Female adults	3.2	1.7	1.5	31.3	95.2	171.7	107.8	412.3	49.7

TABLE 10.14

Calculated and Measured PCB and Dioxin Body Burdens for Female Adolescents and Adult Women

	Body Burden			
	Calculated		Measured	
	PCB (µg/kg bw)	Dioxins (ng TEQ per kg bw)	PCB (µg/kg bw)	Dioxins (ng TEQ per kg bw)
Female adolescents	75.48	3.67	57.12	8.82
Female adults	146.95	7.07	121.63	14.66

Note: bw, body weight.

TABLE 10.15
Measured PCB Body Burdens in Belgian Women Before and After the Contamination Crisis Early in 1999

	PCB 138 (ng/g fat)	PCB 153 (ng/g fat)	PCB 180 (ng/g fat)
1996–1998 106 infertile women (ages 24–42; mean age, 31.9)[a]	69.9	94.5	72.0
Second half of 1999 120 girls (mean age, 17.4)[b]	75.9	101.6	55.5
Second half of 1999 197 women (ages 50–65; mean age, 58.5)[b]	125.4	171.1	123.1
Body burden increase in 1999, after correction for age,[c] as percent of the body burden found from 1996 to 1998 in infertile women	33.6	33.5	10.2

[a] See Pauwels et al. (2000).

[b] See Vlietink et al. (2000).

[c] Correction for age was performed through linear extrapolation based on the measurements done in 1999. This linear extrapolation can be expected to underestimate the body burden at age 31.9 years, as it is likely that a proportionally greater increase in body burden with age will occur between age 17.4 and age 31.9 than between age 31.9 and age 58.5. The real age-corrected increase between the two periods might thus be higher than the one shown in the table.

DISCUSSION

LEVELS OF CONTAMINATION

Background Contamination Levels

Background contamination levels are substantial in Belgium. From May to August 1999, mean PCB concentrations in non-crisis-related food items (but including occasional incidents of isolated contamination) ranged between 41.0 ng/g fat for beef and 84.4 ng/g fat for poultry. Corresponding mean dioxin concentrations ranged between 1.4 pg TEQ per g fat for eggs and 5.7 pg TEQ per g fat for pork. Mean background concentrations of PCBs in cow's milk were 18.2 ng/g fat in 1999 and 29.5 ng/g fat in 2001. These concentrations are high in comparison with background contamination levels for PCBs in U.K. milk, where concentrations of individual congeners ranged between 0.051 and 2.44 ng/g fat (Krokos et al., 1996). Mean dioxin levels in non-crisis-related meat in the second half of 1999 ranged between 1.5 pg TEQ per g fat for pork and 2.9 pg TEQ per g fat for beef. These background concentrations were higher than those found in meat from the United States (0.53–1.10 pg I-TEQ per g fat) (Fiedler et al., 1997).

Contamination Incidents

On the nature of contamination

Schepens et al. (2001) calculated that levels of contamination present in fish meal and vegetable ingredients of animal feed can lead to PCB levels of 16.5 ng/g fat in pork and to 20.2 ng/g fat in chicken. 12.1% of the meat samples contain >50 ng PCB per g fat, and this cannot be explained by background contamination of these main animal feed ingredients. It is most likely that these higher contamination levels result from the incorporation of recycled fats and oils and from waste from slaughtered animals. Very high contamination levels probably result from the admixture of mineral and PCB oils into recycled fats and oils.

Based on the PCDD/PCDF ratio, the PCB/dioxin ratio, and PCB profiles, it was demonstrated that the source of the 1999 incident was transformer oil (Bernard et al., 2002; van Larebeke et al., 2001). In this study, the PCB profiles of animal feed contaminated during the 2000 and 2002 incidents were compared with different types of Aroclor. The animal-feed PCB profile of the 2000 incident in Feluy matched that of Aroclor 1242. This contamination might have originated from an elevator, as this type of synthetic oil is used in hydraulic fluids. The cause of the 2002 contamination episode, however, remains unclear. The PCB profile in animal feed resembles that of Aroclor 1260. This PCB mixture is still present in many of the transformers and capacitors now in use. The source of the contamination might be similar to that of the 1999 crisis because it was demonstrated that the incident-related PCB profile of animal feed during this crisis resembled an Aroclor mixture also containing Aroclor 1260 (Bernard et al., 2002; van Larebeke et al., 2001).

The congener patterns found in the heavily contaminated animal feed samples as shown by van Larebeke et al. (2001) point to the existence of other contamination sources, different from the transformer oil of the 1999 crisis. These PCB profiles are clearly different from the incident-related PCB profile of animal feed. It could be suggested that many smaller unidentified contamination events occurred, some of which resulted in high levels of contamination. That such incidents are most probable is also indicated by the findings of van Larebeke et al. (2001) regarding the occurrence of 1999 samples with high concentrations of PCBs but with a PCB/dioxin ratio that is clearly different from the 50.000/1 ratio characteristic of the 1999 crisis. Because of the stability of the measured dioxin and PCB congeners, these most variable PCB/dioxin ratios point to the existence of other PCB contamination sources, different from the transformer oil implicated in the 1999 crisis.

Comparison of the three PCB and dioxin contamination episodes

Episodes of widespread contamination mean additional exposure and extra contributions to body burdens (van Larebeke et al., 2002). In Figure 10.6, the extent of the PCB contamination of animal feed during the three crises is compared with background contamination during 2001. The highest mean PCB concentrations in animal feed were found during the 2000 crisis. They were approximately 4.5 times higher than during the major crisis of 1999 (3353.9 vs. 776.0 ng/g fat, respectively). The contamination in 2002 resulted in rather low values (129.3 ng/g fat), but the mean concentration was still 4 times higher than background values (35.3 ng/g fat).

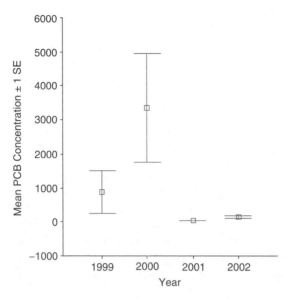

FIGURE 10.6 Mean PCB concentrations and standard errors in animal feed contaminated by the 1999, 2000, and 2002 crises compared to background contamination in 2001.

The 2000 crisis gave rise to elevated PCB concentrations in milk and other food products (155.0 ng PCB per g fat and 794.6 ng PCB per g fat, respectively). The animal feed contamination during the 2002 crisis caused increased PCB levels in chickens (300.0 ng PCB per g fat). Concentrations found in pork fat were comparable to background values (52.8 ng PCB per g fat). It is unclear to what extent the Belgian population was exposed to these elevated PCB levels in food products, as no data exist on the amount of these products contaminated and the amount released for consumption; therefore, it was not possible to estimate the impact of these incidents on human body burdens.

The Scientific Committee on Animal Nutrition (SCAN) has calculated the total dioxin concentration in animal feed for cattle, pork, and poultry (European Commission, 2000). This study is based on all the available published data and additional information obtained by the European Commission from Member States and other sources (South Pacific). Because of the scarcity of reliable data on PCBs, these are not included in this analysis. Mean European dioxin concentrations of 0.18 ng WHO-TEQ per kg dry matter for cattle feed, 0.14 ng WHO-TEQ per kg dry matter for pork feed, and 0.15 ng WHO-TEQ per kg dry matter for poultry feed were found. Values from the South Pacific were slightly lower: 0.16, 0.13, and 0.12 ng WHO-TEQ per kg dry matter for cattle, pork, and poultry feed, respectively. Belgian background dioxin levels in animal feed were not available, but levels during the Belgian incidents were measured. Taking into account a mean fat content in animal feed from 2 to 12% and a dry weight percentage of 89%, dioxin concentrations in animal feed of 2.6 to 15.5 ng TEQ per kg dry weight for the 1999 crisis and 0.5 to 3.0 ng TEQ per kg dry weight for the 2000 crisis (the 2002 crisis was more a PCB crisis than a dioxin crisis) were measured. These values are considerably higher than background concentrations handled by the EU officials (European Commission, 2000).

Although thousands of PCBs and hundreds of dioxin measurements on animal feed, animal fat, and different food items were performed during the 1999 crisis, an important uncertainty still exists regarding the extent to which the Belgian population was exposed to these toxicants. This is due in part to the uncertainty about the extent to which consumed food was contaminated, as sampling of animal fat and food items was not performed in a systematic way but evolved rather haphazardly during the crisis in response to many different needs and pressures, some from national or European regulatory authorities and others commercial in nature. Some of these demands have biased sampling to the more suspect items, others to less suspect products. Further uncertainty about the extent to which the consumed food was contaminated originates from the period of sampling. The results presented in this chapter relate to the food available from the end of May through December 1999. The contamination episode started, however, in January 1999. During January until the end of May, no systematic sampling of the food chain was done. Food items may have been contaminated more often and at higher levels than is evident from the available data.

Comparison of the 1999 crisis with other
non-Belgian contamination episodes

van Larebeke et al. (2001) compared the 1999 crisis with the Yusho (1968, Japan) and Yucheng (1979, Taiwan) incidents and the Seveso accident (1976, Italy). In the Belgian crisis, van Larebeke et al. (2001) estimated that the average Belgian ingested 0.025 mg PCBs and 500 pg TEQ dioxins per kg body weight. They concluded that the exposure during the Belgian incident amounted to only a fraction of that during these three incidents, but far more people were involved. In 1998, a dioxin contamination of animal feed took place in Europe. Around 100,000 tons of citrus pulp pellets (CPPs) from Brazil contaminated with dioxin (up to 32,000 pg I-TEQ per kg) were imported into the European Union (Malisch, 2000). The pulp was used mainly in France, Belgium, The Netherlands, and Germany. These CPPs were used as feeding stuff or feed material and fed mainly to cattle. As a result, increased dioxin levels in milk and meat were found. In Germany, meat samples (beef and veal) were found to contain between 1.72 and 4.26 pg I-TEQ per g fat. A steady increase in dioxin concentrations in cow's milk was also observed; average values were 0.62 pg I-TEQ per g fat before August 1997, 0.89 between September and December, 1.38 between January and February 1998, and up to 7.4 pg I-TEQ per g fat in March (Malisch, 2000). At that time, a provisional maximum level of 500 pg I-TEQ per kg for dioxin in CPPs was set (EC, 1998). During the Belgian crisis of 1999, mean dioxin concentrations of 2.8 pg TEQ per g fat for milk and 5.6 pg TEQ per g fat for beef were measured. The dioxin contamination of animal feed in 1999 gave rise to higher dioxin concentrations in beef than that in 1998, while milk contamination was lower. Another animal feed contamination episode was reported in 1997 in the United States. During a nation-wide survey for dioxins in food products, samples of poultry meat were found to have elevated levels of dioxins. The contamination source proved to be ball clay, an anti-caking agent used in the production of animal feed.

Non-Incident-Related High Values

Occasional incidents of isolated contamination can also lead to high concentrations in food items, and their contribution to body burdens cannot be neglected. This study reports on body burdens based on mean background concentrations of PCBs and dioxins in food products measured after August 1999. These mean concentrations were calculated including high contamination levels due to occasional incidents of isolated contamination. When these values (PCB concentration, >500 ng/g fat; dioxins, >5 pg TEQ per g fat) were excluded from the calculation, mean PCB and dioxin concentrations were noticeably lower:

- *PCBs:* 34.1 vs. 66.3 ng PCB per g fat for poultry, 32.4 vs. 35.8 ng PCB per g fat for beef, 37.2 vs. 40.0 ng PCB per g fat for pork, 32.9 vs. 41.0 ng PCB per g fat for eggs, and 18.2 vs. 18.2 ng PCB per g fat for milk
- *Dioxins:* 2.2 vs. 2.9 pg TEQ per g fat for beef, 2.1 vs. 2.6 pg TEQ per g fat for poultry, and 0.6 vs. 1.5 pg TEQ per g fat for pork

These contamination levels will consequently result in lower body burdens.

INTAKE AND BODY BURDENS

Background Values

In this study, a background intake of dioxins for Belgian adults (19 to 60 years) of 1.58 pg TEQ per kg body weight per day was calculated. Measured body burdens range from 8.82 ng TEQ per kg body weight for female adolescents to 14.66 ng TEQ per kg body weight for adult women. Calculated body burdens (3.67 ng TEQ per kg body weight for adolescents and 7.07 ng/kg body weight for adults), based on current intake levels, are comparable to body burdens actually observed in other countries (2 to 6 ng I-TEQ per kg body weight; WHO-ECEH IPCS, 1998). This agrees with the finding that current intake levels in Belgium are not very different from those in other industrialized countries. Calculated dioxin body burdens were, however, only 41.61% of measured body burdens for female adolescents and 48.23% of actual body burdens of women ages 50 to 65. That measured body burdens are substantially higher than calculated body burdens might stem from the fact that past background intake levels were higher than current ones, from episodes of widespread contamination and from other routes of exposure.

The PCB background intake for Belgian adults was estimated to be 33.0 ng PCB per kg per day. Calculated PCB body burdens resulting from an average Belgian diet with background contamination levels overestimate measured PCB body burdens by 32% for adolescents and by 21% for adults. It is likely that this difference is related to the PCB half-lives that likely overestimate the real half-lives. Considerable uncertainty remains as to the half-lives of PCBs in humans.

It should also be mentioned that babies have particularly high PCB and dioxin body burdens. This is due to the high concentrations of PCBs and dioxins in breast milk, which result in high intake values. Figures 10.4 and 10.5 also show a rapid decline of body burdens after 0.5 years of age. This is due to the change in diet and to short half-lives for PCBs and dioxins in babies.

The Impact of the 1999 Crisis on Body Burdens

During the 1999 crisis, 50 kg of PCBs and 1 g TEQ of dioxins were introduced into the food chain. Assuming that 30% of these amounts was ingested by 10 million Belgian citizens with a mean body weight (children included) of 60 kg, van Larebeke et al. (2002) have calculated that the crisis could have caused a mean PCB body burden increase of 25 µg/kg body weight and an increase in mean dioxin body burden of 500 pg TEQ per kg body weight. Considering that measured PCB and dioxin body burdens (mean for female adolescents and for women ages 50 to 65) were, respectively, about 89.4 µg/kg body weight and about 11.7 ng TEQ per kg body weight at the end of the year 1999, it can be concluded that the crisis resulted in a 28% increase in PCB body burdens and a 4.3% increase in dioxin body burdens (with reference to body burdens measured at the end of the crisis). No data are available to assess the actual increase in dioxin body burden, but measurements of PCB congeners in women before and after the crisis do show an increase of this order of magnitude in PCB body burdens (Table 10.15). It is most probable that a small proportion of the Belgian population was subjected to a much higher intake and consequently a more important increase in body burdens.

Body Burdens in Other Countries

The estimated background intake of dioxins for Belgian adults (19 to 60 years) was 1.58 pg TEQ per kg body weight per day. This value is in the same range as the intake in other countries. MAFF (Department of Health and the Scottish Executive) estimated for the United Kingdom a daily dioxin intake that ranges between 1.0 and 1.5 pg/kg body weight (Ministry of Agriculture, Fisheries, and Food, 1997). In the United States, the estimated dietary intakes by adults in 1995 ranged between 0.48 and 2.4 pg TEQ per kg body weight per day (Schecter et al., 1996). The total dietary PCDD/PCDF intake by the population of Tarragona (Spain) was estimated to be 210 pg I-TEQ per day (Domingo et al., 1999). This coincides with 3.2 pg I-TEQ per kg body weight per day for a mean body weight of 65 kg. Malisch (1998) calculated a mean daily intake of 0.88 pg I-TEQ per kg body weight per day between 1993 and 1996 for the German population. In Germany, the average daily intake for a breast-fed child has been calculated to be 142 pg TEQ per kg body weight per day (Beck et al., 1994). In the United States, a nursing infant may consume an average of 35 to 53 pg TEQ per kg body weight per day in its first year of life (Schecter et al., 1994). In Belgium, due to the high dioxin concentrations in breast milk, the intake of a nursing infant is substantially higher: 206.4 pg TEQ per kg body weight per day.

Dioxin body burdens in Belgium are higher than in most other industrialized countries. Available information derived from numerous studies in OECD countries indicates a dioxin body burden of 2 to 6 ng I-TEQ per kg body weight (WHO-ECEH IPCS, 1998), whereas in Belgium body burdens range from 8.82 ng TEQ per kg body weight for female adolescents to 14.66 ng TEQ per kg body weight for adult women.

Levels of intake of PCBs are similar to those observed in Finland and Italy (Himberg et al., 1993; Zuccato et al., 1999), and PCB body burdens in Belgium are not higher than in some other western European countries (Grimvall et al., 1997; Koopman-Esseboom, 1994).

Health Effects

Acute clinical effects were not reported during the Belgian crisis in 1999. In view of the type of contamination, acute effects such as ischemic heart disease (Kogevinas, 1999), chloracne, or conjunctivitis (WHO, 1995) were also not expected; however, it is most likely that this contamination episode will have delayed effects on the health of exposed individuals. The body burdens prevailing in Belgium are of the same order of magnitude as those that are associated with biological and even adverse effects in animals. According to WHO (WHO-ECEH IPCS, 1998), the lowest dose giving rise to statistically significant health effects following exposure have resulted in body burdens (e.g., 3–73 ng TCDD/kg) in the exposed animals that overlap, at the lower end, the range of body burdens expressed as TEQ that are found in the general population in industrialized countries exposed to background levels of PCDDs, PCDFs, and PCBs (2–6 ng TCDD/kg). The Belgian Health Council has calculated the human estimated daily intakes (EDIs) of dioxins corresponding to lowest-observed-adverse-effect level (LOAEL) values observed in animals exposed to dioxins. For noncarcinogenic effects, these EDIs range between 1.5 and 146 pg per kg body weight per day (Van Poucke and Willems, 1998). In Belgium, the background daily intake of dioxins is 1.59 pg TEQ per body weight. It, therefore, is to be expected that dioxin contamination episodes such as the one in 1999 could lead to intake values at which health effects could occur.

Polychlorinated biphenyls and dioxins are carcinogenic to animals (Cogliano, 1998; IARC 1997), and dioxins have been recognized as carcinogenic to humans (IARC, 1997). Based on different carcinogenic potency estimates, including those of Cogliano (1998) for PCBs and of Becher et al. (1998) for dioxins, van Larebeke et al. (2001) calculated that the 1999 crisis would result in between 44 and 8316 cancer deaths. Important uncertainties exist, in particular, on the carcinogenicity of PCBs, with differences up to a factor 250 (Finley et al., 1997), and of dioxins, with differences up to a factor 100 (Becher et al., 1998; Portier, 2000; Schecter and Olson, 1997).

Noncancer health effect in neonates, infants, and children are important. The dioxin levels in the milk of Belgian women (mean for dioxins, 34.4 pg I-TEQ per g fat; range, 27.3–43.2 pg I-TEQ per g fat) are higher than the threshold value at which thyroid changes occur; therefore, if the body burdens of these mothers increase, thyroid hormone and immunological changes in their babies should be expected. Hemorrhagic disease of the newborn also occurs at concentrations that probably have been reached as a result of the Belgian dioxin incident (van Larebeke et al., 2001). PCBs are also known as neurotoxic compounds that may modulate sex steroid hormones. Steroid hormones play a mediating role in brain development and may influence sex-related behavior, such as childhood play behavior. Indeed, in boys at school age, higher prenatal PCB levels were related with less masculinized play, whereas in girls higher PCB levels were associated with more masculinized play. Higher prenatal dioxin levels were associated with more feminized play in boys as well as girls (Vreugdenhil et al., 2002).

STANDARDS AND REGULATIONS

Animal Feed

In the EU, maximum tolerable levels for dioxin in feed range from 0.75 ng TEQ per kg product for all feed materials of plant origin, animal products (including milk and eggs), and compound feeding stuffs to 6 ng TEQ per kg for fish oil (EC, 2001a). U.S. maximum permitted levels of total PCBs are 0.2 mg/kg product in finished animal feed for food-producing animals and 2 mg/kg product in animal feed components of animal origin, including fishmeal and other by-products of marine origin (21 CFR 509.30; FDA, 1994). Taking into account a mean percentage of fat in animal feed of 2 to 12%, Belgian PCB background values (seven marker PCBs) in animal feed range between 0.0005 and 0.0042 mg/kg product. Maximum tolerated levels in the United States are thus very high. Standards in Belgium are 200 ng/g fat for mixed feed and 250 ng/g fat for feed products of animal origin (Ministerieel Besluit, 2000). These values were calculated based on the seven marker PCBs. Background concentrations of the seven marker PCBs in Belgium are well below those norms (25.2–35.5 ng/g fat).

Food

The Scientific Committee on Food (SCF) has established a tolerable weekly intake (TWI) for dioxins and dioxin-like PCBs of 14 pg WHO-TEQ per kg body weight (SCF, 2001). Although limited information on the occurrence of dioxin-like PCBs is available (the Belgian monitoring programs did not include measurements on these substances), it is most likely that dioxin-like PCBs add substantially to both daily intake and TEQ body burdens (Schecter and Li, 1997). Exposure estimates indicate that a considerable proportion of the population has a dietary intake in excess of the TWI. Certain population groups in Belgium and in other countries could be at higher risk due to particular dietary habits. The reduction of human exposure to dioxins through food consumption is therefore important and necessary to ensure consumer protection. As food contamination is directly related to feed contamination, an integrated approach must be adopted to reduce dioxin levels throughout the food chain — from feed materials through food-producing animals to humans (EC, 2001b); therefore, the Health and Consumer Protection division of

TABLE 10.16

Maximum Levels of PCDD and PCDF (Council Regulation 2375/2001)

Product	Maximum Level (PCDD + PCDF) (pg WHO-PCDD/F TEQ per g fat or product)
Bovine meat	3
Poultry meat	2
Pig meat	1
Sheep meat	3
Fish meat	4 per g fresh weight
Milk	3
Eggs	3

the European Commission has established new maximum limits for dioxins in food in animal feed. No limits currently apply to products such as horsemeat, goat meat, rabbit meat, and eggs from ducks, geese, and quails. Only limited data are available on the prevalence of dioxins in these foodstuffs, and they are of limited significance with regard to the mean intake of most persons. Maximum tolerated levels in food range between 0.75 pg WHO-PCDD/F TEQ per g fat (for vegetable oil) to 6 pg TEQ per g fat (for liver and derived products). Table 10.16 shows the most important maximum levels. van Larebeke et al. (2002) calculated the maximum daily intake of dioxins taking into account the new EU standards and an average Belgian diet. The calculation shows that up to 280 pg WHO-TEQ per day, corresponding to 4 pg/kg body weight per day or to 28 pg/kg body weight per week, can be taken in. This is well above the 1 pg/kg body weight per day that is set by the WHO as a limit for the future and twice the tolerable weekly intake for dioxins and dioxin-like PCBs set by the Scientific Committee on Food at 14 pg WHO-TEQ per kg body weight (EC, 2001b).

Although, from a toxicological point of view, any guideline should apply to the sum of TEQ from dioxins, furans, and dioxin-like PCBs, for the time being the maximum levels are set only for dioxins and furans and not for dioxin-like PCBs, given the very limited data available on the prevalence of the latter. Because no official norm was established for PCB levels in food in 1999, the Belgian authorities had to rapidly set up tolerance levels for PCBs in foodstuffs. A meeting of international experts decided in June 1999 to adopt for poultry meat, eggs, and derived food products the value of 200 ng/g fat (for the seven markers) (EC, 1999). Later, it was decided to apply the same tolerance level to pork and beef products. For milk, the tolerance level was set at a value of 100 ng/g fat, and in 2002 the tolerance level for fish and derived food products was set at 75 µg/kg product. These standards are low in comparison to those set by the U.S. Food and Drug Administration: 3000 ng total PCB per g fat for red meat, which corresponds to about 1000 ng/g fat for the seven PCB markers (Bernard et al., 2002).

CONCLUSION

Dioxin-like compounds are among the biologically active and hormone-disturbing substances whose long-term effects may be insidious and particularly difficult to detect because of the high background levels. These high background levels should go down. Measures are urgently needed to reduce the overall PCB and dioxin burden for the population. Sources known to be important are fish, recycled animal fat, and waste fat that might contain mineral or PCB oils. Recycled animal fat and waste containing PCB oils particularly appear to account for PCB levels above 200 ng/g fat in a few percentages of the meat samples, as shown by background measurements. Individuals exposed to high PCB and dioxin amounts should be traced, and their health status should be monitored. As a precautionary measure, the exposure to these PCBs and dioxins should be decreased by the promotion of chemical and physical hygiene. This form of hygiene is necessary for the primary prevention of cancer and other health problems related to pollution of the environment and the food chain.

ACKNOWLEDGMENTS

We acknowledge help from the Federal Agency of the Safety for the Food Chain (FAVV) in providing the PCB and dioxin data in Belgian food items. This chapter was realized within the framework of the activities of the Focal Point Environmental Health (Steunpunt Milieu en Gezondheid) of the Flemish Community. This work does not reflect the position of the FAVV nor the Focal Point; it reflects only the opinions of the authors.

REFERENCES

Baeyens, W., Windal, I., Leermakers, M., Hanot, V., Degroodt, J.-M., and Goeyens, L. (2002) PCBs and dioxins in North Sea fish and shellfish, in preparation.

Becher, H., Steindorf, K., and Flesch-Janys, D. (1998) Quantitative cancer risk assessment for dioxins using an occupational cohort, *Environ. Health Perspect.*, 106(Suppl. 2): 663–670.

Beck, H., Dross, A., and Mathar, W. (1994) PCDD and PCDF exposure and levels in humans in Germany, *Environ. Health Perspect.*, 102(Suppl. 1): 173–185.

Bernard, A., Broeckaert, F., De Poorter, G., De Cock, A., Hermans, C., Saegerman, C., and Houins, G. (2002) The Belgian PCB/dioxin incident: analysis of the food chain contamination and health risk evaluation, *Environ. Res. A*, 88: 1–18.

Chewe, D., Creaser, C.S., Foxall, C.D., and Lovett, A.A. (1997) Validation of a congener specific method for ortho- and non-ortho-substituted polychlorinated biphenyls in fruit and vegetable samples, *Chemosphere*, 35(7): 1399–1407.

Cogliano, V.J. (1998) Assessing the cancer risk from environmental PCBs, *Environ. Health Perspect.*, 106(6): 317–323.

Dioxin Body Burden Working Group. (2001) *The Belgian PCB–Dioxin Incident 1999*, report presented before the Belgian Health Council, No. 7300/1, Dioxin Body Burden Working Group, Belgium.

Domingo, J.L., Schuhmacher, M., Granero, S., and Llobet, J.M. (1999) PCDDs and PCDFs in food samples from Catalonia, Spain: an assessment of dietary intake, *Chemosphere*, 38(15): 3517–3528.

EC. (1993) *Nutrient and Energy Intakes for the European Community*, Reports of the Scientific Committee for Food, 31st series, Office for the Official Publications of the European Community, Luxembourg.

EC. (1998) European Council Commission Directive 98/68/EC of September 10, 1998, amending Council Directive 74/63/EEC on the fixing of maximum permitted levels for undesirable substances and products in feedingstuffs, *Off. J. Eur. Commun.*, L261/32.

EC. (1999) European Council Commission Decision 1999/449/EC on protective measures with regard to contamination by dioxins of certain products of animal origin intended for human or animal consumption, *Off. J. Eur. Commun.*, L175/70–L175/82.

EC. (2001a). European Council Directive 2001/102/EC of November 27, 2001, amending Council Directive 1999/29/EC on undesirable substances and products in animal nutrition, *Off. J. Eur. Commun.*, L6/45, January 10, 2002.

EC. (2001b) European Council Regulation (EC) 2375/2001 of November 29, 2001, amending Commission Regulation No. 466/2001 setting maximum levels for certain contaminants in foodstuffs, *Off. J. Eur. Commun.*, L321/1–5.

Elskens, M., Pennincks, M., Vandeloise, R., and Vander Donckt, E. (1988) Use of Simplex technique and contour diagrams for the determination of the reaction rate constants between glutathione and thiram in the presence of NADPH, *Int. J. Chem. Kinet.*, 20: 837–848.

European Commission. (2000) Opinion of the Scientific Committee on Animal Nutrition on the Dioxin Contamination of Feedingstuffs and Their Contribution to the Contamination of Food of Animal Origin, Health and Consumer Protection Directorate — General (http://europa.eu.int/comm/food/fs/sc/scan/out55_en.pdf).

FDA. (1994) 21 CFR 509.30, Unavoidable Contaminants in Animal Food and Food-Packaging Material: Temporary Tolerances for Polychlorinated Biphenyls, http://www.access-data.fda.gov/scripts/cdrh/cfdocs/cfcfr/CFRSearch.cfm?FR=509.30.

Fiedler, H., Cooper, K.R., Bergek, S., Hjelt, M., and Rappe, C. (1997) Polychlorinated dibenzo-*p*-dioxins and polychlorinated dibenzofurans (PCDD/PCDF) in food samples collected in southern Mississippi, U.S.A., *Chemosphere*, 34(5–7): 1411–1419.

Finley, B.L., Trowbridge, K.R., Burton, S., Proctor, D.M., Panko, J.M., and Paustenbach, D.J. (1997) Preliminary assessment of PCB risks to human and ecological health in the lower Passaic River, *Toxicol. Environ. Health*, 52(2): 95–118.

Frame, G.M., Cochran, J.W., and Boewadt, S.S. (1996) Complete PCB congener distributions for 17 Aroclor mixtures determined by 3 HRGC systems optimized for comprehensive, quantitative, congener-specific analysis, *J. High Resol. Chromatogr.*, 19: 657–668.

Gallagher, D., Heymsfield, S.B., Heo, M., Jebb, S.A., Murgatroyd, P.R., and Sakamoto, Y. (2000) Healthy percentage body fat ranges: an approach for developing guidelines based on body mass index, *Am. J. Clin. Nutr.*, 72(3): 694–701.

Grimvall, E., Rylander, L., Nilsson-Ehle, P., Nilsson, U., Stromberg, U., Hagmar, L., and Ostman, C. (1997) Monitoring of PCBs in human blood plasma: methodological developments and influence of age, lactation and fish consumption, *Arch. Environ. Contam. Toxicol.*, 32: 329 –336.

Himberg, K., Hallikainen, A., and Louekari, K. (1993) Intake of polychlorinated biphenyls (PCBs) from the Finnish diet, *Z. Lebensm. Unters. Forsch.*, 196(2): 126–130.

IARC. (1997) *IARC Monographs on the Evaluation of Carcinogenic Risks to Humans*, Vol. 69, *Polychlorinated Dibenzo-Para-Dioxins and Polychlorinated Dibenzofurans*, International Agency for Research on Cancer, Lyon, France.

Jacobs, M.N., Covaci, A., and Schepens, P. (2002) Investigation of selected persistent organic pollutants in farmed Atlantic salmon (*Salmo salar*), salmon aquaculture feed, and fish oil components of the feed, *Environ. Sci. Technol.*, 36(13): 2797–2805.

Kogevinas, M. (1999) Cohort studies of occupationally and environmentally exposed populations, *Organohalogen Comp.*, 44: 353–356.

Koopman-Esseboom, C., Huisman, M., Weisglas-Kuperus, N., Van der Paauw, C.G., Tuinstra, L.G.M.Th., Boersma, E.R., and Sauer, P.J.J. (1994) PCB and dioxin levels in plasma and human milk of 418 Dutch women and their infants: predictive value of PCB congener levels in maternal plasma for fetal and infants' exposure to PCBs and dioxins, *Chemosphere*, 28: 1721–1732.

Kreuzer, P.E., Csanady, G.A., Baur, C., Kessler, W., Papke, O., Greim, H., and Filser, J.G. (1997) 2,3,7,8-Tetrachlorodibenzo-*p*-dioxin (TCDD) and congeners in infants: a toxicokinetic model of human lifetime body burden by TCDD with special emphasis on its uptake by nutrition, *Arch. Toxicol.*, 71(6): 383–400.

Krokos, F., Creaser, C.S., Wright, C., and Startin, J.R. (1996) Levels of selected ortho and non-ortho polychlorinated biphenyls in UK retail milk, *Chemosphere*, 32(4): 667–673.

Leonards, P.E.G., Lohman, M., de Wit, M.M., Booy, G., Brandsma, S.H., and de Boer, J. (2000) RIVO Rapport CO34/00, Actuele situatie van gechloreerde dioxines, furanen en polychloorbifenylen in visserijproducten: Quick-en Full-Scan, RIVO, Wageningen, The Netherlands.

Lovett, A.A., Foxall, C.D., Creaser, C.S., and Chewe, D. (1997) PCB and PCDD/DF congeners in locally grown fruit and vegetable samples in Wales and England, *Chemosphere*, 34(5–7): 1421–1436.

Malisch, R. (1998) Update of PCDD/PCDF intake from food in Germany, *Chemosphere*, 37(9–12): 1687–1698.

Malisch, R. (2000) Increase of the PCDD/F-contamination of milk, butter and meat samples by use of contaminated citrus pulp, *Chemosphere*, 40(9–11): 1041–1053.

Ministerieel Besluit. (2000) Ministerieel Besluit tot wijziging van het ministerieel besluit van 12 februari 1999 betreffende de handel en het gebruik van stoffen beschermd voor dierlijke voeding. C-2000/16122. *Belgisch Staatsblad.*, 24.05.2000: 17372–17378.

Ministry of Agriculture, Fisheries, and Food (1997) *Dioxins and Polychlorinated Biphenyls in Foods and Human Milk*, Joint Food Safety and Standards Group Food Surveillance Information Sheet No. 105, http://archive.food.gov.uk/maff/archive/food/inf-sheet/1997/no105/105dioxi.htm.

Needham, L.L., Gerthoux, P.M., Patterson, D.G., Jr., Brambilla, P., Turner, W.E., Beretta, C., Pirkle, J.L., Colombo, L., Sampson, E.J., Tramacere, P.L., Signorini, S., Meazza, L., Carreri, V., Jackson, R.J., and Mocarelli, P. (1997/1998) Serum dioxin levels in Seveso, Italy, population in 1976, *Teratog. Carcinog. Mutagen*, 17(4–5): 225–240.

Pauwels, A., Covaci, A., Weyler, J., Delbeke, L., Dhont, M., De Sutter, P., D'Hooghe, T., and Schepens, PJ. (2000) Comparison of persistent organic pollutant residues in serum and adipose tissue in a female population in Belgium, 1996–1998, *Arch. Environ. Contam. Toxicol.*, 39: 265–270.

Portier, C. (2000) Risk ranges for various endpoints following exposure to 2,3,7,8-TCDD, *Food Addit. Contam.*, 17(4): 335–346.

RIVM Milieucompendium. (2000) *Rijksinstituut voor Volksgezondheid en Milieu*, Centraal Bureau Voor de Statistiek, The Netherlands.

SCF. (2001) *Opinion of the Scientific Committee on Food on the Risk Assessment of Dioxins and Dioxin-like PCBs in Food*, European Commission CS/CNTM/DIOXIN/20 final, Scientific Committee on Food, Brussels, Belgium.

Schecter, A. and Li, L. (1997) Dioxins, dibenzofurans, dioxin-like PCBs, and DDE in U.S. fast food, 1995, *Chemosphere*, 34(5–7): 1449–1457.

Schecter, A. and Olson, J.R. (1997) Cancer risk assessment using blood dioxin levels and daily dietary TEQ intake in general populations of industrial and non-industrial countries, *Chemosphere*, 34(5–7): 2569–2577.

Schecter, A., Startin, J., Wright, C., Kelly, M., Papke, O., Lis, A., Ball, M., and Olson, J.R. (1994) Congener-specific levels of dioxins and dibenzofurans in U.S. food and estimated daily dioxin toxic equivalent intake, *Environ. Health Perspect.*, 102(11): 962–966.

Schecter, A., Cramer, P., Boggess, K., Stanley, J., Olson, J.R., and Kessler, H. (1996). Dioxin Intake from U.S. Food: Results from a New Nationwide Survey, paper presented at the 16th Symp. on Chlorinated Dioxins and Related Compounds, Amsterdam, August 12–16, 1996.

Schepens, P.J.C., Covaci, A., Jorens, P.G., Hens, L., Scharpé, S., and van Larebeke, N. (2001) Surprising findings following a Belgian food contamination with polychlorobiphenyls and dioxins, *Environ. Health Perspect.*, 109(2): 101–103.

Shirai, J.H. and Kissel, J.C. (1996) Uncertainty in estimated half-lives of PCBs in humans: impact on exposure assessment, *Sci. Total Environ.*, 187: 199–210.

Silver, H.K., Kempe, C.H., and Bruyn, H.P., Eds. (1983) *Handbook of Pediatry*, 14th ed., Lange Medical Publications, Los Altos, CA.

Stichting Nederlands Voedingsstoffenbestand (1993) NEVO tabel, Voorlichtingsbureau voor de Voeding, Den Haag

Van den Berg, M., Birnbaum, L., Bosveld, A.T.C., Brunström, B., Cook, P., Feeley, M., Giesy, J.P., Hanberg, A., Hasegawa, R., Kennedy, S.W., Kubiak, T., Larsen, J.C., van Leeuwen, F.X., Liem, A.K., Nolt, C., Peterson, R.E., Poellinger, L., Safe, S., Schrenk, D., Tillitt, D., Tysklind, M., Younes, M., Waern, F., and Zacharewski, T. (1998) Toxic equivalency factors (TEFs) for PCBs, PCDDs, PCDFs for humans and wildlife, *Environ. Health Perspect.*, 106: 775–792.

van Larebeke, N., Hens, L., Schepens, P., Covaci, A., Baeyens, J., Everaert, K., Bernheim, J.L., Vlietinck, R., and De Poorter, G. (2001) The Belgian PCB and dioxin incident of January–June 1999: exposure data and potential impact on health, *Environ. Health Perspect.*, 109(3): 265–273.

van Larebeke, N., Covaci, A., Schepens, P., and Hens, L. (2002) Food contamination with polychlorinated biphenyls and dioxins in Belgium: effects on the body burden, *J. Epidemiol. Commun. Health*, 56(11): 828–830.

Van Poucke, I. and Willems, J.L. (1998). Voorstel voor een getolereerde dagelijkse inname van dioxinen en dioxine-achtige stoffen, rapport ten voordele van de Hoge Gezondheidsraad, Hoge Gezondheidsraad, Zelbestuurstraat 4, B1070 Brussels, Belgium; see also http://www.health.fgov.be/CSH_HGR/Nederlands/Advies/dioxinen_en_PCB.htm.

Vlietinck, R., Schoeters, G., Van Loon, H., and Loots, I. (2000) Eindrapport van het onderzoek Milieu & Gezondheid: ontwikkeling van een concept voor de opvolging en risico — evaluatie van blootstelling aan leefmilieupolluenten en hun effecten op de volksgezondheid in Vlaanderen, http://www.wvc.vlaanderen.be/gezondmilieu/onderzoeken/koepel/index.htm.

Voedingscentrum. (1998) *Zo eet Nederland: Resultaten van de Voedselconsumptiepeiling 1997–1998*, Voedingscentrum, The Hague.

Vreugdenhil, H.J.I., Slijper, F.M.E., Mulder, P.G.H., and Weisglas-Kuperus, N. (2002) Effects of perinatal exposure to PCBs and dioxins on play behavior in Dutch children at school age, *Environ. Health Perspect.*, 110(10): A593–A598.

WHO. (1995) *Concern for Europe's Tomorrow: Health and Environment in the WHO European Region*, European Center for Environment and Health, Wissenschaftlifche Verlagsgesellschaft mbH, Stuttgart, Germany.

WHO. (1996) *WHO-Coordinated Exposure Study: Levels of PCBs, PCDDs and PCDFs in Human Milk*, Environmental Health in Europe, No. 3, World Health Organization, European Centre for Environment and Health, Bilthoven.

WHO-ECEH IPCS. (1998) *Assessment of the Health Risk of Dioxins: Re-evaluation of the Tolerable Daily Intake (TDI)*, WHO Consultation, May 25–29, Geneva, Switzerland, WHO European Centre for Environment and Health, International Programme on Chemical Safety.

Wolff, M.S. and Schecter, A. (1991) Accidental exposure of children to polychlorinated biphenyls, *Arch. Environ. Contam. Toxicol.*, 20(4): 449–453.

Zuccato, E., Calvarese, S., Mariani, G., Mangiapan, S., Grasso, P., Guzzi, A., and Fanelli, R. (1999) Level, sources and toxicity of polychlorinated biphenyls in the Italian diet, *Chemosphere*, 38(12): 2753–2765.

Index

A

abamectin, 221–222
acceptable daily intake (ADI), 128
acephate, 217
acetic acid, 219
  bacteria, 7, 10, 11
Acetobacter, 11
acetohydroxy acids, 6
acetoin, 6, 12
Acetomonas, 2, 10
acetylation, 219
acetylcholine, 53, 201, 219, 222
  mimics of, 217, 222
acetylcholinesterase, 137
  inhibition of, 217–221
Acinetobacter, 12
acrolein, 140
actin, 27
actin filaments, 27
adenosine diphosphate (ADP), 157, 198
adenosine triphosphate (ATP), 15, 22, 29,
      137, 138, 139, 157, 158
adenylate cyclase toxins, 198
ADI, *see* acceptable daily intake
ADP, *see* adenosine diphosphate
ADPR, *see* adenosine diphosphate–ribose
Advisory Committee on Immunization
      Practices (ACIP), 115
Aerobacter, 7
aflatoxins, 2
  aflatoxin M$_1$, 271
aglycone, 140
AHH, *see* arylhydrocarbon hydroxylase
albumin, alcohol and, 22
alcohol
  absorption modification, 22–23
  as food, 21–24
  as toxin, 24–33
  biphasic effects, 23
  calories of, 21
  cellular immunity, and, 26
  cytokines, and, 26

diet modification, and, 22
effect on immunogenic barrier, 26–27
effect on intestinal barrier, 25
effect on non-immunogenic intestinal
      barrier, 27–30
folate deficiency, and, 23
gut leakiness and, 30
humoral immunity, and, 26
-induced barrier dysfunction,
      consequences of, 30–33
intestinal permeability, and, 19–35
metabolism, dietary modification of,
      23–24
motor vehicle accidents, and, 20–21
neutrophil function, and, 27
obesity, and, 22
thermal injury, and, 26
alcohol dehydrogenase (ALDH), 140–141
alcoholic liver disease (ALD), 30, 31–33, 34
  endotoxemia, and, 32–33
  endotoxin, and, 31–32
  Vibrio parahaemolyticus, and, 176
ALD, *see* alcoholic liver disease;
      approximate lethal dose
ALDH, *see* alcohol dehydrogenase
Aldicarb, 218
aliphatic organophosphates, 217–218
amberjacks, 56
amino acids, nitration of, 29
β-aminopropanoic acid, 131
aminotransferases, serum, hepatitis A and,
      99
amitriptyline, as treatment for ciguatera fish
      poisoning, 81
amylase, 2–4
anamnestic shellfish poisoning (ASP), 46
anaphylotoxins, 207
anilinopyrimidines, 226
anticholinesterases, 218
anti-ciguatoxin (anti-CTX), 64, 66
anti-endotoxin antibodies, 206